HOW to EAT

AUTUMN BATES

a SIMPLE, BALANCED APPROACH *for* OPTIMAL WELLNESS

(VB)

VICTORY BELT PUBLISHING INC.

LAS VEGAS

First published in 2026 by Victory Belt Publishing Inc.

ISBN-13: 978-1-628605-72-3

Cover design by Yordan Terziev and Boryana Yordanova

Interior design by Kat Lannom and Justin-Aaron Velasco

Illustrations by Kat Lannom

Cover photo and lifestyle photography by Nicole Parmele and Sandy Barba

Printed in Canada

TC 0126

TABLE *of* CONTENTS

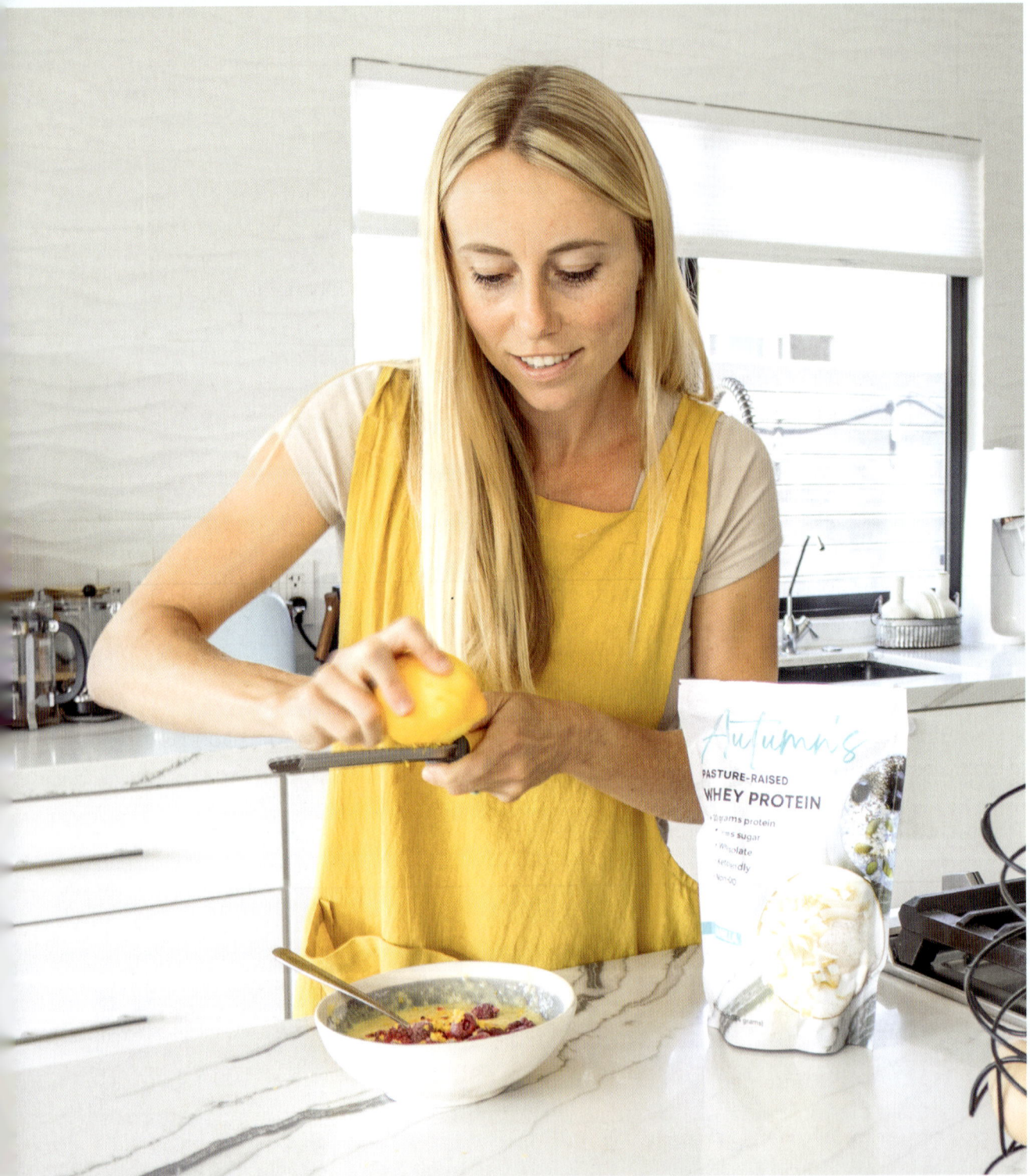

INTRODUCTION

ABOUT ME

I grew up in a relatively "ahead of its time" healthy household. My dad is a chiropractor, and my mom made home-cooked meals with an emphasis on organic produce. Every day, she would serve me eggs, oatmeal, or french toast on whole-grain bread for breakfast while prepping my peanut butter and honey sandwich with carrot slices, hummus, and homemade fruit "leather" to bring to school for lunch. From as early as I can remember, my dad was loading us up with vitamins as well: sublingual B12, chlorella, cod liver oil, Celtic sea salt, and digestive enzymes. He even had us taking collagen supplements when it was still considered the "poor man's protein."

One day, my mom read a book that focused on eating a plant-forward, vegetarian diet. The book convinced her that cutting out animal-based foods was the best thing she could do for the health of our family. So, from 1995 to about 2005, we didn't eat meat. We still shopped at the farmers market, ate locally, used rice milk instead of dairy milk, and ate low-sugar foods (like the horrible "high-fiber" cereals of the time that became soggy as soon as you added milk to them), but we had a new focus of eliminating meat because that's what we were told was healthy.

I remember thinking that my diet was healthier than my peers' because of these changes. Which, in a lot of ways, it was. I was always excited to sleep over at one of my friends' houses because her dad would make us pancakes that we topped with butter and "sprinkled" with cane sugar before rolling them up into little taquitos to eat. This little "sprinkle" of sugar often turned into about ¼ cup per pancake. As a nine-year-old, I loved it. But even then, I had the body awareness to know that I felt nauseous and ill after eating those sugar bombs.

But in very real ways, my diet was incredibly lacking. I was low in vitamin B12 and dangerously low in vitamin D3. I was very skinny despite eating everything in sight, and my gut health seriously suffered. My stomach would make embarrassing bloaty digestive noises during class (always when the room was silent, to my horror) as a result of my poor gut health. I would experience blood sugar crashes that resulted in "hanger," I was always hungry, and my anxiety skyrocketed.

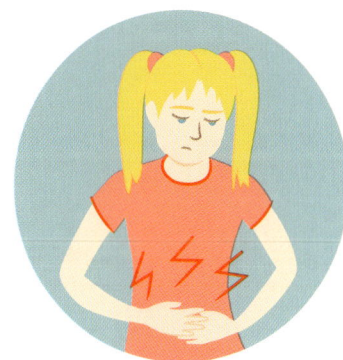

As I entered high school, my family reintroduced meat to help cover these deficiencies, but my bloating and severe anxiety continued. At one point in college, the abdominal pain escalated to the point that I had my boyfriend (now husband) take me to the emergency room because I thought I had appendicitis.

With my dad as a main influence in my life, I always subscribed to a chiropractic philosophy about how the body works: "The power that made the body heals the body, from above down, inside out." It was because of this thought process that I knew something was wrong with my diet and possibly my lifestyle. All of these "healthy" ways of eating and living were obviously not working for my body. I needed to make a change. Learning how became the focus of my higher education.

This pursuit of knowledge led me to graduate at the top of my class with a bachelor's degree in nutrition and dietetics and a master's in nutrition and human performance. I became a Certified Clinical Nutritionist and a Certified Personal Trainer. I spent a summer studying the Mediterranean diet with a combined cultural and scientific emphasis. I read hundreds of books on biochemistry and nutrition. I experimented with nearly every diet and cleanse, like vegan, juice cleanses, raw food, gluten-free, carnivore, keto, and Paleo. I even tried colonics at one point, hoping *that* would finally help support my gut. And still, after all of that studying and experimentation, I felt lost about how to heal my body and provide it with the nutrients it needed to thrive.

To give you a little insight into this type of formal nutrition schooling, there is a heavy focus on two extremes: broad and arguably unscientific dietary guidelines (think of the old-school food pyramid) and individual nutrients, pathways, and mechanisms. There isn't a lot of practical instruction on how to eat in a way that promotes optimal health (and not just prevents deficiencies).

Through my own research, I discovered something called the migrating motor complex (MMC) and finally felt like I'd started to make some real progress. The MMC is a gut-cleaning pathway that is turned on when we don't eat. When activated, it flushes out food and bacteria that could cause bloating or other gut health issues if left behind. It takes a full 3 hours and 45 minutes of "fasting" between meals to complete one cycle of cleaning. At the same time, I also "relearned" that certain foods turn on hormones in the body that reduce hunger and prevent the urge to snack between meals. After nearly a decade of formal education, it's like something finally clicked in my brain, and so many pieces of the nutrition puzzle fell into place.

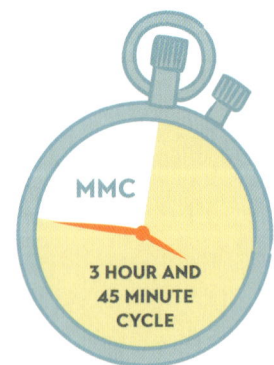

MMC

3 HOUR AND 45 MINUTE CYCLE

Our bodies have a natural system that prevents gut health issues; we just rarely turn it on because we're used to eating in a way that makes us constantly hungry and requires snacking. This fit with my philosophy that the body can take care of itself as long as it is provided with the proper fuel to do its thing. It all finally made sense.

For years, I had only part of the equation. I did a great job of eating my micronutrient- and fiber-packed veggies, but I missed out on the foods that raise hormones to shut off hunger and allow for this natural gap between meals: quality sources of protein and fat.

I didn't need to meticulously track every single thing that went into my mouth or go through the complicated steps of food sensitivity reintroduction or stick to rigid nutrition protocols. I just needed to learn the basics of how to eat.

It was almost too simple. But holy moly, did it work.

After I readjusted my meals to focus on protein, fat, and fiber, my gut started to heal. I was able to go four hours without feeling hungry, which allowed my MMC to turn on and do its thing. My sleep improved, my anxiety dropped, my mood lifted, and bloating became a non-issue. I was also finally seeing results from my workouts that I had never seen before. I was getting stronger, and my body fat dropped while my muscle mass increased. I felt *good* like I had never felt before.

I needed to tell the world.

In 2018, I left my full-time job at a popular fitness and nutrition website to start a blog and a YouTube channel of my own. I wanted full control over the message so that I could share what I knew would be life-changing information for millions.

It started small but grew rapidly. Even in an oversaturated market of health, nutrition, and weight loss, this message was novel (despite its simplicity) and started to spread like wildfire.

At the time of this writing, my YouTube channel has over 1,000 videos with several million views a month. My private Facebook group has over 22,000 members, all eagerly supporting one another throughout their journeys. Each person has their own story to share about how everything finally clicked and they finally feel good again.

Unlike so much in the contentious world of nutrition, this message is positive. It doesn't require you stick to a specific dietary protocol (like carnivore or plant-based). It doesn't even force you to count calories (in fact, it actively steers you away from doing so). Instead, this message empowers you to fuel your body, feel satisfied from your meals, and let your body do its thing. You just need a basic understanding of how the body works, and you're off to the races.

In our community, we have people from all types of backgrounds, ranging from plant-based folks to meat eaters. There are stay-at-home moms, retired men, post-menopausal women, and serious athletes, all using this same philosophy to achieve their varied goals. Because once you have a basic understanding of "how to eat," making minor adjustments to your meals to serve your individual goals becomes incredibly easy. You've already nailed down 95 percent of the equation, so the last 5 percent becomes simple to navigate.

This empowerment has attracted people around the world to finally see progress with their weight loss (or, more specifically, fat loss) and enjoy delicious meals in the process. It's simple, science-backed, and flexible. And it very likely will change your life too.

WHY WE NEED TO LEARN "HOW TO EAT"

All other animals have a clear notion of what they need to eat. Lions know that they need to hunt gazelles, whereas koalas know they need eucalyptus leaves to keep hunger at bay. But as omnivores, we humans have so many options available to us that we can become confused about what we *need* to eat in order to thrive.

Within the last hundred years or so, the food industry has made things even more confounding by adding hyper-palatable ultra-processed foods to the mix. To help counter this confusion, we've tried to study nutrition and biochemistry in such minute detail that we've arguably made things even more baffling for the average consumer (and even the average healthcare practitioner).

Because of this information overload, there are now many different types of dietary protocols that you could follow, with zealots preaching the benefits of each diet.

The truth is, most of these diets have their place for some people. For example, the carnivore diet seems to work particularly well for those with severe autoimmune or food sensitivity issues. Those who have celiac disease obviously benefit from following a strict gluten-free diet. Type 2 diabetics have found success by greatly limiting carbs or even following a keto-style diet. But not everyone needs to follow these specific (and sometimes overly restrictive) protocols in order to find wellness and weight-loss success.

A lot of people fall into the trap of jumping from one diet to the next, like I did in college, because they haven't been taught the basics of what the body needs to feel strong, healthy, and happy. We leap from zero understanding of food to applying nuanced dietary protocols that we don't fully understand (or probably need). So, inevitably, when one diet feels too restrictive for the small benefit that we experience, we abandon ship and try a different diet instead (or perhaps give up on health and wellness entirely).

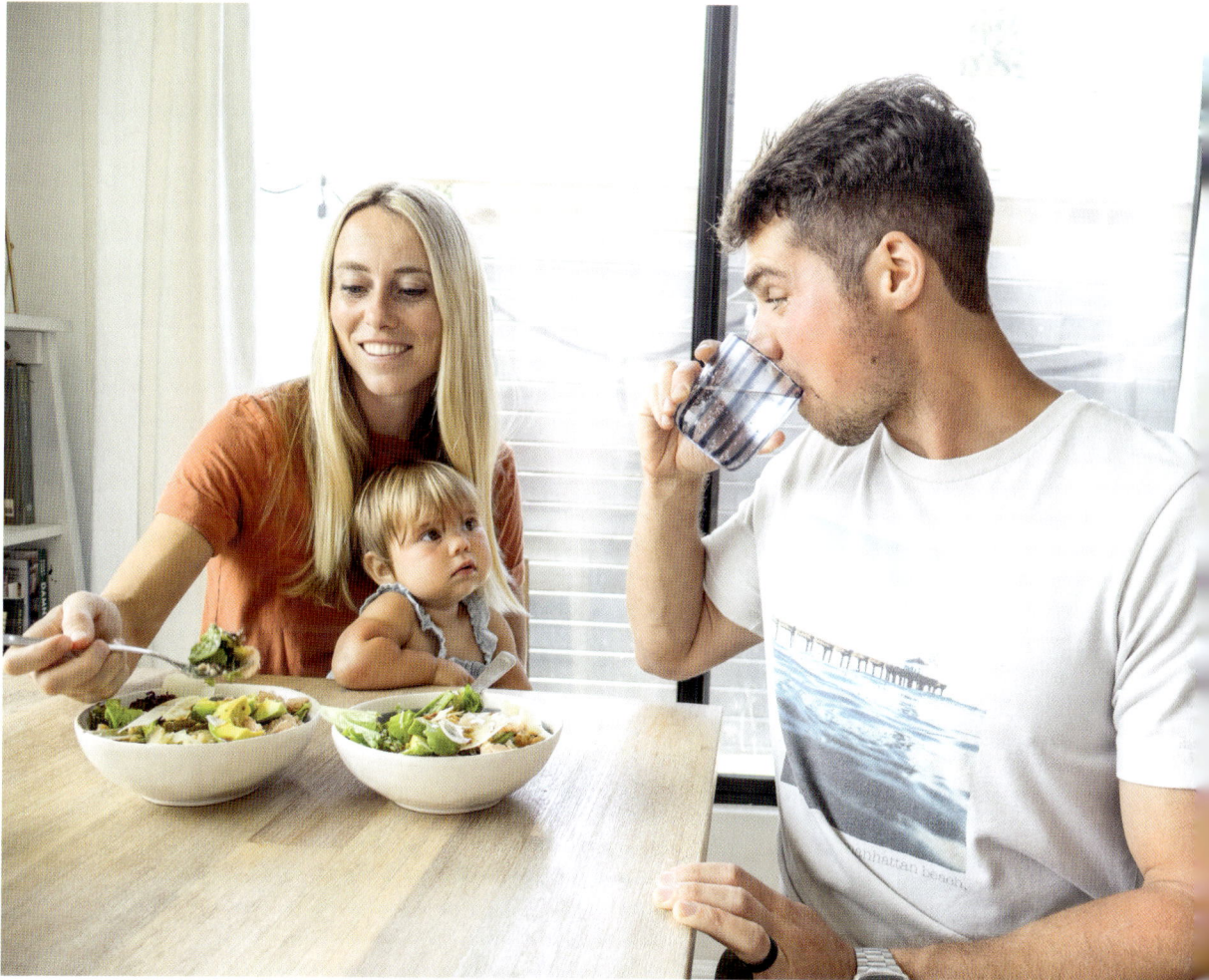

Instead, we need to bring it back to the "basics." Learning how food impacts your body and what you need to fill your plate with to support health, wellness, and natural weight loss eliminates the need for many of these more restrictive nutritional strategies.

Learning how to eat also provides you with food freedom that you've likely never experienced. You can eat delicious cheeses, meats, legumes, sauces, veggies, fruits, dairy, nuts, seeds, and even some grains while still supporting your health and wellness goals.

There is certainly a case for some people to make additional dietary changes, like limiting carbs or eliminating dairy or gluten, but without the context of understanding "how to eat," these changes are pointless and could even be harmful to your short- and long-term health and wellness goals.

As I always say in my videos, it's time to tap into fat-burning mechanisms, eat meals you love, and *finally* feel good again.

ABOUT THIS BOOK

This book is likely quite different from other nutrition books you've read. Nowhere will you see calorie counts, because, quite frankly, this information is not helpful for most people's goals and could actually derail your progress. If you're a chronic calorie counter, it might feel like you're letting up control and might incentivize you not to use these strategies. But let me follow that up with a quick question: If counting calories has worked for you without fail, then why are you reading this book? There's a reason why about 95 percent of diets fail. Nearly every one of them relies on reducing calories as the primary focus.

I'm not saying that "calories don't matter," but rather that this extreme focus on calories as the main method of weight loss is not contributing to long-term, sustainable results (as we'll get into in chapter 1).

Instead, we're tapping into a much more reliable resource: the body's own ability to regulate hunger and burn body fat as fuel. This might sound "woo-woo," but I promise you, we'll be getting into the science behind how this works and the simple steps you can take to navigate this resource. If you need a little encouragement, just check out the stories from folks in my community, beginning on page 12. Exactly zero of them count calories, and they are seeing incredible results.

In order to get the most out of this book, I highly recommend reading chapters 1 and 2 before making any dietary changes. You will learn about the hormones in your body that shut off hunger and boost your metabolism. You will then learn how to fill your plate with the types of foods that support gut-health and weight-loss (or, more specifically, body-recomposition) goals. From there, you'll gain insight into addictive foods that hack your brain and cause overeating. You'll also learn how to make adjustments to your meals depending on specific health, activity, or lifestyle factors.

These tools are science-backed and used by thousands of people around the world as the basis of their weight-loss and wellness journeys. By making a minimal time investment to learn "how to eat," you'll get back wellness dividends you never even imagined possible.

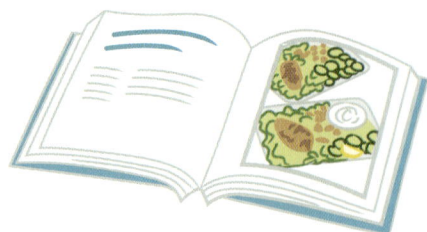

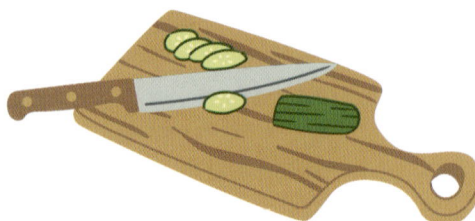

HOW TO USE THE RECIPES

As you'll learn throughout this book, protein, fat, and fiber should be the cornerstones of each meal. These food groups help raise satiety hormones, shut off hunger, reduce cravings, and maintain muscle mass throughout a weight-loss journey. Because each of them is so important, every meal should have a balance of all three. Every recipe in this book has a minimum of 30 grams of high-quality protein, has between two and four servings of high-quality fat, and uses at least one fiber-containing ingredient.

Unless otherwise noted, the recipes also prioritize carbohydrates with a low to medium glycemic load to provide the highest nutrient density while minimizing blood sugar spikes.

Most of the recipes are entire meals; however, some focus on a particular protein or veggie/fiber component. In those cases, you will find recommended protein or veggie pairings for these recipes to make sure you get protein, fat, and fiber at every meal.

You will not find any snack recipes in this book. Snacking promotes eating between meals, which shuts off the MMC, our important gut-cleaning pathway. Plus, when we eat enough protein, fat, and fiber at mealtimes, snacking becomes irrelevant because satiety cues are so high. I've found that it's best to view the urge to snack between meals as a sign that you likely didn't eat enough protein, fat, or fiber at your last meal. With this information, you can bump up your serving size the next time you eat to help counter hunger between meals. However, there is a bit of a learning curve to this, so I have provided quick protein-rich snack ideas that you can reach for if/when you accidentally undereat at a meal (see pages 44 and 45).

This book also includes some better-for-you desserts. There will always be occasions for a sweet treat, like a birthday, anniversary, or celebration. In these cases, sharing a dessert can be an important part of community and bonding with others. For this reason, I've included some desserts that use fewer addictive ingredients so that you can enjoy a tasty treat and still easily jump back to your usual protein, fat, and fiber–based meals.

All of the recipes in this book are designed to taste great, be relatively simple to make, and be crowd-pleasers for friends and family alike. Food isn't just fuel; it's also part of what builds our culture. If you don't love your meals, you won't stick with what you're doing. I encourage you to seek out some of your favorites, but try some new recipes too. Food is one of the great joys in life, so have fun on your new, tasty adventure!

FROM THE COMMUNITY

I'll start with my own success story, because I really do practice what I preach.

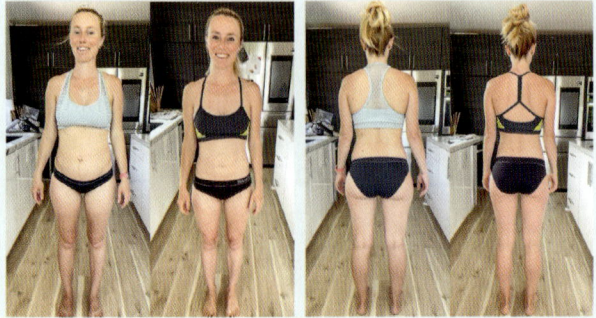

I feel strong and in better shape than I ever have in my life (which isn't something I expected after having my first baby!).

I think there's something to be said about "starting over." Starting from "scratch" allowed me to really build a healthy base from the beginning and incorporate strategies as my body was ready for them. Even though the progress was slow in the beginning, it was a maintainable schedule. I wasn't hungry. I didn't have to count calories. I was eating delicious food. I was energized, and my sleep was improving. I was moving my body in a way that felt good. Overall, I just felt good again! And isn't that really what the goal is, anyway?

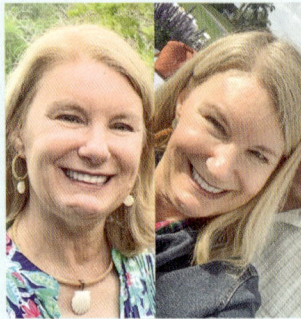

"Since my friends and I are all over 50 and through menopause, ...our metabolisms are slower, and just cutting meals/calories is NOT enough. Most of all, [Autumn's approach] was healthy... I felt GREAT within 4 days, and at the end of the program, I was down 6 pounds—from 121.5 to 115.5—and at 5 ft 2 in...you can see it in my face."

—LAURA

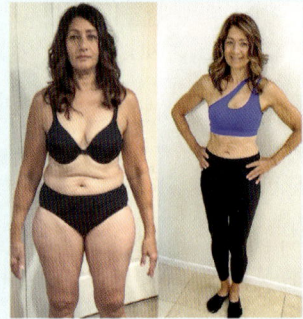

"I turned 57 this past March, and I have never felt better. This June (2022) will be a year that I have kept my weight off without any effort. I started at 167, and today I go from 120 to 123-ish. I have so much energy..."

—JEANNETTE

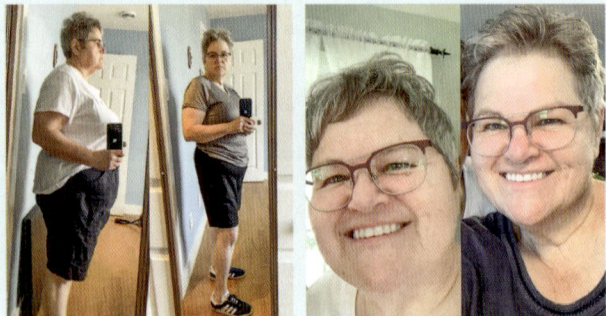

"Contrary to other ways of losing weight, I do not rely on willpower to get through, and I have amazing results. I am no longer in a battle with food. I eat foods that tell my body to use fat as fuel. It is as simple as that."

—GUYLAINE

"What started as a quick weight-loss goal for me turned into a lifestyle. I became conscious of how good my body felt when I fueled it the right way, and I wanted to keep feeling that way. The choices I made were not for some external source, not just to check a box, but for my own well-being. When my nutrition is on point, I function better, and my body and mind feel good. Plus, Autumn's recipes are delicious, so that helps!"

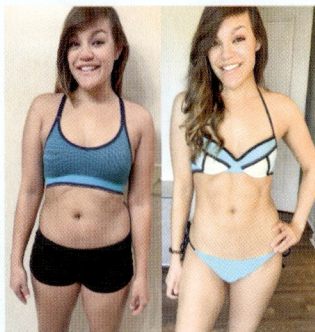

—MONICA

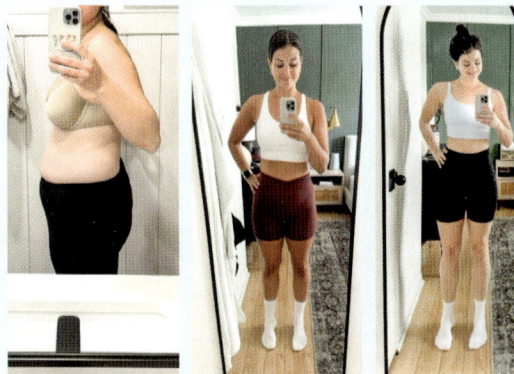

"It's been a year now, and I went from 185 to 155 pounds. From a size 14 to an 8–10. I'm now slimmer and healthier than before I had kids... Thank you, Autumn, for everything, and for all the Autumn Elle Nutrition peeps on Facebook! I am never going back to my old habits again!"

—JOELLE

"In the past, I tried many programs to 'tone up,' tried cutting out food groups, and tried counting calories to lose weight and be healthy, but I could never stay consistent. It wasn't until I found Autumn and began practicing her protocols that I finally learned how to eat delicious meals that helped me feel and look my best (without the need to track my calories or macros!).

"What I love most about Autumn's tips, strategies, and meal plans is that she taught me not to be married to any particular food group or protocol, as our body and wellness goals change with time. Instead, she taught me how to fill my plate with nutrient-dense foods that help me reach my goals, depending on what my goals may be at the time. I feel like I've found food freedom and fluidity, as I no longer constantly worry about food, and in the process, I've lost body fat, improved my fertility, and gained muscle!

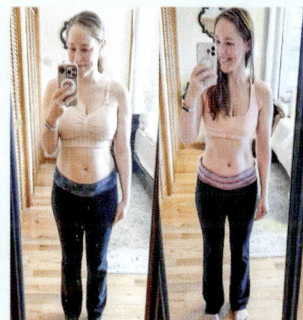

"Thank you, Autumn!!!!"

—KATY

CHAPTER 1

HORMONES, BLOOD SUGAR, FOOD ADDICTION, and SATIETY

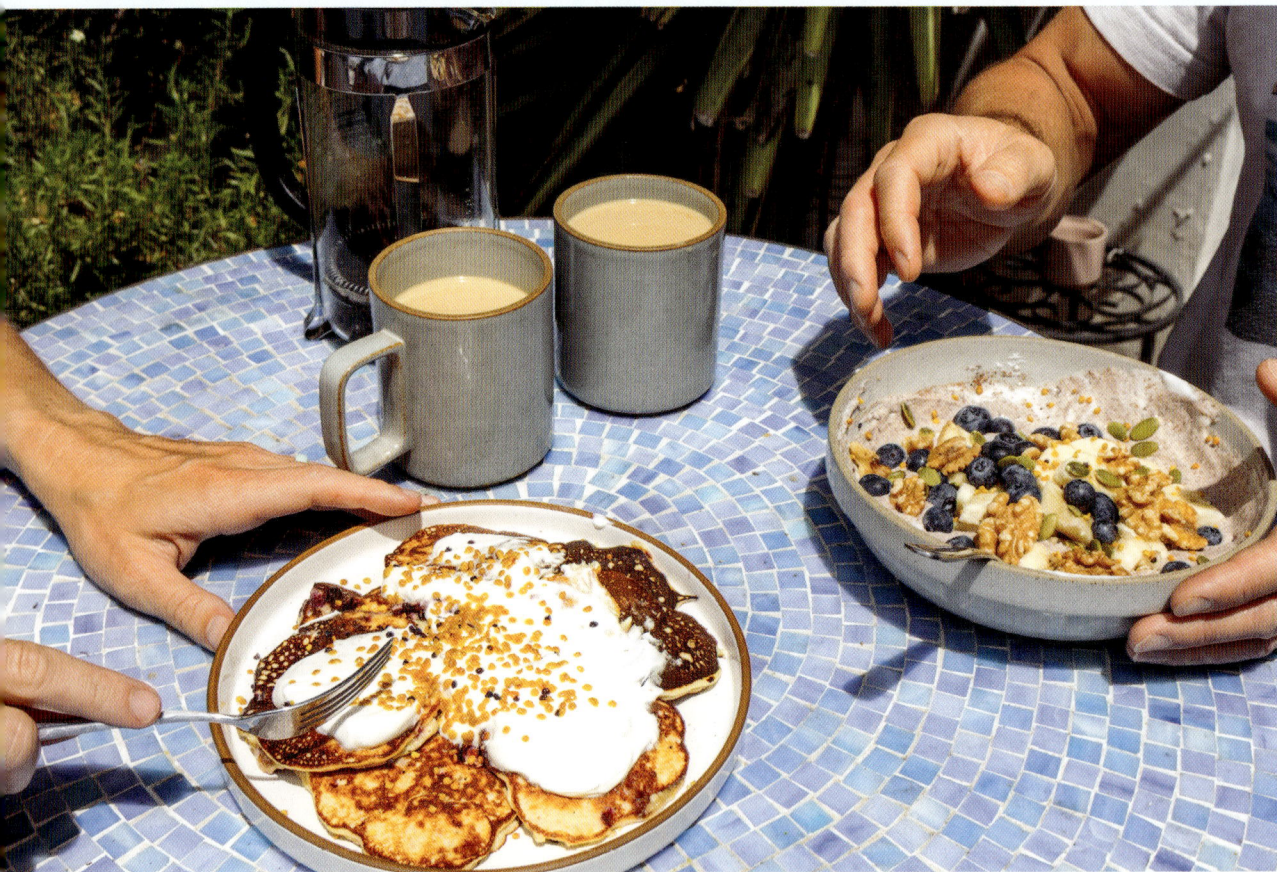

To understand how to eat, you first need to know how your body responds to food. Some ingredients make you feel full and satisfied, while others can cause overeating and addiction-like spirals. When you prioritize the foods that turn on your natural satiety cues, you're able to eat the amount your body needs without counting calories and still burn fat.

Before I continue, I need to clarify the meaning of one key word: satiety. I talk a lot about this key concept, so it's important that you understand it. Satiety is the feeling of satisfaction after a meal. When you feel satiated, you feel full, but not too full. This feeling is the result of satiety hormones that are raised after eating protein, fat, and fiber, including (but not limited to) peptide YY, CCK, and GLP-1. When levels of these hormones are high, your brain gets the message that you're full and don't need to keep eating.

Most people confuse satiety with excessive fullness. Excessive fullness or bloating is *not* satiety; it is the result of eating foods that do not raise satiety hormones. Because these foods don't tell your brain to stop eating, it's easy to overeat. As a result of this overeating, your stomach feels overly stretched, you might experience gastric upset or bloating, and you become sluggish or lethargic. Even though you have overeaten and might feel sickly full, you might also still feel "hungry" because you didn't eat enough protein, fat, or fiber, and your satiety hormones are low.

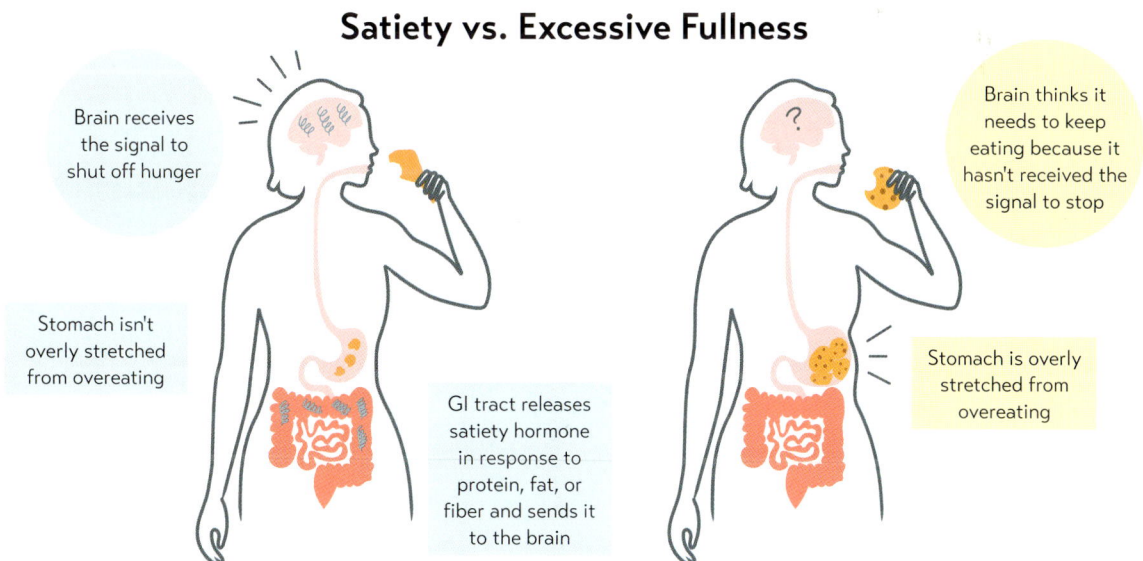

Satiety vs. Excessive Fullness

Brain receives the signal to shut off hunger

Stomach isn't overly stretched from overeating

GI tract releases satiety hormone in response to protein, fat, or fiber and sends it to the brain

Brain thinks it needs to keep eating because it hasn't received the signal to stop

Stomach is overly stretched from overeating

NOTE: When you eat food low in protein, fat, or fiber, it keeps hunger turned on, which then causes you to overeat and feel excessively full.

For example, I can easily eat an entire box of mac and cheese that's intended to feed two or three people. Even though this meal provides about 900 calories, I'm still hungry (albeit bloated) afterward because the mac and cheese lacks the nutrients needed to raise satiety hormones. Many people fall into this same trap of eating the wrong foods that don't support satiety and therefore shy away from the concept of eating until satisfied. Ironically, when you eat foods that raise satiety hormones, it's difficult to "overeat." You feel full, but not excessively full. You're satisfied.

The goal with every meal should be to eat enough of the foods that raise satiety hormones. The foods that do so are quality sources of protein, fat, and fiber.

In addition to boosting satiety hormones, you want to make sure you're eating meals that stabilize your blood sugar levels. Stable blood sugar levels help keep cravings in check. Cravings are different from hunger. You can crave certain foods without actually feeling hungry or needing nourishment. Plus, cravings are nearly always for foods that do not support a weight-loss or wellness goal, such as baked goods or chocolate. Foods rich in protein, fat, and fiber help keep blood sugar levels stable. Ultra-processed, high-sugar, and certain high-carbohydrate foods can cause very unstable blood sugar levels. When you experience unstable blood sugar levels, your body starts ramping up cravings for sweet and starchy foods such as chocolate, chips, crackers, or cookies, which can further perpetuate the cycle of unstable blood sugar.

The final piece of the puzzle is avoiding or greatly limiting foods that are engineered to be overeaten. Studies have found that ultra-processed foods have addictive qualities that are on par with substances like alcohol and tobacco. Imagine telling an alcoholic that they should limit their intake to a few glasses per day rather than abstain entirely—probably not the best advice. Including addictive foods throughout the day means you can no longer rely on your satiety hormones to naturally and effortlessly keep your food intake in check. If you include these in your daily life, you are forced to add a level of discipline to your diet that is normally unnecessary because you are now battling something that resembles addiction. I'll dive more into this concept in chapter 2.

To tackle each of these pieces—satiety, stable blood sugar, and limiting ultra-processed foods—you need a basic understanding of what your food is made of and how it impacts your body. Let me reintroduce you to protein, fat, and carbohydrates. You're likely already familiar with these three macronutrients to some extent, but you're about to see them in a whole new light. You're going to learn how to use each of them to work with your body's natural satiety hormones, effortlessly achieve your goals, and love what you're eating in the process.

PROTEIN

Protein is the king of satiety. It raises key satiety hormones, such as peptide YY, CCK, and even GLP-1—yup, the same GLP-1 found in popular pharmaceuticals that people use to lose weight. Protein is so good at shutting off hunger that people who focus on eating adequate amounts of it often lose weight without intentionally controlling calories. One study had overweight participants follow an "ad libitum" higher-protein diet. This means that the participants were allowed to eat as much as they desired as long as a certain percentage of those calories came from protein. On average, participants lost over 8 pounds of pure body fat during a twelve-week period without intentionally reducing their calorie intake.[1]

In addition to boosting satiety, protein is necessary for maintaining muscle mass while losing weight. This is an important consideration even if you aren't a fitness fanatic, because muscle mass is crucial to a healthy metabolism. The more muscle you have, the more energy your body needs for fuel each day.

Protein is so important that eating the same number of total calories but higher amounts of protein can have a drastic impact on weight-loss and health outcomes. In fact, studies comparing higher-protein diets to other diets with the same number of total calories have found that the higher-protein option resulted in more fat loss, higher resting metabolism, and greater muscle mass.[2]

Typical calorie-restricted diets that don't account for protein can result in significant muscle loss and therefore decreases in metabolism. This slower metabolism then leads to a weight-loss plateau and forces the individual to eat even less to continue seeing weight-loss progress...until the next plateau occurs. And the cycle continues until the metabolism is so slow that it's impossible to keep eating less. At this point, most people give up dieting because they are taking in so few calories that it's no longer sustainable. As they start to eat even *slightly* more (think just a few hundred calories per day), they regain weight rapidly and usually end up heavier than they were before starting their weight-loss journey.

However, when you're able to retain muscle mass while losing weight, your body can better target primarily body fat and keep the metabolism high. In fact, research shows that a higher protein intake helps prevent the weight regain that's so common with other weight-loss methods.[3]

Standard Low-Calorie Diet Outcome

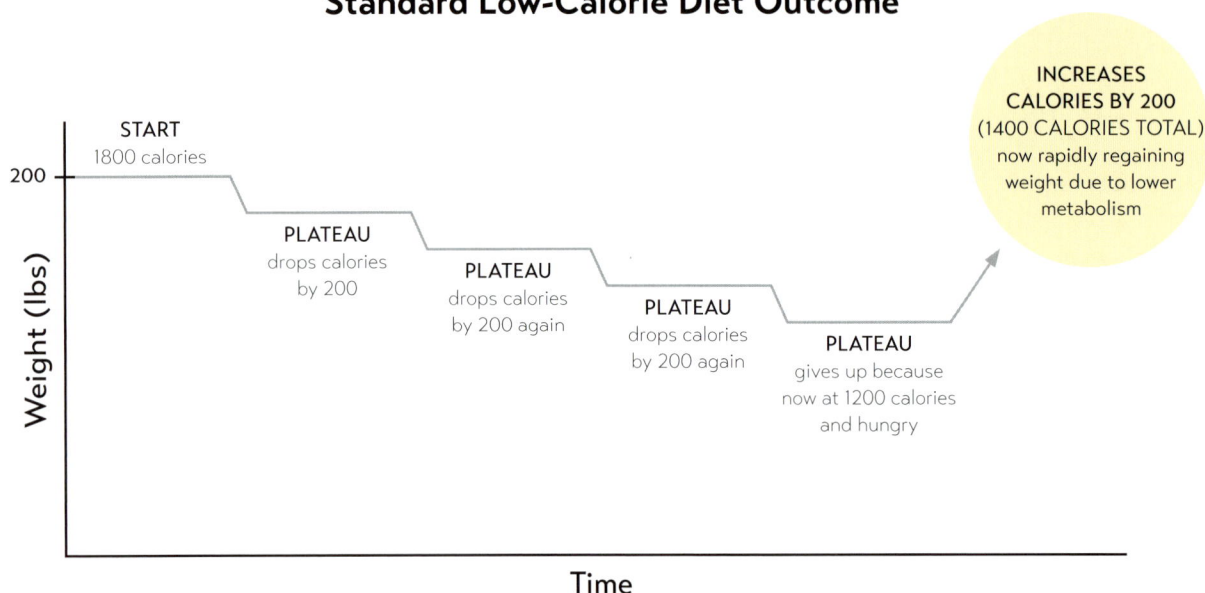

START
1800 calories

PLATEAU
drops calories
by 200

PLATEAU
drops calories
by 200 again

PLATEAU
drops calories
by 200 again

PLATEAU
gives up because
now at 1200 calories
and hungry

**INCREASES
CALORIES BY 200**
(1400 CALORIES TOTAL)
now rapidly regaining
weight due to lower
metabolism

200

Weight (lbs)

Time

Lower muscle mass can also contribute to serious health issues such as osteoporosis and type 2 diabetes. When you keep your muscle during the weight-loss process, your metabolism stays active and healthy while you maintain bone health and insulin sensitivity.

In addition to boosting satiety hormones and maintaining muscle, protein helps promote gut health and stable blood sugar levels. Eating enough protein slows down the GI tract to allow for more efficient absorption of nutrients. As a result, carbohydrates are absorbed more gradually as well, which can keep blood sugar levels stable and prevent crashes.

The combination of boosted satiety hormones and slower absorption of nutrients also makes it easier to naturally space meals out and prevent snacking. Remember the migrating motor complex that helps clean the GI tract and prevent bloating that I mentioned on page 6? It's only turned on when you aren't eating. By eating enough protein, you're able to naturally prevent the urge to eat for about four hours, which, interestingly, is nearly the exact length of time it takes to complete one cleaning cycle with the migrating motor complex. So, when you eat enough protein, you also promote gut health and help prevent bloating.

All of these amazing benefits are contingent on two things: the quantity and quality of the protein you eat. You can't receive the muscle-sparing, fat-burning, and gut and bone health–promoting benefits of protein if you aren't eating enough of it and if you aren't eating the right types.

First, let's talk quantity.

HOW MUCH PROTEIN TO EAT

Current research shows that we need 0.73 gram of high-quality protein per pound of body weight per day to optimize for health and wellness goals.[4]

How Much Protein Do You Need?

Current weight* x 0.73 = **Grams of protein per day**

Example: **150 pounds** x 0.73 = **109.5 grams of protein per day**

*If your BMI is higher than 30, use your ideal weight rather than your current weight. You can find online calculators to figure out your BMI.

Now, if you were to stumble across the USDA *Dietary Guidelines for Americans*, you might be confused, because they recommend half this amount of protein. However, keep in mind that the guidelines are meant to prevent deficiencies, not to promote optimal health and body composition. Recent research has found that to reap the benefits of protein, you need to double the USDA protein recommendation. From personal experience as well as from working with people around the world, I can verify that this higher level of protein does a much better job of achieving those health and wellness objectives.

As we age, the amount of protein we need *increases* by an estimated 25 percent.[5] Around the age of forty, we begin to lose muscle and bone at a much faster rate. To offset this rapid loss, the body needs more protein from meals. Ignoring protein as you age can be disastrous to health outcomes. A multitude of studies have found that a low-protein diet in older adults significantly increases frailty, which results in increased risk of sarcopenia (loss of muscle, strength, and function) and lower strength and energy levels. Increasing protein intake helps reverse this functional decline, reduce in-hospital and overall complication rates, and increase lean body mass and strength.[6]

Ideally, you would calculate how much protein you need to eat in a day (using the figure at the top of this page) and evenly split this total among three meals. However, if you find this kind of math a bit overwhelming, I've found that most people benefit from hitting 30 grams of protein at every meal. This is likely a significant jump from the amount you've been eating and therefore can help you reap the benefits of more protein without having to break out a calculator and figure out your specific needs. Once you've gotten the hang of hitting 30 grams, you can advance to figuring out your own individualized protein needs and making adjustments down the line. Not sure what 30 grams of protein looks like? Check out page 23 for a breakdown of 30 grams of protein from a variety of sources.

NOTE: To my friends who live outside the US: Because you use grams and not ounces to measure your food, it's important not to mix up the weight of your *food* with the grams of protein in that food. For example, a cooked chicken breast weighing 113 grams contains 35 grams of protein. Unless you're using a pure protein powder, the weight of your food *will not* equal the amount of protein you're getting from it. Don't make the mistake of eating 35 grams of chicken thinking that you're getting 35 grams of protein!

Scan this QR code to use the free protein calculator on my website:

WHAT KIND OF PROTEIN TO EAT

Just like calories, not all protein is created equal. Quality is as important as quantity.

Many studies have confirmed that animal-based proteins provide the most benefit. One study compared a group of omnivores to a group of vegetarians eating the same amount of protein. The omnivore group had significantly more muscle mass than the vegetarian group.[7] This is because animal-based proteins have a better balance of essential amino acids and are easier for the body to absorb and use than plant proteins.

We track protein quality with something called the Digestible Indispensable Amino Acid Score (DIAAS). Organizations such as the Food and Agriculture Organization (FAO) suggest using DIAAS to support claims about protein quality, such as "high quality" and "a good source of protein"; however, it hasn't been universally adopted yet. Protein-rich foods with a DIAAS of greater than 1 are considered "high quality."

Those that score between 0.75 and 0.99 are considered "good quality." Any food that receives a score of less than 0.75 is deemed "poor quality" and cannot make a protein claim.

DIAAS
A Measurement of Protein Quality

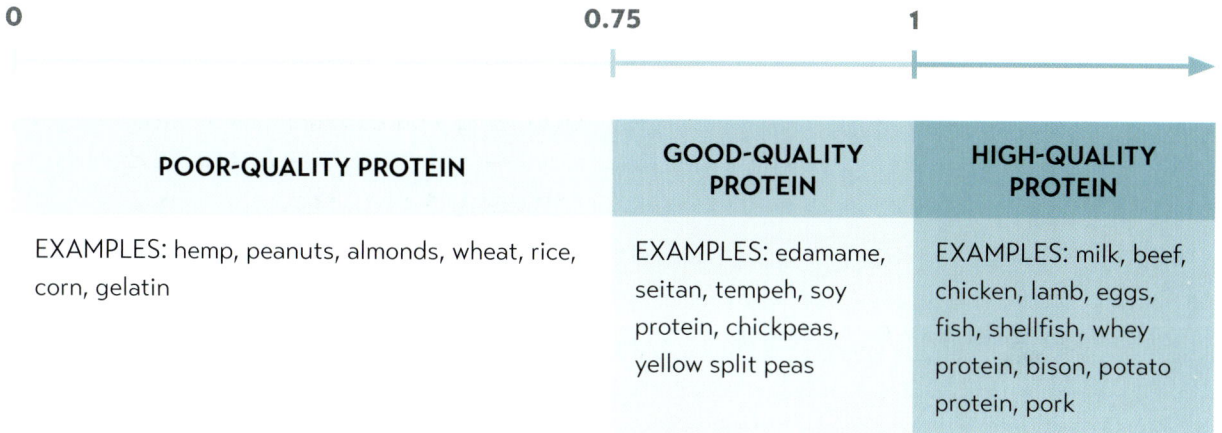

0	0.75	1

POOR-QUALITY PROTEIN	GOOD-QUALITY PROTEIN	HIGH-QUALITY PROTEIN
EXAMPLES: hemp, peanuts, almonds, wheat, rice, corn, gelatin	EXAMPLES: edamame, seitan, tempeh, soy protein, chickpeas, yellow split peas	EXAMPLES: milk, beef, chicken, lamb, eggs, fish, shellfish, whey protein, bison, potato protein, pork

All animal foods other than bone broth and powdered collagen peptides have a score of greater than 1 and therefore are excellent proteins to eat. They are easy for the body to break down, absorb, and use for various functions. As a result, they are also the most effective at boosting satiety hormones, preventing muscle loss, and keeping hunger at bay.

Older adults specifically greatly benefit from prioritizing high-DIAAS proteins. Because older adults already have higher protein needs and a generally lower ability to break down and absorb protein, it's crucial for them to focus on easy-to-chew animal-based proteins such as ground beef, dairy products, eggs, and whey protein powder.

There are some plant-based proteins that fall into the category of "good quality" that you can focus on if your diet is primarily plant based.

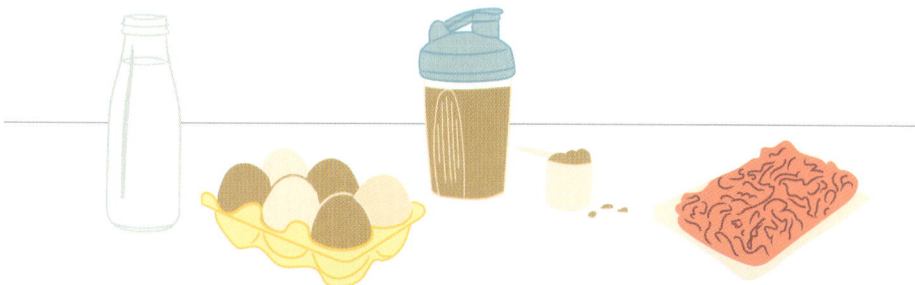

HIGH-QUALITY AND GOOD-QUALITY PROTEINS

The following is a list of the high- and good-quality proteins from animal- and plant-based sources. The third category combines various low-quality proteins in specific proportions to raise the overall DIAAS and make the end result a "good-quality" protein. Although these are here for reference, I recommend sticking to animal-based proteins if possible. They are the most bioavailable and micronutrient-dense sources. If you prefer to eat a primarily plant-based diet, then you will get the most protein benefit by sticking with the foods in the second column as your primary sources. The proteins in the third column are to be used as a last resort, as they are much lower-quality sources.

ANIMAL-BASED PROTEINS

- Beef (any cut)
- Bison (any cut)
- Chicken (any cut)
- Pork (any cut)
- Fish (any type—salmon, sardines, anchovies, tilapia, etc.)
- Lamb (any cut)
- Venison (any cut)
- Crab
- Lobster
- Oysters
- Shrimp
- Eggs
- Cow milk
- Goat milk
- Sheep milk
- Kefir (from any of the milks above)
- Cheese (from any of the milks above)
- Cottage cheese
- Greek yogurt
- Skyr
- Halloumi
- Paneer
- Egg white protein powder
- Whey protein isolate powder

PLANT-BASED PROTEINS

- Edamame
- Seitan
- Tempeh (fermented soy)
- Tofu
- Plant-based yogurt with added protein
- Pea protein powder
- Potato protein powder
- Soy protein powder
- Chickpeas
- Split yellow peas (borderline, DIAAS 0.73)

COMBINED PLANT-BASED PROTEINS[8]*

- Fava beans/corn/soy (10/20/70)—combined DIAAS 0.85
- Soy/oats (90/10)—combined DIAAS 0.92
- Oats/lupin/soy (10/10/80)—combined DIAAS 0.91
- Oats/lupin (7/93)—combined DIAAS 0.76
- Fava beans/corn/potato (15/20/65)—combined DIAAS 1.00
- Corn/potato (25/75)—combined DIAAS 1.00
- Corn/soy (15/85)—combined DIAAS 0.88

*These are listed in ratios that maximize the DIAAS of each combination of protein sources. For example, a meal that is made up of 10 percent fava beans, 20 percent corn, and 70 percent soy has a combined DIAAS of 0.85. These combinations are less likely to be used by the home cook and more likely to be used by manufacturers when developing plant-based meat and protein alternatives.

If your diet is plant based, it's crucial to prioritize the proteins that have a good DIAAS; otherwise, you will not reap the full protein benefits. It's also important to be aware of the carbohydrate-to-protein ratio in the plant-based proteins you choose. Most have very little protein compared to the total carb count. A great example is a white potato, which has a fantastic DIAAS of 1. However, to get 30 grams of protein, you would need to eat the equivalent of 6.5 potatoes, which also contributes over 200 grams of high–glycemic load carbohydrates. This massive amount of carbohydrates will result in significant blood sugar spikes and crashes. Not to mention that eating more than 5 whole potatoes at one meal simply isn't realistic.

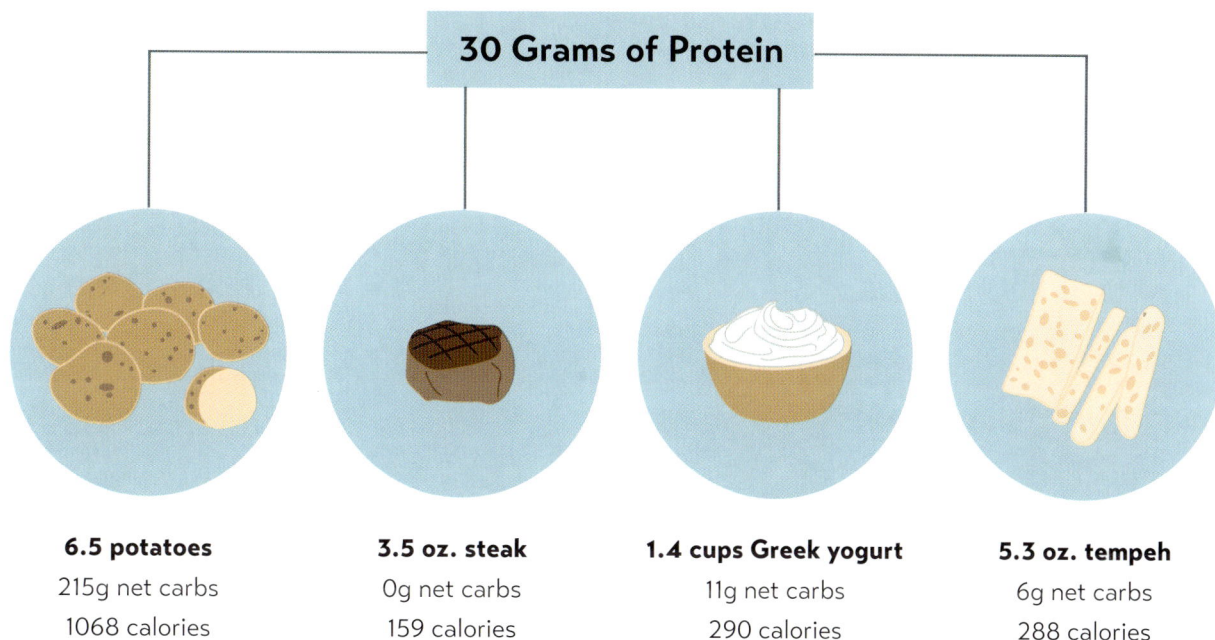

30 Grams of Protein

6.5 potatoes	**3.5 oz. steak**	**1.4 cups Greek yogurt**	**5.3 oz. tempeh**
215g net carbs	0g net carbs	11g net carbs	6g net carbs
1068 calories	159 calories	290 calories	288 calories

Although you can combine plant-based proteins to raise the DIAAS of a meal, doing so requires specific attention to ratios and still results in high carbohydrate levels. Refer to the previous page for the DIAAS list and ratios for various plant-based protein combinations. If all of this seems overwhelming, you can find my plant-based and vegetarian tips on pages 57 to 59.

The foods that have the highest DIAAS are also the most nutrient-dense and healthiest foods available. A 2022 study analyzed all foods to find which ones are highest in critical nutrients, such as iron, calcium, vitamin B12, and vitamin A. These are nutrients in which people are commonly deficient and can lead to serious negative health outcomes when underconsumed. The study found eleven foods that rank especially high in all of these categories: beef, cow milk, eggs, dark leafy greens, bivalves, mutton and lamb, canned small fish with bones, organ meats, crustaceans, small dried fish, and goat. The study also named eight honorable mentions: cheese, goat milk, pork, yogurt, fresh fish, pulses, teff, and canned fish without bones.[9] If you cross-reference these foods with the DIAAS list on page 21, you'll notice that nearly all of them are incredibly rich sources of high-quality protein.

Foods High in Iron, Calcium, Vitamin B12, and/or Vitamin A

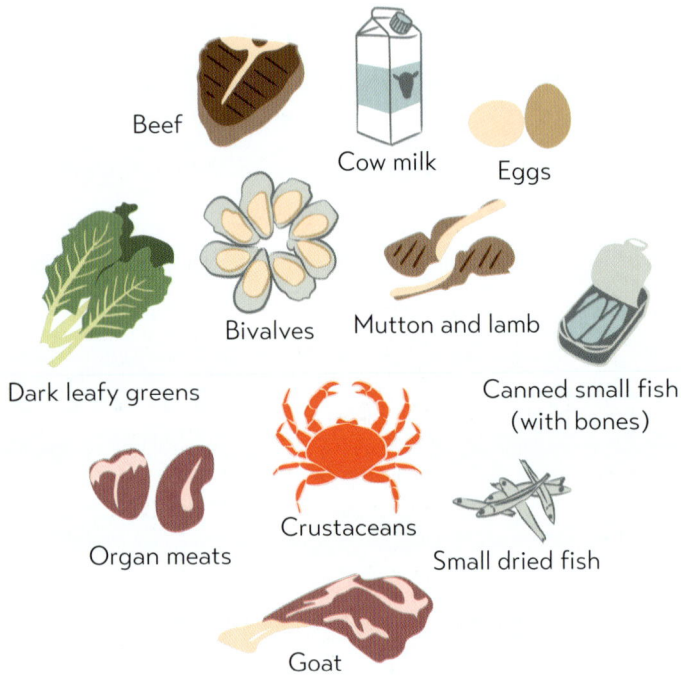

Beef

Cow milk

Eggs

Dark leafy greens

Bivalves

Mutton and lamb

Canned small fish (with bones)

Organ meats

Crustaceans

Small dried fish

Goat

Honorable Mentions

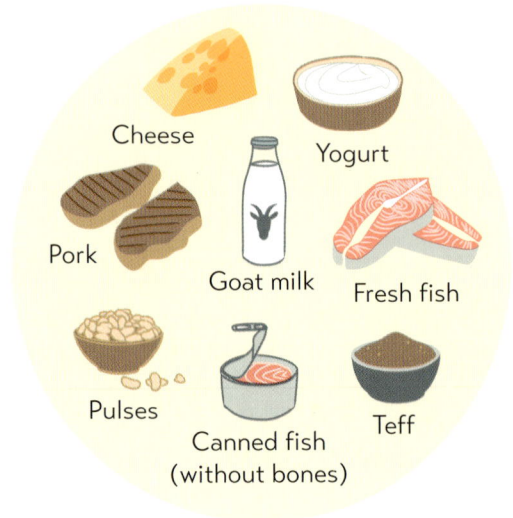

Cheese

Yogurt

Pork

Goat milk

Fresh fish

Pulses

Canned fish (without bones)

Teff

FINAL THOUGHTS ON PROTEIN

To keep things simple, focus on eating animal-based or vegetarian sources of protein and try to get at least 30 grams at every meal. To support both weight loss and long-term wellness, every meal needs to be centered around high-quality protein. This vital macronutrient should never be an afterthought.

FAT

If protein is king, then fat is the queen. Protein is the most efficient tool to help keep the metabolism healthy while losing weight, but fat is also needed to boost satiety and prevent nutrient deficiencies.

Just like protein, fat helps prevent hunger and stabilize blood sugar levels by raising satiety hormones and slowing the absorption of food from the GI tract. Fat tends to have a bigger impact on the satiety hormone cholecystokinin (CCK), whereas protein dominates the hormone peptide YY. Having a balance of both protein and fat helps boost satiety across the board.

Studies comparing equal-calorie diets that were either low in fat or low in carbs found that the low-carb (and therefore higher-fat) group lost more visceral fat (fat stored around the organs in your abdomen, which is often linked to a higher risk of chronic disease) and total body fat than the low-fat group.[10]

Higher-quality fat intake also seems to improve blood sugar and fasting insulin levels.[11] Structuring your meals around blood sugar–stabilizing protein and fat can help balance your blood sugar levels, leading to less severe insulin spikes when you eat carbs. It can also eventually allow for more flexibility with the amount and type of carbs you're able to eat without gaining weight or facing negative health consequences. (I dive into this concept in the "Carbohydrates" section that begins on page 31.)

Fat on its own does not have the same satiety-inducing results that protein has. In fact, when fat is combined with sugar or refined carbs, it can actually *bypass* normal satiety cues and turn on something called the "bliss point." In research, the bliss point is the "perfect" combination of fat, sugar, and salt that the food industry uses to create highly craveable foods.[12] These foods tend to be ultra processed and very hard to stop eating once you start. Think of treats like ice cream, croissants, candy, and cookies. All of these have a high fat content in the form of butter, seed oil, or dairy paired with a high sugar or processed flour content. It's not the fat *per se* that's the problem. It's not even the sugar that's necessarily the problem, but rather the combination of fat and sugar in the absence of protein. This is why it's incredibly important to combine protein with high-quality fat and low–glycemic load carbohydrates to avoid this addictive "bliss point." But just like with protein, the type of fat matters.

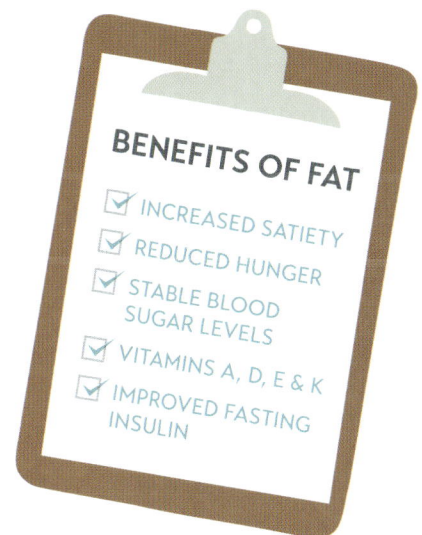

BENEFITS OF FAT

☑ INCREASED SATIETY
☑ REDUCED HUNGER
☑ STABLE BLOOD SUGAR LEVELS
☑ VITAMINS A, D, E & K
☑ IMPROVED FASTING INSULIN

One review found that monounsaturated and omega-3 fats had the biggest impact on the satiety hormone GLP-1.[13] Foods that are naturally rich in monounsaturated fats include almonds, avocados, hazelnuts, macadamia nuts, olives, olive oil, peanuts, and pistachios. The foods highest in quality omega-3 fats include anchovies, cod liver oil, herring, mackerel, salmon, salmon roe, and sardines.

Even though monounsaturated and omega-3 fats are often highlighted, certain saturated fats have their place too, particularly when we're talking about dairy.

Scientists have been baffled for years over something they call the "Dairy Fat Paradox." Common sense would lead us to believe that full-fat dairy products would be worse for weight loss because they're higher in calories. But over the last few decades, studies have consistently found that those who ate full-fat dairy products were much less likely to become obese than those who opted for low-fat dairy.[14] The theory is that full-fat dairy is rich in protein as well as fat, making it much more satiating than low-fat varieties and therefore resulting in natural weight maintenance.

FERMENTED AND AGED DAIRY

The amount of fat, carbs, and protein can vary in dairy. When looking to optimize for a fat-loss goal, it's important to choose the highest-quality protein and preferably fermented dairy sources. Fermentation breaks down lactose (milk sugar) through the action of bacteria and yeasts added to milk. This lowers the glycemic load of the dairy product and makes it more blood sugar stabilizing. Fermentation also makes dairy much easier to digest for those who are lactose intolerant because the lactose has been broken down by the bacteria, making fermented dairy products very low in lactose. Aged dairy products, such as most cheeses, have a similar benefit, as the lactose is broken down through a combination of enzymes naturally found in milk and bacteria added to assist in the aging process. These higher-protein and fermented or aged dairy products include cottage cheese, Greek yogurt, and cheddar, Parmesan, and Swiss cheeses. Just remember to always choose the full-fat option! Don't forget about the Dairy Fat Paradox! Other dairy products that are higher in lactose and/ or lower in protein, such as milk, kefir, and regular yogurt, are still good options to include in your meals, but they aren't as ideal as the higher-protein alternatives.

Fat is not only important for satiety and weight loss; it's also crucial for preventing nutrient deficiencies. Certain nutrients are only found in or can only be absorbed with fat. If you don't eat enough fat, then you can quickly become deficient in important nutrients for short- and long-term health.

Some key nutrients include the following.

VITAMIN K2

Vitamin K2 is different from the plant-based vitamin K1. K2 helps get calcium out of arteries and into bones. This role makes K2 key for preventing calcification of the arteries while simultaneously promoting strong, healthy bones. Without vitamin K2, calcium would be left in the arteries, potentially causing damage that could lead to cardiovascular disease. Because K2 helps direct calcium to its proper location, studies have found that it also helps prevent bone loss[15] and tooth loss.[16]

Vitamin K2 is less widely available than vitamin K1. It is found mostly in full-fat dairy products (fermented dairy is even higher in K2), egg yolks, and natto. Low-fat dairy products have substantially lower levels of K2. This is because K2 resides in the fat, so when you remove the fat, you also remove the K2.

Growing up, I didn't eat much dairy or meat, which meant I was low in vitamin K2 and calcium. Sadly, I also ended up developing dozens (yes, dozens) of cavities even though I didn't eat a lot of sugar. This is speculation, but I would bet that the lack of full-fat dairy products in my diet as a kid led me to spend way too much time at the dentist.

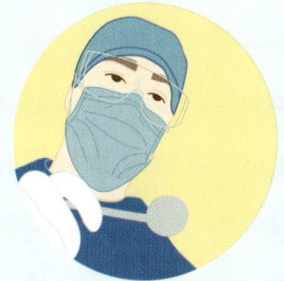

VITAMIN A

Vitamin A plays an important role in immune function, bone health, vision, and reproduction. Technically, your body can make vitamin A if you get beta carotene from plant-based sources such as carrots, but the conversion of beta carotene to vitamin A is very low and not efficient. This means you need sources of vitamin A in your diet as well. This is called pre-formed vitamin A. Some of the best sources of pre-formed vitamin A include liver, cod liver oil, milk, cheese, and eggs.

OMEGA-3

Omega-3 is an essential fatty acid. This means that the body can't make it, so you *need* to get it from food. You can get omega-3 in three forms: EPA, DHA, and ALA.

EPA and DHA are found exclusively in animal foods like fatty fish. ALA is mostly found in plant-based foods like chia seeds, flax seeds, hemp seeds, and walnuts. Each form has different benefits, and it's important to get a mix of all three. EPA and

DHA are both great for reducing inflammation and promoting heart health, but DHA is particularly important during pregnancy. One study found that increasing DHA consumption helped reduce preterm births by 40 to 64 percent.[17] EPA and DHA have also been found to improve various inflammatory conditions ranging from post-exercise muscle soreness[18] to swollen joints due to rheumatoid arthritis.[19] Fish oil, which contains both EPA and DHA, has been shown to reduce waist circumference independent of weight loss.[20] ALA is converted to either EPA or DHA in the body, but this conversion is very poor. Only a small percentage of ALA is converted to EPA or DHA; the rest is stored or used as an energy source.

Ideally, you want a mix of all three sources of omega-3 for the best benefits. This means eating meals throughout the week that contain salmon, sardines, anchovies, oysters, shrimp, seaweed, hemp seeds, chia seeds, flax seeds, and walnuts.

OMEGA-6

Omega-6 is the other essential fatty acid that the body can't create, so you need to get it from food. Whole-food sources of omega-6 include chicken, nuts, seeds, whole grains, soybeans, peanuts, and avocados. Omega-6 fats get a bad reputation for being "inflammatory," but they are still critical to your health. These fats are used to signal that your body needs to ramp up the immune response or increase inflammation when you're sick or injured. If you didn't have omega-6 fats, then you wouldn't be able to recover from these states of stress. You would have a delayed immune response when you got sick, your body wouldn't be able to recover efficiently from simple scratches or wounds, and you would have an increased risk of getting infected with a bug or virus.

The problem with omega-6 is when it's eaten out of balance to the anti-inflammatory omega-3. Researchers have suggested that an omega-6 to omega-3 ratio of 5:1 is ideal for optimal health and balanced inflammatory levels.[21] However, most people have a ratio of 20:1, a significantly higher level of omega-6. It's theorized that this imbalance could increase the risk of inflammatory diseases and metabolic syndrome.

If you're eating whole-food sources of omega-6 (such as almonds, sunflower seeds, and chicken) while balancing them with whole-food sources of omega-3 (like salmon, hemp seeds, and walnuts), then you're unlikely to hit this significant imbalance. However, if your diet is high in concentrated and highly processed forms of omega-6, such as soybean oil, corn oil, fried foods, processed snacks, prepackaged baked goods, and margarine, then it's easy to sneak toward that 20:1 ratio. When looking for the best fats to support a balanced inflammatory response, stick to whole-food sources of both omega-3 and omega-6 and avoid highly processed versions.

FIBER FATS

In addition to the nutrients primarily found in fat, some whole-food fats are fantastic sources of fiber. I call these "fiber fats." The following fats are also rich in fiber:

- Almonds
- Avocados
- Cacao nibs
- Chia seeds
- Flax seeds
- Olives

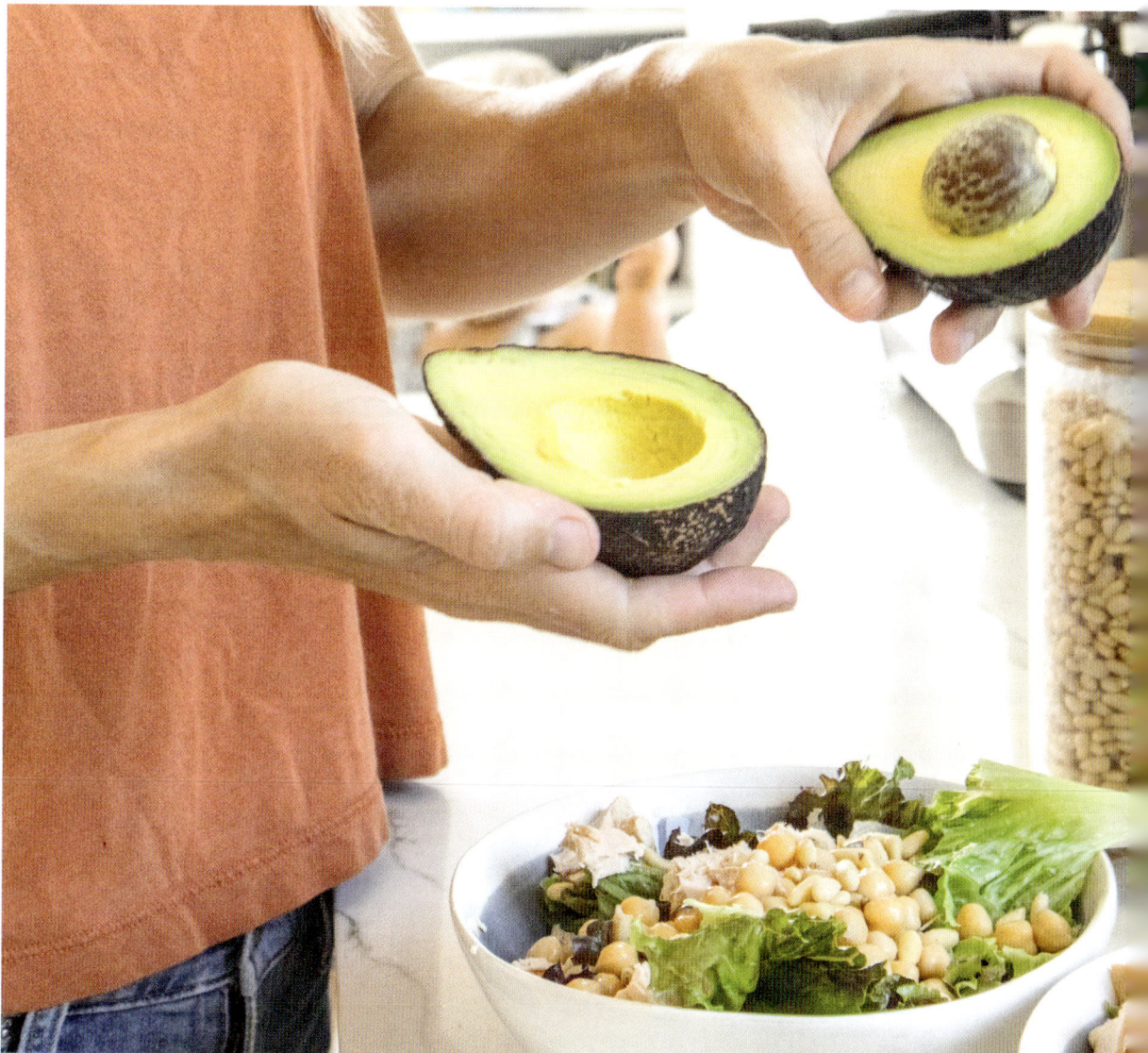

FATS TO AVOID

Although good-quality fat is incredibly important for health and weight loss, there are certain fats that are harmful for health and weight-loss goals.

Studies have found that the ultra-processed fats used in ultra-processed foods cause overeating and addiction-like behavior, especially when combined with ultra-processed carbs.[22] You often find this combination in candy, "energy" or "protein" bars, fried foods, fast food, cereal, and conventional baked goods. The fats most often used in these highly processed foods are vegetable oil, corn oil, soybean oil, safflower oil, and sunflower oil. When choosing the best fats to support weight loss and wellness, it's important to choose whole-food varieties while minimizing (or completely removing) these highly processed seed oils. See the following table for more on how fats are processed.

THE TYPE OF PROCESSING MATTERS		
WHOLE FATS	**PROCESSED FATS/OILS**	**ULTRA-PROCESSED FATS/OILS**
Whole fats are foods that are naturally high in fat and have not been pressed, rendered, shaken, or chemically altered in any way. These fats nearly always come naturally packaged with either protein, some carbs, or fiber. They include avocados, olives, milk, sunflower seeds, walnuts, almonds, meat, fish, chicken, and eggs. These are great fats to prioritize because they provide other important nutrients and micronutrients.	Whole fats are pressed, shaken, or rendered to create an oil or fat. This type of processing is minimal and does not require chemicals to extract the fat. These fats are great to use for cooking or in dressings and marinades. Examples: Olives (pressed) → olive oil Heavy cream (shaken) → butter Avocados (pressed) → avocado oil Beef fat (rendered) → tallow Almonds (ground) → almond butter	Ultra-processed fats and oils have undergone some type of chemical processing. You would not be able to extract the fat by simply pressing, shaking, or rendering the original food source. Often, these fats and oils are high in inflammatory omega-6 fatty acids. They also tend to be oxidized during processing, which can increase inflammation in the body. This category includes grapeseed, soybean, safflower, canola, corn, and "vegetable" oil. Example: Soybeans (pressed, purified, refined, and sometimes chemically altered and extracted with solvents) → soybean oil

Thankfully, when you stick to mostly whole-food sources, it's easy to avoid highly processed fats that can work against a health or weight-loss goal.

FINAL THOUGHTS ON FAT

Without an adequate intake of high-quality fats, you would miss out on maximizing satiety hormones and preventing nutrient deficiencies. Interestingly, some of the best sources of fat are also rich in protein. They include fatty fish, beef, lamb, pork, chicken (with the skin on), eggs, and dairy products. By eating whole-food sources of high-quality protein that are also rich in fat, you can cover nearly all of your nutrient needs while also preventing hunger and food cravings.

Exactly how much fat you should eat is based on your activity level, hunger, sugar cravings, and even food preferences. We'll dive into exactly how to structure your meals as well as how much fat to eat in chapter 2.

CARBOHYDRATES

Now, we get to the final piece of the puzzle: carbohydrates.

Depending on which nutritional circle you've been running in, carbohydrates can have a pretty bad reputation, and not without reason. Carbs are the easiest foods to process into hyperpalatable versions. When compared to protein and fat, carbs are the least able to raise satiety hormones and shut off hunger. They are also the basis of nearly all of the highly processed foods that line grocery store shelves and have been tied to a wide array of health concerns, such as type 2 diabetes,[23] heart disease,[24] cancer,[25] and Alzheimer's.[26] To top it all off, carbs are the main food type that raises blood sugar levels, which means you need to be extra conscious of the types of carbs you're eating if you're looking to balance blood sugar.

But carbohydrates in their whole-food form can be very nourishing and supportive of health and weight-loss goals. They also can be packed with important micronutrients for health and longevity, such as folate, B vitamins, potassium, and vitamin C. When choosing carbohydrates, you want to select those that contain the most micronutrients while also being the most blood sugar stabilizing.

THE THREE TYPES OF CARBS

The three main categories of carbohydrates to be aware of are sugars, starches, and fiber.

Sugars are the simplest form and are rapidly absorbed into the bloodstream from the GI tract. Sugars are found in nutrient-dense foods such as blueberries and lemons and in nutrient-poor foods such as high-fructose corn syrup and cane sugar.

Although sugar is present in all sorts of foods, how it's packaged matters. Whole foods such as fruit also contain fiber and water. It also takes more effort to chew these foods before you can swallow them. From there, that food needs to be further broken down by enzymes in the small intestine before the body can access and absorb those sugars. This process helps slow the absorption and therefore keeps blood sugar levels stable. Sugary drinks and candy are much higher in sugar and contain little or no fiber. They also require minimal or zero effort to chew and digest. Because they've already undergone processing outside of the body, the body doesn't need to use as many resources to break them down before absorbing the sugars. This causes the body to absorb the sugar rapidly and leads to very unstable blood sugar levels.

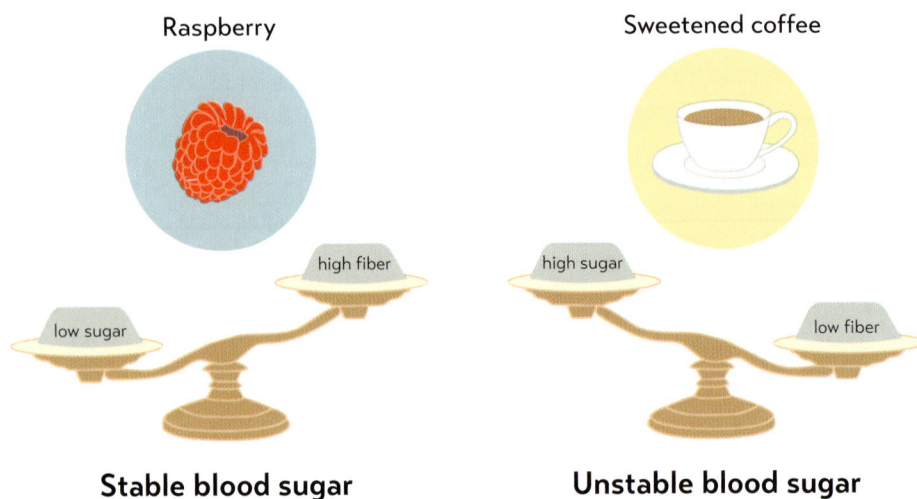

Raspberry

Sweetened coffee

high fiber

low sugar

high sugar

low fiber

Stable blood sugar

Unstable blood sugar

Then we have starches, which are chains of sugars strung together. These are found in foods like sweet potatoes, grains, beans, and lentils, but they're also present in highly processed foods like chips, bread, crackers, cereal, and baked goods. Because starch is bound in a chain, a little extra digestion is required in the GI tract to break it down before it can enter the bloodstream. Ultimately, though, it all breaks down into sugar. Some starches break down very quickly and therefore cause a large blood sugar spike, whereas others break down slowly and have a minimal impact on blood sugar. For most health and weight-loss goals, you want to stick with starches that break down slowly to help balance blood sugar levels and reduce hunger and cravings.

The third type is fiber. Fiber is a type of carbohydrate that the body doesn't break down into energy. Instead, fiber passes through the GI tract and exits during a bowel movement. We technically don't *need* fiber because it doesn't have any nutritional value. But it does help with stabilizing blood sugar. In fact, it's the fiber content of a food that determines how quickly or slowly the sugars and starches are absorbed into the bloodstream. Fiber acts as a physical barrier that your body must get around before it can use the starches and sugars in the food. Higher-fiber foods usually require more digestion before the body can start breaking down the starches and sugars, which slows their absorption into the bloodstream. This is why naturally higher-fiber foods such as avocados, chia seeds, and raspberries help stabilize blood sugar levels and prevent hunger and cravings.

In addition to stabilizing blood sugar levels, fiber can help raise satiety hormones. A type of fiber called soluble fiber in foods such as nuts, artichokes, beans, and fruit is fermented in the colon and creates short-chain fatty acids that raise the satiety hormone GLP-1.[27] When combined with quality sources of protein and fat, fiber can help curb hunger naturally and make achieving a weight-loss goal nearly effortless.

The types and amount of carbs you eat will largely depend on your wellness goal. The carbs that a type 2 diabetic should eat look much different than the carbs that would support a casual athlete. It's your job to understand which carbs are best for different intended outcomes. On top of that, you need to know that as your goals change, your carbohydrate types and amount likely should change too.

Rather than counting carbs or sticking to a keto or low-carb diet, I've found that having a basic understanding of how carbs impact the body is much more helpful for sustainable, long-term results. The best way of understanding carbs is with the glycemic load.

GLYCEMIC LOAD

As you have learned throughout this chapter, for optimal health and weight-loss results, you want to stabilize your blood sugar levels as much as possible. This means you want to fill your plate with carbohydrates that minimize blood sugar spikes.

You may have heard of the glycemic index, which measures how much 50 grams of carbs of a certain food will impact blood sugar. Although this index is a good first step, it's not the most ideal measurement to track because it doesn't account for realistic serving sizes. Fifty grams' worth of carbs from a food is not always indicative of real-life portions.

For example, the following all have 50 grams' worth of carbs:

- 120 cups of spinach
- 16 cups of cauliflower
- 14 cups of broccoli
- 6 cups of strawberries

- 2¼ medium-sized sweet potatoes
- 3¾ slices of white bread
- 1⅔ cups of cooked whole-wheat pasta
- 1¼ cups of cooked white rice

Clearly, most people are not eating 120 cups of spinach or 16 cups of broccoli. However, it's easy to eat 1¼ cups of cooked white rice. This means the glycemic index for some foods might be artificially inflated, whereas for others it might be unrealistically low.

To get a more accurate idea of how foods impact blood sugar, we'll be using glycemic load (GL). This takes the glycemic index and multiplies it by the actual amount of carbohydrates that are eaten at a time.

$$\frac{\text{Glycemic index of a food} \times \text{Net carbs in a food}}{100} = \text{GL}$$

- **Foods that score less than 10 are considered low GL.** Low-GL foods have a minimal impact on blood sugar levels and therefore are helpful for supporting weight-loss and wellness goals. Low-GL foods tend to be higher in fiber and important vitamins and minerals that support the body.

- **Foods that score between 11 and 19 are considered medium GL.** Medium-GL foods are still relatively blood sugar stabilizing, especially if you are physically active. However, they do tend to result in higher blood sugar spikes than low-GL foods and therefore are not ideal for those who are carb sensitive or insulin resistant (see the sidebar on the next page). Medium-GL foods are usually higher in carbohydrates than low-GL foods but still tend to have some fiber and important vitamins and minerals.

- **Foods that score higher than 20 are considered high GL.** These can have a significant impact on blood sugar levels and tend to cause the biggest spikes and falls in blood sugar. High-GL foods are often low in fiber and very high in carbohydrates. They also tend to be quite low in important vitamins and minerals compared to lower-GL foods. Typically, all processed foods fall into the high-GL category; however, some natural foods land in this category as well.

ARE YOU CARB SENSITIVE?

People who are carb sensitive or insulin resistant have high fasting blood sugar, have high fasting insulin, or are type 2 diabetic. You might be carb sensitive if you notice that you have a difficult time losing weight or you gain weight easily. I have a free quiz on my website to help you determine if you're carb sensitive; scan the QR code for the quiz.

Some foods, such as leafy greens and broccoli, have a low glycemic load regardless of how much of them you eat. For others, the GL will vary greatly depending on the amount you consume. Chickpeas are a great example. Cooked chickpeas are considered low GL when you eat a cup or less of them. However, when the amount increases to 2 cups, chickpeas jump into the medium-GL category. This is why you'll find serving sizes for some foods in the glycemic load chart that follows. Any food that doesn't have a serving size listed has a very low GL regardless of how much of it you eat.

LOW GLYCEMIC LOAD

This category should be included in all of your meals, regardless of your goal. These carbs typically have the most fiber and highest micronutrient content.

- Apricots
- Artichokes
- Asparagus
- Bean sprouts
- Beets
- Bell peppers
- Blackberries
- Bok choy
- Broccoli
- Brussels sprouts
- Cabbage
- Carrots
- Cauliflower
- Celery
- Cucumbers
- Daikon
- Eggplant
- Garlic
- Green beans
- Hearts of palm
- Jicama
- Leafy greens
- Leeks
- Mushrooms
- Onions
- Radishes
- Raspberries
- Snow peas
- Sprouts
- Sugar snap peas
- Swiss chard
- Tomatoes
- Turnips
- Water chestnuts
- 4 cups okra
- 3 plums
- 2½ cups strawberries
- 2 cups cherries
- 2 peaches
- 1½ cups cooked mung beans
- 1½ cups watermelon
- 1 apple
- 1 citrus fruit
- 1 cup blueberries
- 1 cup cooked beans (black, kidney, white, etc.)
- 1 cup cooked chickpeas
- 1 cup cooked lentils
- 1 small pear
- ¾ cup cantaloupe
- ¾ cup grapes
- ¾ cup honeydew
- ½ small banana

MEDIUM GLYCEMIC LOAD

Your intake of this category will depend on your goals. Refer to pages 37 and 38 to see if or how much you should eat from this category.

- Any food listed in the Low Glycemic Load category that is eaten in quantities larger than the suggested serving size
- 2 slices sourdough bread (62 grams total)
- 2 small slices whole-wheat bread (preferably sprouted and naturally fermented)
- 1¼ cups fresh corn kernels
- 1½ cups cooked buckwheat noodles
- 1 cup cooked bulgur
- 1 cup cooked kamut

- 1 cup cooked quinoa
- 1 cup cooked whole-wheat pasta
- 1 cup cooked wild rice
- 1 cup cooked yam
- 1 small boiled potato (160 grams)*
- 1 small sweet potato (80 grams)
- ¾ cup cooked couscous
- ½ cup cooked brown rice
- ½ cup cooked rolled oats

*You can bring down the glycemic load of boiled potatoes significantly by eating them after they have cooled completely.

HIGH GLYCEMIC LOAD

Your intake of this category will depend on your goals. Refer to pages 37 and 38 to see if or how much you should eat from this category.

- Any food listed in the Medium Glycemic Load category that is eaten in quantities larger than the suggested serving size
- Cereal
- Chips
- Cider
- Cocktails with added sugar
- Cooked millet

- Cooked rice noodles
- Cooked white rice
- Corn or flour tortillas
- Dried fruit
- Flour (other than coconut or almond flour)
- Fruit juice
- Sugar, such as honey, agave nectar, coconut sugar, cane sugar, and maple syrup*

*Technically, a lot of added sugars aren't very high glycemic load in amounts up to 2 tablespoons. However, due to the low satiety level and highly addictive nature of sugar, I usually group added sugars in the high-GL category. An exception is small amounts used infrequently in an otherwise low-GL meal (such as a low-GL baked good). I strongly advise against consuming any drink with added sugar, as this will greatly spike its glycemic load due to the lack of fiber or chewing.

When choosing the type of carbs to fill your plate with, you need to consider your goals:

- **Weight Loss:** If your goal is to lose body fat and maintain muscle, then it's ideal to stick to only low–glycemic load carbohydrates. These are going to provide the most nutrient bang for your carbohydrate buck. They're also going to be the most blood sugar stabilizing and therefore the best at preventing hunger and cravings. Stick to the low-GL category on page 35 if your primary goal is fat loss.

- **Muscle Gain or Athletic Performance:** Athletes tend to have much more muscle mass than non-athletes, which means they have a bigger "sugar sponge." This gives them more flexibility with the amount and types of carbs they can eat while keeping their blood sugar levels stable. Athletes and those looking to increase muscle mass also tend to struggle to eat enough food to support their significantly higher metabolism and lean mass. Protein, fat, and fiber should still be the basis of meals when the goal is to increase muscle or achieve athletic performance because this combination provides the necessary building blocks and essential nutrients for recovery and energy creation. However, if you simply add more fat or more fiber-rich foods on top of this baseline, then you will get too full before you are able to hit your nutrient needs. Because people in this category struggle to eat enough food in general, they tend to benefit from including medium–glycemic load and some high–glycemic load foods, which are inherently less satiating and therefore allow them to eat more. Depending on the individual, this might be one to two servings of higher-GL foods per meal in addition to protein, fat, and fiber. These foods should never replace protein, fat, and fiber; rather, they should be added to a meal. Finding the right proportions will take some trial and error, but monitoring performance and strength is a great way to determine whether you're on the right track. If your performance is improving, then you're probably getting the proper balance for your body. However, if your performance is struggling or you aren't gaining muscle mass and you know you're getting enough protein, then it might be time to up your servings of higher-GL foods.

- **Managing Carb Sensitivity or Insulin Resistance:** If you struggle with weight gain from eating any type of carbohydrates, or you know that you're insulin resistant, then it's important to stick to the most blood sugar–stabilizing, low–glycemic load foods possible and not venture beyond those. Some people in this category might be hyper-reactive to even the low-GL category. In this case, limiting simple sugars from fruits to one serving per day tends to be helpful.

- **Maintenance or General Health:** Assuming that you aren't carb sensitive and you're active throughout the week, this category can include one to three servings of medium–glycemic load foods per day. Depending on your exercise level, occasional high–glycemic load foods can be included with two to three servings per week; however, these need to be limited due to the massive impact they have on blood sugar and their higher potential for addictive behavior.

- **Age 50+:** As you get older, insulin resistance tends to go up, which means that the carbs your body used to tolerate probably won't work for you anymore. This isn't the case for everyone in their fifties or older. If you are quite active and focused on building or maintaining muscle mass, you probably are still able to eat the same types of carbs you've always eaten. However, if you've noticed that you suddenly are gaining weight while eating the foods you've always eaten, you might be experiencing some age-related insulin resistance. With this in mind, prioritizing low–glycemic load foods will help keep your blood sugar levels stable without further driving up insulin resistance.

The piece of the puzzle that most people (including many health professionals) tend to miss is that you need to be adaptable. As you can see, each of the categories is goal dependent. If you are currently working toward a weight-loss goal, then you likely will do best with low-GL foods. But eventually, you're going to require maintenance of your goal rather than continued fat loss. This is when it's important to shift gears and focus on the tools that are tailored for general health and maintenance. Or maybe you've hit your goal, and now you want to try to gain a little muscle. At this point, you need to use the strategies that are directed toward that endeavor.

What works for you now is probably not going to work for you in the future because as you change, so do your goals. The problem I've run into is that people are wary of change, especially if they've had great success already. But if you don't adapt your strategy to fit your current aims, then you won't achieve your new goals. Always be honest with yourself and take a few minutes to assess where you are in your journey. If you've hit your weight-loss goal, great! Take the steps to make sure you can maintain your results by switching to the maintenance strategies. Or if you are working to increase muscle for your health, that's awesome! Don't be afraid to test out some high-GL foods to support that goal.

Remember, if your goals change, then your meals should too.

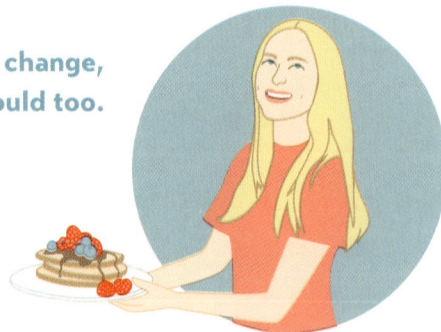

REFERENCES

[1] Weigle, David S., Patricia A. Breen, Colleen C. Matthys, et al. "A High-Protein Diet Induces Sustained Reductions in Appetite, Ad Libitum Caloric Intake, and Body Weight Despite Compensatory Changes in Diurnal Plasma Leptin and Ghrelin Concentrations." *American Journal of Clinical Nutrition* 82 (2005): 41–48.

[2] Wycherley, Thomas P. et al. "Effects of Energy-Restricted High-Protein, Low-Fat Compared with Standard-Protein, Low-Fat Diets: A Meta-Analysis of Randomized Controlled Trials." *American Journal of Clinical Nutrition* 96, no. 6 (2012): 1281–1298. doi:10.3945/ajcn.112.044321

[3] Moon, Jaecheol, and Gwanpyo Koh. "Clinical Evidence and Mechanisms of High-Protein Diet-Induced Weight Loss." *Journal of Obesity & Metabolic Syndrome* 29, no. 3 (2020): 166–173. doi:10.7570/jomes20028

[4] Wu, Guoyao. "Dietary Protein Intake and Human Health." *Food & Function* 7, no. 3 (2016): 1251–1265. doi:10.1039/c5fo01530h

[5] Nowson, Caryl, and Stella O'Connell. "Protein Requirements and Recommendations for Older People: A Review." *Nutrients* 7, no. 8 (2015): 6874–6899. doi:10.3390/nu7085311

[6] Coelho-Júnior, Hélio José et al. "Low Protein Intake Is Associated with Frailty in Older Adults: A Systematic Review and Meta-Analysis of Observational Studies." *Nutrients* 10, no. 9 (2018): 1334. doi:10.3390/nu10091334

[7] Aubertin-Leheudre, Mylène, and Herman Adlercreutz. "Relationship Between Animal Protein Intake and Muscle Mass Index in Healthy Women." *British Journal of Nutrition* 102, no. 12 (2009): 1803–1810. doi:10.1017/S0007114509991310

[8] Herreman, Laure, Paul Nommensen, Bart Pennings, and Marc C. Laus. "Comprehensive Overview of the Quality of Plant- and Animal-Sourced Proteins Based on the Digestible Indispensable Amino Acid Score." *Food Science & Nutrition* 8, no. 10 (2020): 5379–5391.

[9] Beal, Ty, and Flaminia Ortenzi. "Priority Micronutrient Density in Foods." *Frontiers in Nutrition* 9 (2022). https://doi.org/10.3389/fnut.2022.806566

[10] Gower, Barbara A., and Amy M. Goss. "A Lower-Carbohydrate, Higher-Fat Diet Reduces Abdominal and Intermuscular Fat and Increases Insulin Sensitivity in Adults at Risk of Type 2 Diabetes." *Journal of Nutrition* 145, no. 1 (2015): 177S–183S. doi:10.3945/jn.114.195065

[11] Samaha, Frederick F. et al. "A Low-Carbohydrate as Compared with a Low-Fat Diet in Severe Obesity." *New England Journal of Medicine* 348 (2003): 2074–2081.

[12] Rao, Pingfan et al. "Addressing the Sugar, Salt, and Fat Issue the Science of Food Way." *NPJ Science of Food* 2 (2018): 12. doi:10.1038/s41538-018-0020-x

[13] Bodnaruc, A. M., D. Prud'homme, R. Blanchet, et al. "Nutritional Modulation of Endogenous Glucagon-Like Peptide-1 Secretion: A Review." *Nutrition & Metabolism (London)* 13, no. 92 (2016). https://doi.org/10.1186/s12986-016-0153-3

[14] Crichton, Georgina E., and Ala'a Alkerwi. "Whole-Fat Dairy Food Intake Is Inversely Associated with Obesity Prevalence: Findings from the Observation of Cardiovascular Risk

Factors in Luxembourg Study." *Nutrition Research (New York, N.Y.)* 34, no. 11 (2014): 936–943. doi:10.1016/j.nutres.2014.07.014

[15] Ma, Ming-Ling et al. "Efficacy of Vitamin K2 in the Prevention and Treatment of Postmenopausal Osteoporosis: A Systematic Review and Meta-Analysis of Randomized Controlled Trials." *Frontiers in Public Health* 10 (2022): 979649. doi:10.3389/fpubh.2022.979649

[16] Chuai, Yuanyuan et al. "Association of Vitamin K, Fibre Intake and Progression of Periodontal Attachment Loss in American Adults." *BMC Oral Health* 23 (2023): 303. https://doi.org/10.1186/s12903-023-02929-9

[17] Yelland, L. N. et al. "Predicting the Effect of Maternal Docosahexaenoic Acid (DHA) Supplementation to Reduce Early Preterm Birth in Australia and the United States Using Results of Within Country Randomized Controlled Trials." *Prostaglandins, Leukotrienes, and Essential Fatty Acids* 112 (2016): 44–49. doi:10.1016/j.plefa.2016.08.007

[18] Corder, Katherine E. et al. "Effects of Short-Term Docosahexaenoic Acid Supplementation on Markers of Inflammation after Eccentric Strength Exercise in Women." *Journal of Sports Science & Medicine* 15, no. 1 (2016): 176–183.

[19] Dawczynski, C. et al. "Docosahexaenoic Acid in the Treatment of Rheumatoid Arthritis: A Double-Blind, Placebo-Controlled, Randomized Cross-Over Study with Microalgae vs. Sunflower Oil." *Clinical Nutrition (Edinburgh, Scotland)* 37, no. 2 (2018): 494–504. doi:10.1016/j.clnu.2017.02.021

[20] Du, Shichun et al. "Does Fish Oil Have an Anti-Obesity Effect in Overweight/Obese Adults? A Meta-Analysis of Randomized Controlled Trials." *PloS One* 10, no. 11 (2015): e0142652. doi:10.1371/journal.pone.0142652

[21] Bishehkolaei, Maral, and Yashwant Pathak. "Influence of Omega N-6/N-3 Ratio on Cardiovascular Disease and Nutritional Interventions." *Human Nutrition & Metabolism* 37 (2024): 200275. https://doi.org/10.1016/j.hnm.2024.200275

[22] Gearhardt, Ashley N. et al. "Social, Clinical, and Policy Implications of Ultra-Processed Food Addiction." *BMJ (Clinical Research Ed.)* 383 (2023): e075354. doi:10.1136/bmj-2023-075354

[23] Delpino, Felipe Mendes et al. "Ultra-Processed Food and Risk of Type 2 Diabetes: A Systematic Review and Meta-Analysis of Longitudinal Studies." *International Journal of Epidemiology* 51, no. 4 (2022): 1120–1141. doi:10.1093/ije/dyab247

[24] Juul, Philippa et al. "Ultra-Processed Foods and Cardiovascular Diseases: Potential Mechanisms of Action." *Advances in Nutrition* 12, no. 5 (2021): 1673–1680. https://doi.org/10.1093/advances/nmab049

[25] Cordova, Reynalda et al. "Consumption of Ultra-Processed Foods and Risk of Multimorbidity of Cancer and Cardiometabolic Diseases: A Multinational Cohort Study." *The Lancet* 23 (2023): 100771.

[26] Claudino, Paola A. et al. "Consumption of Ultra-Processed Foods and Risk for Alzheimer's Disease: A Systematic Review." *Frontiers in Nutrition* 14 (2024). https://doi.org/10.3389/fnut.2023.1288749

[27] See note 13.

CHAPTER 2

BUILDING YOUR MEALS

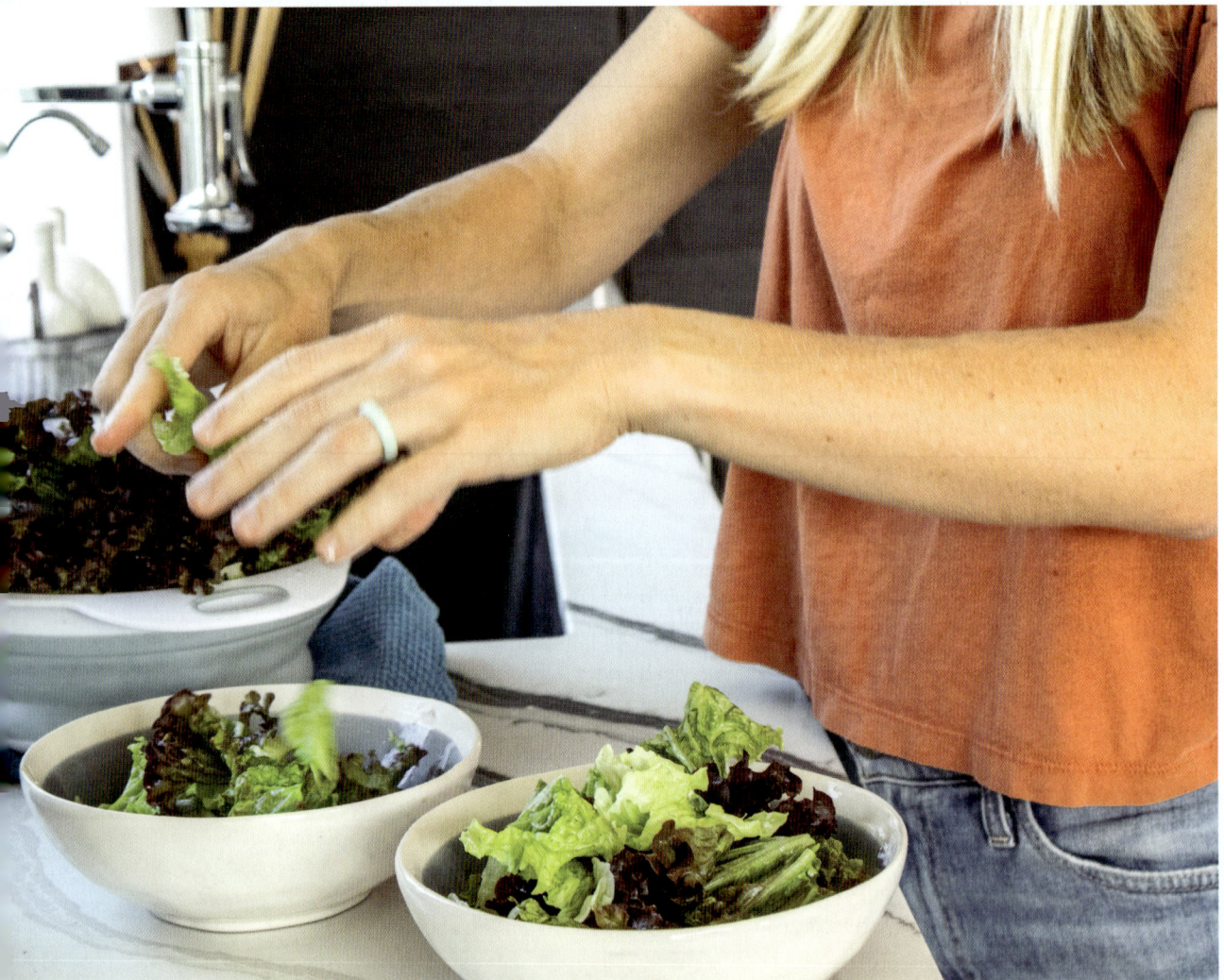

Now that you have an understanding of the building blocks of what your body needs to feel full and satisfied, it's time to put them onto a plate. In this chapter, you'll learn how often and how much you should eat to maximize satiety and wellness and achieve your fat-loss goals while still fitting it into your busy lifestyle and your food preferences.

MEALS, NOT SNACKS

If you were trying to make absolutely sure that you didn't get hungry throughout the day, you would probably pack a ton of snacks in your bag and plan to eat every few hours. You wouldn't be alone in this thinking, either. If you browse nearly any weight-loss website or even the USDA's dietary guidelines, you would be told to aim for six to eight small meals throughout the day to ensure "stable blood sugar levels" and to help prevent hunger. But interestingly, this is a terrible strategy for preventing hunger, and I can prove it.

Researchers have dug into the question of meal frequency to see which frequency *actually* makes us feel fuller longer and prevents cravings. One study had groups of overweight or obese individuals eat either six or three meals per day. The groups were further split up into "normal" protein groups (14 percent of total calories) and "high" protein groups (25 percent of total calories). In total, there were four groups:

- Normal protein with three meals
- Normal protein with six meals
- High protein with three meals
- High protein with six meals

Although meal frequency and protein intake differed, the groups ate the same number of total calories. The study found that those eating three meals per day with higher protein experienced lower late-night desire to eat, fewer preoccupying food thoughts, and greater evening and late-night fullness.[1]

Another interesting fact is that Americans are significantly more likely to snack compared to people in other countries. A 2022 poll found that 65 percent of Americans identify themselves as snackers, whereas only 30 percent of the French people surveyed said they snacked between meals.[2] When you realize that the current obesity rate in the US is over 42 percent and in France it's only 17 percent,[3] you might start asking some serious questions about our snacking habits. Of course, much more than meal frequency goes into obesity rates, but it's a major contributing factor, as it's obviously something that you either do or don't do every single day.

When you split your eating into three larger meals instead of six smaller ones, you're able to fully tap into the power of satiety hormones that prevent hunger and cravings. This cannot be achieved with smaller, more frequent meals.

STRATEGIC SNACKING FOR SOME PEOPLE

Even though snacking is generally not a good idea for most people, some can benefit from strategically adding in one or two snacks per day. This can include athletes, growing kids, those who are pregnant or breastfeeding, and those who generally have a difficult time eating enough in a day to fulfill their needs. These types of people have significantly increased nutritional needs that are often higher than what satiety hormones will allow for. Because snacking helps you eat *more*, it can be a useful strategy for these folks.

Also, there will inevitably be times when you accidentally undereat and need a quick bite to hold you over until your next meal. The following are 25 tasty ideas with at least 10 grams of protein that you can lean on in a pinch. Just remember to adjust your future meals to be more satiating, because even high-quality snacks can work against your weight-loss or wellness goals if eaten consistently.

Autumn-Approved Snacks:

- 0.75 ounce pork rinds (I like the brand 4505)
- 1 or 2 beef sticks
- 1 ounce baked Parmesan "chips" (like Parm Crisps)
- 1 ounce beef jerky with ¼ cup nuts
- 1 scoop protein powder shaken with 8 ounces whole milk or almond milk
- 1 scoop vanilla protein powder blended into coffee
- 1 slice cauliflower toast (I like the brand Outer Aisle) with ½ avocado
- 1 slice deli cheese and 1 slice deli meat rolled up together
- 1 string cheese with ½ apple
- 1.3 ounces sliced aged cheese (like Parmesan or Swiss)
- ½ cup cottage cheese with ½ cup berries
- ½ cup cottage cheese with sliced cucumbers and black pepper
- ½ cup Greek yogurt with ½ cup berries
- 2 egg bites (homemade or store-bought)
- 2 hard-boiled eggs
- 2 ounces soft cheese (like goat or Brie) with 1 piece low-glycemic fruit
- 2- to 3-ounce pouch tuna or salmon
- ¾ cup edamame dipped in tamari or soy sauce
- Cottage Cheese Deviled Eggs (page 211)

- Cottage Cheese Protein Cookie Dough*
- Greek Yogurt Dessert Bowl (page 240)
- Mini charcuterie board: 1 ounce cheese, 2 or 3 slices salami, ¼ cup olives, and a handful of baby carrots
- Protein Hot Chocolate*

- Protein Mug Cake*
- Quickie chia pudding (mix together 2 tablespoons chia seeds, ½ cup almond milk, and 1 scoop vanilla protein powder and let sit for 30 minutes before eating)

These recipes can be found on my blog (autumnellenutrition.com/blog).

Think of it like your gas tank. If you add only a few dollars' worth of fuel to your car, you're going to need to stop at a gas station almost every time you drive somewhere. But if you make sure to fill your tank completely whenever it's low, you get the benefit of driving for hundreds of miles before you need to even think about stopping. Same goes for your body. Fill it up with the right type of food every time you eat, and you get the benefit of not having to eat as often.

Small, Frequent Meals   vs.   **3 Full Meals**

CCK   Peptide YY   GLP-1

Peptide YY   GLP-1   CCK

Meal 1   Meal 2   Meal 3   Meal 4   Meal 5   Meal 6

Meal 1   Meal 2   Meal 3

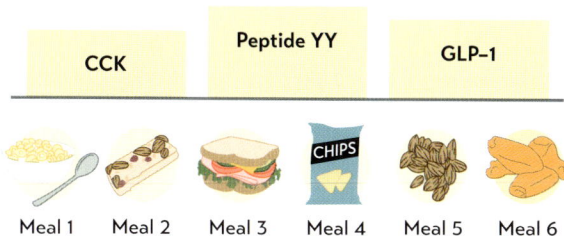

6 small meals result in smaller bumps of satiety hormones. This means you will feel hungry again faster, usually within 1 to 2 hours.

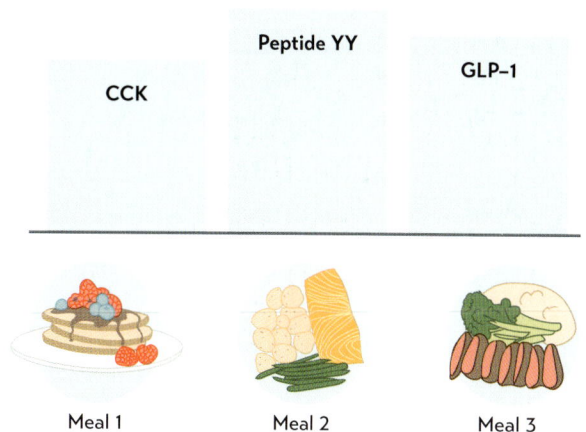

3 larger meals result in larger rises of satiety hormones. This means you won't feel hungry again for another 3 to 5 hours.

Eating enough protein, fat, and fiber to adequately raise satiety hormones shuts off the desire to eat and stabilizes blood sugar levels to help prevent cravings. But if you eat smaller meals throughout the day (or when you "graze"), you never raise those satiety hormones enough to feel satisfied. Smaller meals are also typically lower in protein and higher in carbohydrates, which can lead to unstable blood sugar levels. This results in feeling slightly (or very) hungry throughout the day. It could also lead to signs of low blood sugar, such as headaches, nausea, or mood changes (like the dreaded "hanger"). Due to increased hunger and unstable blood sugar levels, your cravings change too. Rather than wanting a high-protein meal that would help break the cycle of hunger and cravings, you typically reach for something high in sugar or processed carbohydrates to try to quickly raise your blood sugar levels. This is why people often graze on chips, crackers, sugary "protein" bars, granola, cereal, pretzels, or dried fruit when they don't eat enough to sustain a three-meal structure. Because these common snack foods are high in sugar or processed carbohydrates, they don't raise satiety hormones (again), which perpetuates the cycle of needing to eat more processed foods within an hour or so.

But even if you focus on eating whole foods and split them up into six or more meals, you can still run into the same issue of not adequately raising satiety hormones enough to feel satisfied and prevent hunger shortly after eating. A common example is snacking on fruit and/or nuts between meals. These are healthy, whole-food ingredients, but they don't contain enough protein to raise satiety hormones and prevent hunger from quickly returning. (In fact, nuts specifically can be a "trigger" food for many, but we'll get into that later in this chapter.) This is why paying attention to filling your plate with both *enough* and the *right type* of food is crucial for achieving and maintaining health and weight-loss goals.

The benefits of eating less frequently span a multitude of health parameters. Eating enough protein, fat, and fiber to feel satisfied at meals can

- **Reduce hunger:** By boosting peptide YY, CCK, and GLP-1, these foods naturally shut off hunger and the desire to eat for three to five hours or so.

- **Turn on the migrating motor complex:** Because you aren't snacking, the gut-cleaning process called the migrating motor complex can switch on. This sweeps out left-behind food and bacteria that often lead to bloating if left unchecked.

- **Improve gut health:** Gut health issues like SIBO (small intestine bacterial overgrowth) are often linked to a disrupted or disturbed migrating motor complex. By not snacking, you can turn on the important gut-cleaning process that promotes overall gut health.

- **Reduce inflammation:** What happens in your gut is usually seen in the rest of your body. Constant eating doesn't allow your GI tract to get enough rest or repair. This can result in increased gut inflammation in the form of issues like IBS, leaky gut, or SIBO, which can impact other inflammatory conditions throughout the body.[4] Healing the gut can help you make substantial progress toward healing the rest of your body. Removing snacks is a major tool in that process.

- **Boost metabolic flexibility:** When you snack, you get stuck on the blood sugar roller coaster that shuts off efficient fat burning. However, stabilizing blood sugar levels allows the body to more easily turn to fat stores for fuel instead. This ability to easily switch back and forth between carb and fat fuel sources is called metabolic flexibility.

If frequent low-calorie, lower-protein meals are a problem, why are they constantly hyped? It comes back to the commonly recommended breakdown of protein, fat, and carbs in a meal. The USDA guidelines emphasize a higher-carb diet with 45 to 65 percent of calories coming from carbohydrates, or 225 to 325 grams of carbs per day (assuming someone is eating 2,000 calories a day). Blood sugar–stabilizing low– and medium–glycemic load carbs are much lower in total carbohydrates, and it would be *very* difficult to get enough volume from just these categories of foods to hit those numbers. The only way to eat *this many* carbs is to eat quite a lot of starchy, higher–glycemic load foods, which are inherently less blood sugar stabilizing than their lower-GL counterparts. This is where recommendations for pasta, rice, and cereals take center stage to hit this high recommendation for carbs.

VOLUME MATTERS

The following is how much you would need to eat of either all low–glycemic load foods or all higher–glycemic load foods to hit around 235 grams of net carbs (near the low end of the USDA recommended intake). As you can see, it's difficult if not impossible to eat enough food from exclusively low-GL ingredients when you're aiming for such a high carb count. It's much easier when you're eating high-GL foods, even from "whole-grain" sources. This is one of the reasons these high-GL foods are often promoted despite being less beneficial for satiety, body composition, and nutrient density.

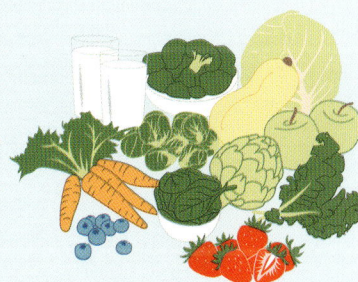

Low Glycemic

- **Low Glycemic:** 10 cups spinach, 5 cups strawberries, 4 cups broccoli, 4 carrots, 4 cups kale, 3 cups cabbage, 2 apples, 2 cups Brussels sprouts, 2 cups butternut squash, 2 cups milk, 1 artichoke, 1 cup blueberries

- **High Glycemic:** 2 slices whole-wheat bread, 2 cups whole-wheat pasta, 1½ cups oatmeal, 1½ cups white rice, 1½ whole-wheat tortillas

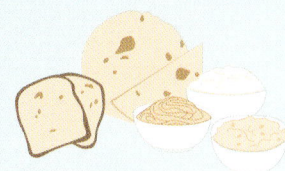

High Glycemic

But as you learned on page 34, those foods can lead to a large blood sugar crash and the resultant hunger and cravings shortly thereafter. Rather than having three larger high-carb meals, it's often recommended to stick to smaller, more frequent meals to "get ahead" of this blood sugar crash and "prevent hunger." In reality, this approach doesn't balance blood sugar levels; it just continues the blood sugar roller coaster. Eating frequently is a necessity with this meal structure due to lower satiety hormones and more unstable blood sugar levels.

Although the standard guidelines opt for this arguably unsustainable approach, researchers and clinicians alike are finding that eating three satisfying meals rich in protein, fat, and fiber results in much better weight-loss and wellness progress.

Small, "normal" protein, higher-carb meals

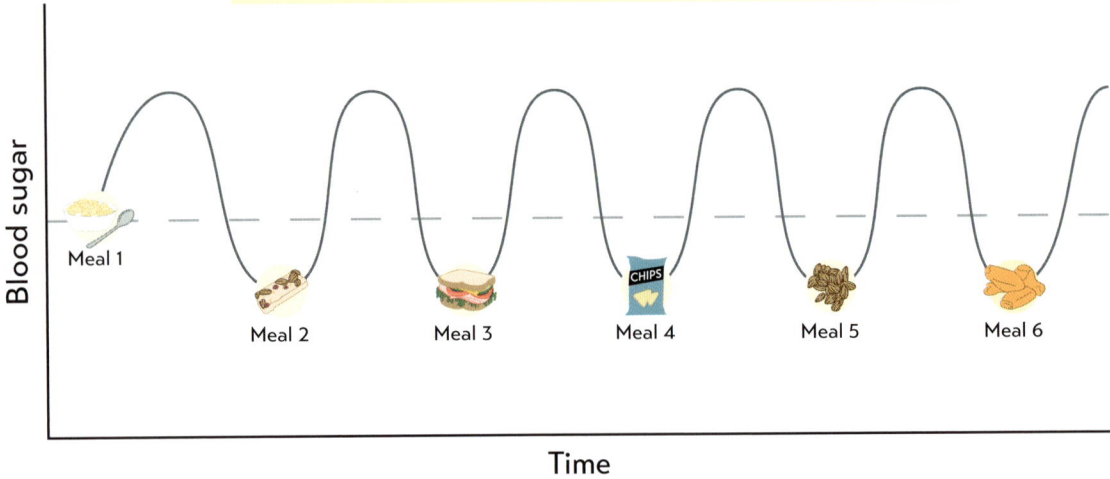

Larger, "higher" protein, fat, and fiber meals

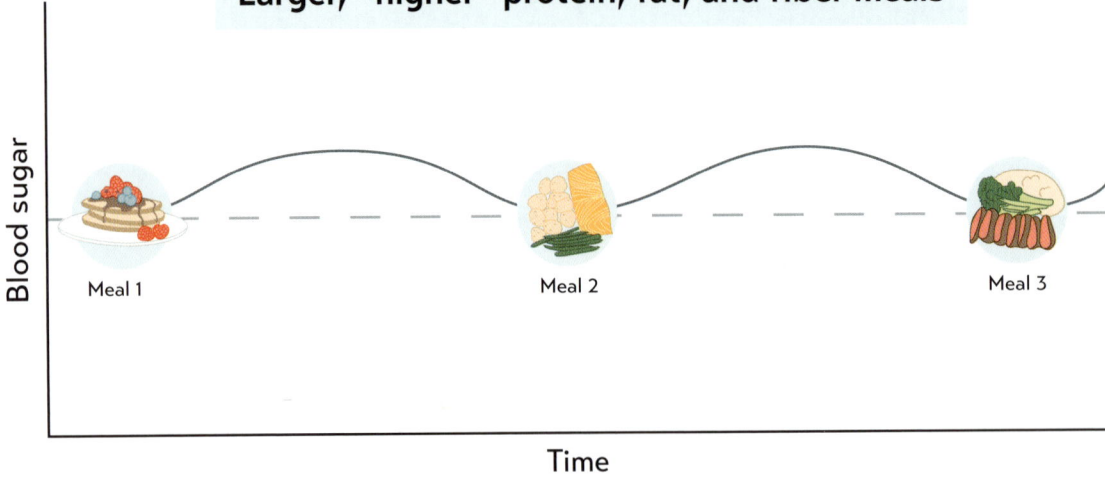

INTERMITTENT FASTING

As you can see, eating less frequently can be an incredible health and weight-loss tool, which is one of the main reasons intermittent fasting has gained massive popularity as an eating pattern. The benefits of three meals can be further amplified with a well-structured intermittent fast, such as a 12-, 14-, or 16-hour fast. In fact, this is one of the main tools I used to help heal my gut from extremely painful and persistent bloating.

Even though intermittent fasting is a fantastic tool, it's really important to do it the right way. A common mistake I often see is that people either simply skip one meal or fast for way too long. These poor approaches can lead to increased hunger, muscle loss, and at times even fat gain. This is why I created the 21 Day Intermittent Fasting Program that thousands of people have used over the last seven years to help them achieve their goals with the proper use of intermittent fasting. If you want to grab my best-selling program, you can find it at autumnellenutrition.shop.

Hopefully by now you can see the immense benefit of eating three full and satiating meals per day. So let's talk about how you go about building a plate that supports that goal.

BUILDING YOUR PLATE

For maximum satiety-boosting benefits, you want a roughly even split between high-quality protein, fats, and low–glycemic load carbohydrates. This of course will vary depending on your specific needs (see pages 37 and 38 for details), but this even split is a great starting place for most goals. Some people, such as athletes, will need to add an additional component of starchy carbs.

Just because you're looking for an even split of the three food types at most meals doesn't mean that they will *look* even. For example, fat is much denser than fiber-rich foods. This means a serving of a high-fat food like avocado will be smaller than a serving of a very low-fat food like spinach. Rather than tracking everything you eat (which is unsustainable at best and could lead to a poor relationship with food at worst), you can get an idea of what typical serving sizes look like for each type of food.

Let's start with protein.

PROTEIN

I always recommend starting with protein. Your meal should be centered around protein. The star of the show, if you will. But that doesn't mean it needs to be center stage visually. A great example is chili. It's super easy to "hide" significant amounts of ground beef in a big bowl of steaming chili. However you serve it, protein should make up roughly a third of your meal.

A good rule of thumb is to aim for 30 grams of protein per meal (or at least 90 grams of complete protein per day). This equates to 4 ounces of *cooked* protein at each meal (12 ounces total for the day). Or you can swap meat, fish, or chicken for a vegetarian source such as 1½ cups of skyr, 1¼ cups of cottage cheese, or five eggs. (Find the full list of protein amounts below.) You can also use my protein calculation on page 19 to determine a number more specific to your needs. Whichever you choose, you *must* formulate each meal around protein. Otherwise, it's easy to miss your protein mark and get hungry.

The following is a list of foods that have 30 grams of protein (listed in *cooked* weight). This list is not exhaustive but gives you an idea of some of the most common foods I've been asked about over the years. You can always do a quick search of a food on the Cronometer app if you want to know how much of it you need to eat to hit 30 grams of protein.

Animal-based sources:

- Bacon*, 3 ounces
- Beef, 4 ounces
- Bison, 4 ounces
- Chicken, 3.5 ounces
- Fish, 4.2 ounces
- Goat, 4.75 ounces
- Kangaroo, 5 ounces
- Lamb, 4.75 ounces
- Pork loin, 3.75 ounces
- Sausage*, 7 ounces
- Shellfish, 5.5 to 6 ounces
- Venison, 4 ounces

Vegetarian sources:

- Cottage cheese, 1¼ cups
- Eggs, 5
- Greek yogurt, 1½ cups
- Halloumi, 4.5 ounces
- Hard cheese, 4.5 ounces
- Kefir (from whole milk)*, 33 ounces
- Paneer, 5 ounces
- Skyr, 1¼ cups
- Whey protein powder, 1½ servings
- Whole milk*, 33 ounces

*I wouldn't recommend making these foods the main protein of a meal, as you would need to eat a *lot* of them to hit 30 grams. Instead, use these to complement other protein-rich foods, such as blending whole milk or kefir into a smoothie that also contains protein powder or Greek yogurt.

Plant-based sources:

- Chickpeas, 2¼ cups
- Edamame**, 9 ounces
- Firm tofu**, 9 ounces
- Green peas, 3¾ cups
- Plant-based Greek-style yogurt with added protein (usually soy)**, 1½ cups
- Potato protein powder, 1½ servings
- Seitan**, 5 ounces
- Split peas, 1½ cups
- Tempeh, 5.25 ounces

**These are some of my least favorite plant-based proteins because they either provide little to no nutrient value or contain significant levels of antinutrients (like phytates and lectins) that block the body's ability to absorb important minerals.

Here are my top tips for adding protein to a meal:

- **Most cuts of meat, fish, or chicken provide three servings (30 grams of protein each) per pound when measured raw.** This comes out to about ⅓ pound of animal-based protein per serving. So, if you're planning a meal for four people, you'll need 1⅓ pounds of raw meat, fish, or chicken.

- **Don't look at the "serving size" in a recipe. Look at how much protein is in the ingredient list and increase the protein if needed.** I do this whenever I'm trying out a new recipe. Unfortunately, a lot of recipes in other cookbooks skimp on the protein source in favor of grains or veggies. I always scan the ingredient list for the protein (for example, chicken, salmon, beef, or cottage cheese) and recalibrate the recipe based on that number. For example, if a recipe says it serves four but calls for only ½ pound of beef, I up the beef to 1⅓ pounds and keep everything else the same to serve four with the proper protein intake.

- **Be aware of the shrinking protein effect.** Protein shrinks when it's cooked because it loses water. Protein isn't lost during cooking; it just gets more concentrated. For example, 3 ounces of cooked chicken has roughly the same amount of protein as 4 ounces of raw chicken. If you're weighing a protein to get an idea of how much you need to eat, always weigh it *cooked* unless you know how much protein is in the *raw* form. Most food trackers and nutrition labels provide the protein of a food based on the cooked weight, not the raw.

- **Plan for leftovers; don't rely on eating "what's left over."** Very few people accurately plan for lunch. Most often, I see clients save whatever they have left over from dinner to eat for lunch the next day. However, if you didn't cook extra protein to account for leftovers, then you're probably eating too little protein at both dinner *and* the next-day lunch. So, if you plan on having lunch from a leftover dinner, cook an extra ⅓ pound of raw protein and put it to the side before you eat dinner.

- **Measure *all* protein sources at least a few times before you start eyeballing.** I'm a big fan of eyeballing it. You should never feel tied to a kitchen scale, because it is tedious to use and simply isn't necessary most of the time. However, there's a time and place for a food scale. When you're first learning how much protein you need to eat at every meal, a scale can be useful for giving you an idea of what that amount looks like. Measure each source a few times, and then feel free to eyeball it after that.

- **"Hide" protein if you find it hard to eat a lot of it.** Especially if you're new to eating animal-based protein, you might find it difficult to eat more of it. I've found that sneaking it into "pasta" dishes, like my Slow-Cooked Bolognese (page 159), or chilis, like my loaded Beef Chili (page 130), helps hide the meat and makes it much easier to eat.

- **Switch up your protein sources.** Each protein has different benefits. Dairy is super high in calcium and vitamin K2. Eggs are insanely high in choline. Beef is a great source of iron. Salmon and sardines are fantastic for omega-3s. Switching up your protein sources throughout the day and the week helps you get a broader range of nutrients. It also helps prevent food fatigue and getting tired of your meals. I love to break it up like this: dairy at breakfast, eggs at lunch, and meat, fish, or chicken at dinner.

- **Don't skimp on breakfast.** Breakfast tends to be the lowest-protein meal, even when you think you're eating "high-protein" foods. Eggs, bacon, sausage, and yogurt are all common first meal choices, but each is sneakily low in protein. One egg has only 5 to 6 grams of protein. You need to eat three breakfast sausage links for just 9 grams of protein. And regular yogurt has only 5 to 7 grams of protein per cup. Check out my delicious breakfast ideas for how to take typical breakfast ingredients and up the total protein content to 30 grams or more.

- **Be aware of protein quality.** This is specifically something my plant-based and vegetarian friends need to be conscious of. Check out my plant-based and vegetarian tips on pages 57 to 59 for details. If you're sticking to primarily animal-based proteins, then you don't need to be concerned about protein quality, as nearly all types are considered high DIAAS (see pages 20 to 24 for more on the DIAAS scale).

- **Know your total, then split it into three.** If you choose to calculate your protein requirement to get a more specific idea of what your body needs, that's great! Once you have your total number, divide it by three to determine how much protein you need at every meal. For example, if you need 120 grams of protein per day, then you should eat 40 grams at every meal.

- **Err on the side of more rather than less.** Assuming you're getting most of your protein from whole-food sources, it's difficult to overdo it. Protein is so satiating that most people tend to err on the side of eating less rather than more. If you find that you're feeling a little hungry after your meal, go for some extra protein first to make sure you're getting enough.

Next up, let's talk fiber and carbohydrates.

FIBER AND CARBOHYDRATES

Even though my slogan is "protein, fat, and fiber," I've found that when creating a meal, it's easier to consider the carbohydrate/fiber next, as this will dictate the type of fat you should use in that meal.

When working toward a weight-loss goal, I've found the best results by sticking to low–glycemic load carbs (see page 35 for the list). If you stick to this category exclusively when choosing your carbs, then you can eat as much of them as you like. Many of the low-GL carbs also sneak in some fiber—although some have much more fiber than others. Either way, by eating foods from the low-GL column, you can get nutrient-dense carbs with some fiber too. The two caveats are those borderline low/medium-GL carbs and fruit.

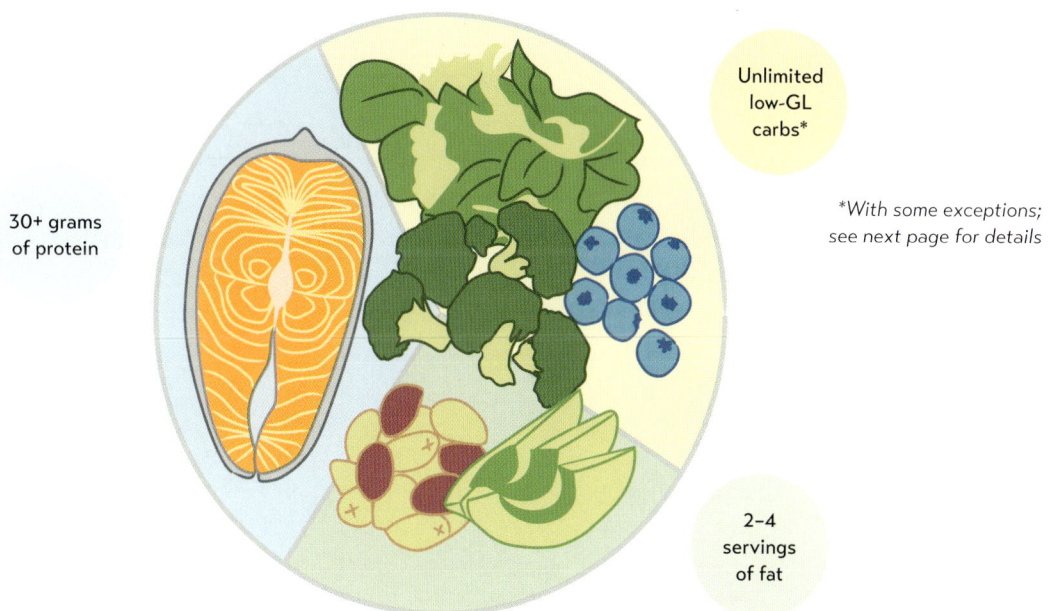

Unlimited low-GL carbs*

With some exceptions; see next page for details

30+ grams of protein

2–4 servings of fat

On the glycemic load charts on pages 35 and 36, there are specific amounts listed for some foods (for example, 1 cup chickpeas). To keep these foods low glycemic load, adhere to the designated serving size. Eating more of one of those foods could bring it into the medium-GL category and possibly hinder a weight-loss goal.

NOTE: If you love veggies but have a hard time eating enough protein, make sure you don't fill up on carbs and fiber while sacrificing your protein intake. If necessary, eat your protein *first* and then move on to veggies so you don't accidentally undereat protein.

The other major caveat is fruit. Although most fruits are low glycemic load, they can be problematic for some people because of the sugar content. For this reason, I generally recommend sticking to one or two servings of fruit at each meal. If you are very carb sensitive, then this limit should be dropped to one serving per meal with an additional focus on the highest-fiber fruits, such as blackberries, raspberries, and strawberries.

You can see how determining your carb choice will also help you determine your fat choice. For example, if you want to have skyr or Greek yogurt (protein) paired with raspberries and blueberries (carbs) for breakfast, then you probably don't want to have olives and rendered bacon fat as the fat. It wouldn't exactly go well in terms of taste.

So, once you've figured out your protein and carb/fiber choices, it's time to add the fats.

FAT

Each person's fat needs will vary based on their activity level and possibly other health-related concerns. The range that I usually recommend is two to four servings of fat per meal. Because fat is an energy source, those who are very active will likely need four servings in order to feel satisfied. On the flip side, if you are sedentary, then two servings is probably going to be enough to make you feel full and raise your satiety hormones.

There will be a bit of trial and error in finding the specific fat amounts that work for you, and this amount can change depending on where you are in your weight-loss or wellness journey. For example, I've found that those first starting their weight-loss journey with 20-plus pounds of body fat to lose tend to do very well and feel quite satiated with two servings of fat at each meal. However, as they get closer to their goal and have less body fat to pull from, they start to feel hungrier. Assuming protein and carbohydrate intake have stayed the same, this would be an excellent time to bump up the servings of fat to three per meal and assess how you feel.

But in the beginning, it's great to start with two servings with the knowledge and freedom to increase your fat intake by one to two servings if needed.

Going back to the Greek yogurt and fruit bowl example, you might want to add 3 tablespoons of toasted coconut flakes and 2 tablespoons of walnuts for your two servings of fat. (Which sounds delicious, I might add.)

The following is a list of high-quality fats and their serving sizes. Keep it as a reference for the start of your journey. However, I promise that it starts to become second nature, and soon enough, you won't even need the chart!

HIGH-QUALITY FATS	
FOOD	**SERVING SIZE**
Avocado	½
Cheese	1 ounce
Nuts	2 tablespoons
Nut, seed, or coconut butter	1 tablespoon
Avocado, coconut, or olive oil	1 tablespoon
Butter or ghee	1 tablespoon
Coconut flakes	3 tablespoons
Tallow	1 tablespoon
Cacao butter	1 tablespoon
Sour cream	3 to 4 tablespoons
Heavy cream	1 tablespoon
Full-fat Greek yogurt or cottage cheese*	1 cup
Eggs*	2
Fatty fish*	4 ounces
Most animal proteins (skin on)*	4 ounces

These are considered both proteins and fats.

But just like with carbs, there are some caveats with fat. Sometimes you don't need to add any fat at all because the proteins you're choosing are already quite high in fat. This is particularly true if you're including only two servings of fat at each meal.

Common high-fat proteins include

- Cheese
- Halloumi
- Lamb
- Most sausages
- Paneer
- Whole eggs
- Whole milk

When eating these naturally higher-fat proteins, you typically do not need to add more fat to the meal. The exceptions are if you are highly active or if you've combined some of these higher-fat proteins with leaner ones (such as eggs and ground beef).

When creating meals, I highly recommend putting them together in this order: protein, low–glycemic load carbs, and fat. This will ensure that you prioritize the ingredient that will make you the most satisfied while being able to adjust your fat content to your hunger level.

WHAT ABOUT DESSERTS?

I've found that scheduling "treat meals" can be quite helpful for long-term results. When you allow for the occasional treat, you can participate in celebrations like a birthday party or wedding. However, when working toward a weight-loss goal, it's important to limit desserts to no more than two per week. Some people might find that they need to remove them altogether while they get their sweet tooth in check. Head to pages 68 and 69 for my top tips for how to incorporate a treat meal.

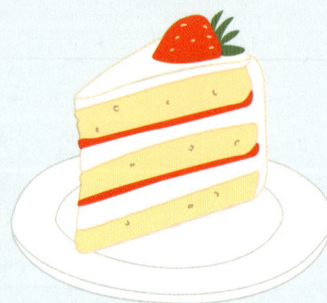

PLANT-BASED AND VEGETARIAN TIPS

As discussed in chapter 1, quality *really* matters when it comes to choosing the right protein to see the best body recomposition and weight-loss results. It also *really* matters for ensuring that your body is adequately fed and receiving the proper micronutrients for long-term health.

If your diet is primarily plant based, it's important to know that your high-quality sources of protein are going to be quite limited. I understand that this can be difficult, especially as someone who was vegetarian for the first half of my life. I wish I could tell you that you can get enough protein by just eating a bunch of veggies and not taking note of very specific foods, but I would be lying to you. I want you to live your healthiest life, so if you choose to be plant based, you must be very observant of your protein sources.

Check out the list of the top plant-based sources on page 22. Tempeh is one of the best sources for most meals, as it's a fermented soy product. Due to the fermentation, it has significantly lower amounts of antinutrients than regular soy. It's also the densest whole-food source of plant-based protein, so you won't have to eat a ridiculous amount to hit your protein needs.

The following are some of my top tips for vegans:

- **Avoid highly processed fake meats.** Take a second and look at the ingredients on the label of one of those products. If you can't even recognize half of the ingredients as food, then you should skip it. Although "fake meats" are convenient, there are much more nutrient-dense alternatives to choose from.

- **Watch your carb intake.** Most plant-based proteins are very high in carbs. For example, to get 30 grams of protein from chickpeas, you're also getting 65 grams of net carbs. That's a lot. Try balancing these higher-carb proteins with lower-carb options, like tempeh or edamame.

- **Choose Ezekiel bread.** Ezekiel bread is made from a variety of sprouted grains, legumes, and seeds, making it a more complete protein than typical bread. It's also low glycemic load. Two slices give you 10 grams of protein to work with too. Just don't rely on eating a ton of bread, as it can quickly rack up the carb count and raise your glycemic load.

- **Make "Greek yogurt" bowls.** Some brands are now offering plant-based Greek-style yogurt by adding protein powder after fermentation. The brand Kite Hill has an option that can be used in place of traditional dairy-based Greek yogurt or skyr.

- **Experiment with crumbled tempeh in place of ground meat.** I use a lot of ground meat because it's fast, easy, and relatively inexpensive. For a lot of my recipes that use ground meat, you can swap in crumbled tempeh.

- **Try nutritional yeast.** Adding 2 tablespoons of nutritional yeast to a meal gives it a cheesy flavor and adds 5 grams of protein. It appears to be high DIAAS as well.

- **Account for missing nutrients.** When avoiding animal products, there are quite a few important nutrients that you'll need to supplement. Examples include B12, heme iron, vitamin A, choline, and vitamin K2. A deficiency in these key nutrients can lead to a plethora of skeletal, immune, and mental health concerns down the line.[5] Make sure you're working with a nutritionist or functional medicine doctor who is well versed in plant-based nutrition and can guide you with your supplement intake.

If you are vegetarian but not vegan, you have much more flexibility with your protein choices. By adding in dairy and eggs, you are able to significantly increase the nutrient density of your meals. However, it's still crucial to pay attention to the amounts you're eating.

Here are some of my top tips for vegetarians:

- **You still may need to supplement nutrients like vitamin B12 and iron.** Work with a nutritionist or functional medicine doctor who is well versed in vegetarian nutrition and can guide you with your supplement intake.

- **Eggs are your best friend.** Eggs are incredibly versatile and rich in a variety of micronutrients. They also are pretty cheap! You can make them into so many different meals to help prevent food fatigue. Try making egg bites, poached eggs, egg salad, frittatas, omelets, or scrambled eggs to switch things up.

- **Not a fan of eggs?** You can sneak them into recipes like protein pancakes! Try my recipe on page 97.

- **Get familiar with Greek yogurt, skyr, cottage cheese, and halloumi.** These high-protein dairy products can be used in a variety of different meals. Greek yogurt, skyr, and cottage cheese are great for breakfast bowls, in smoothies, or as a topping for protein pancakes. Halloumi is an excellent swap for grilled chicken and cooks up in minutes. For inspiration, check out my recipe using halloumi on page 207.

- **Use a high-quality whey isolate protein powder.** You can easily sneak in more protein with a high-quality protein powder. I developed my zero-sugar, pasture-raised whey protein powder to taste *amazing* in recipes such as protein pancakes, protein waffles, smoothies, yogurt bowls, and chia pudding. In fact, our community loves it so much that we've sold out of each flavor on more than one occasion. Grab a bag or two on my website, autumnellenutrition.shop.

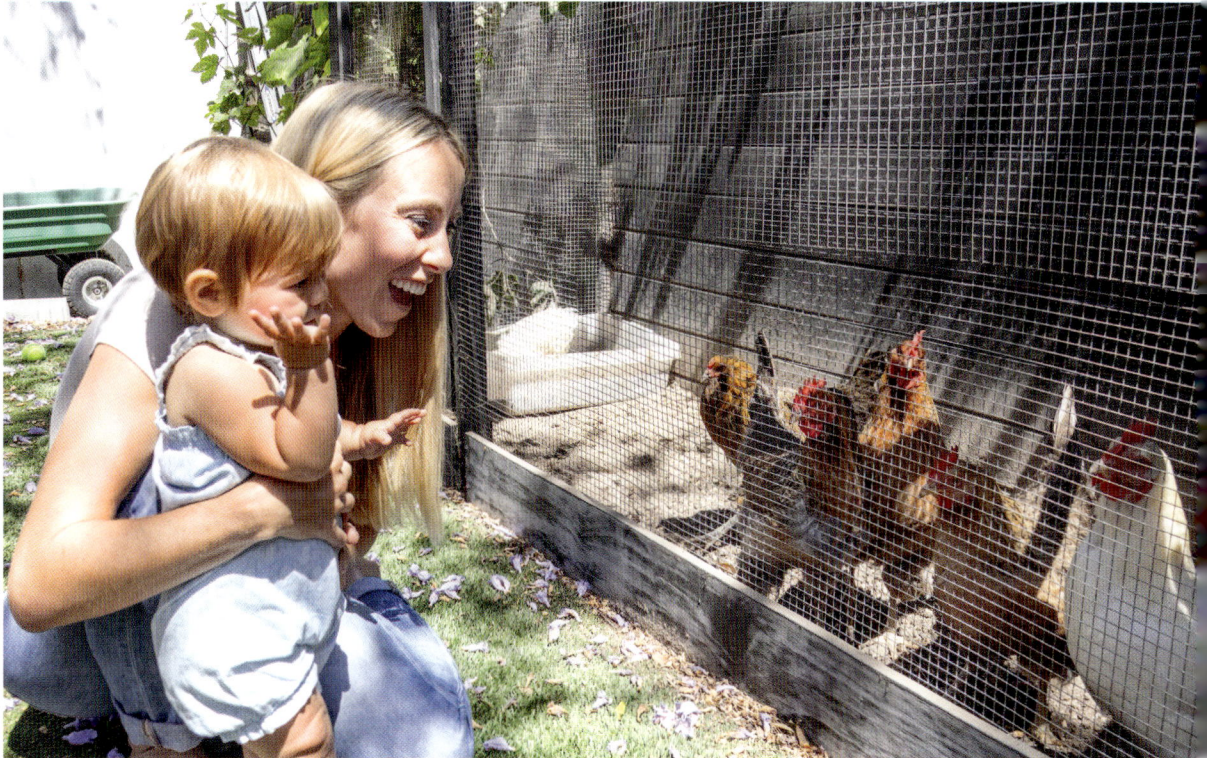

CUES YOU'VE EATEN ENOUGH (OR NEED TO EAT MORE)

Very few people trust in their body's ability to let them know when they've eaten enough. It's not a totally unwarranted concern, either, given that we are surrounded by hyperpalatable and processed foods that are designed to hijack our satiety hormones and force our bodies to "forget" how to regulate hunger.

But the good news is that nearly all cases of "overeating" are due to eating too much of the *wrong* foods, not too much food in general. When you eat protein, fat, and fiber, your body is able to tap into internal satiety cues that prevent overeating. The trouble is learning to trust these cues again, especially if you're used to a lifetime of restricting your intake and always feeling a little bit hungry.

So, if you aren't sure what to look for, these are the common signs you've either eaten enough, too little, or too much. Please note that the signs you've eaten enough or too little *only* apply to well-balanced meals rich in protein, fat, and fiber. They do not apply to hyperpalatable foods. On the same note, the signs you've eaten too much really only apply to hyperpalatable or "trigger" foods. See the next section for more on addictive and trigger foods.

SIGNS YOU'VE EATEN ENOUGH

- **You don't feel the need to eat for three to five hours.** This is due to rising satiety hormones after eating protein, fat, and fiber.

- **Eating between meals might seem undesirable.** When your brain receives the message that you're full, it shuts off appetite, making any food between meals seem undesirable.

- **It's easy to pass up a treat.** Those who start eating enough protein, fat, and fiber are often surprised that the candy bowl at the office or the pizza shop on the way home from work is no longer tempting. This is from the action of satiety hormones.

- **You don't feel the need to eat something sweet after a meal.** This one can take a little time to adjust to, as some sugar cravings are driven by stress and comfort rather than just hunger. However, you might notice that your post-meal sugar cravings are significantly lower or nonexistent.

- **Your energy levels are stable.** Due to stable blood sugar levels, you shouldn't experience a sudden spike and crash in energy levels. Instead, your energy levels should remain steady throughout the day.

- **Your mood is stable.** On that same note, because you aren't experiencing blood sugar crashes, you won't experience the sudden mood swings that result from those crashes.

- **You don't feel bloated.** Bloating after a meal is commonly from eating too much of the wrong food. We'll get into that shortly. When you eat enough protein, fat, and fiber, you should feel full but not overly stuffed.

- **You probably will "think" you've eaten too much.** If you're used to restricting your intake, then you'll very likely feel like you've eaten way too much because you aren't hungry after the meal. It takes time to change this mental state around hunger and satiety, but know that it is a common feeling that many people have experienced. Those who stick with it are always pleasantly surprised when they see that they have lost weight even though they haven't felt hungry.

If you've found you have eaten enough and you check these boxes, great! Keep doing what you're doing. But always look out for signs that you have not eaten enough so you know to add extra protein, fat, or fiber at your next meal.

SIGNS YOU *HAVE NOT* EATEN ENOUGH

- **You're hungry within one to two hours.** Satiety hormones when fully activated should keep you feeling full and satisfied for three to five hours. Feeling hungry shortly after a meal is a huge red flag that you have not eaten enough.

- **You still feel a little hungry right after a meal.** This is from satiety hormones not rising enough to trigger lasting satiety. Check out the figure on page 45 for a visual example.

- **You have the urge to "eat a little something sweet" after the meal.** When you don't eat enough, your body searches for a fast source of energy to replace what it hasn't received through the meal. The fastest source of energy is sugary and starchy foods, meaning the body will ramp up cravings for foods like chocolate, chips, crackers, or candy.

If you haven't eaten enough, then this is a great learning opportunity to assess what you need to change with your next meal. Ask yourself these questions in this order:

1. **Was the meal too low in protein? Did you hit at least 30 grams of protein?** If so, calculate your protein needs (see page 19) and determine if you need substantially more protein per meal. If you do, make sure to up your protein to the new amount at each meal. In the meantime, you can have a higher-protein snack between meals to hold you over. See pages 44 and 45 for a list of good snack options.

2. **Was the meal too low in fat?** Remember, you have two to four servings of fat to work with (although some people who are very active might need even more). If you've assessed your protein intake and it's fine, then try adjusting your fat intake and see if you feel more satisfied.

3. **Was your meal too low in fiber or low–glycemic load carbs?** If you ate enough protein and fat, try upping your fiber by 1 cup or more. Remember, low-GL carbs can be scaled up or down as much as you desire. Refer to page 35 for a list of foods that fall into this category.

4. **Do you need to add a starchy carbohydrate?** If you are very active or working toward a muscle mass goal, you might need to add a medium– to high–glycemic load carb to aid in muscle recovery. Remember not to sacrifice protein, fat, or low-glycemic carbs for the starch! It should be added to the meal, not replace parts of it.

5. **Are you stressed? Have you gotten poor sleep?** Both stress and insufficient sleep can raise hunger and cravings. Try going for a walk outside to reduce stress levels, and go to bed earlier to improve sleep quantity and quality.

A SATIETY HACK

During my second postpartum weight-loss period, I found that adding 1 cup of beans to my lunch or dinner significantly increased satiety due to their very high fiber content. So, if you struggle with satiety even after you've upped your protein, then including beans for the fiber might be a helpful hack.

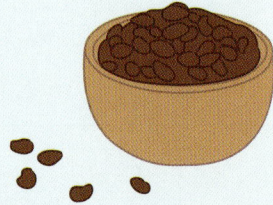

SIGNS YOU'VE EATEN TOO MUCH OF THE WRONG FOODS

- **You feel bloated.** Bloating is the result of the stomach becoming overly stretched or bacteria fermenting the food and "farting" it back into your GI tract. It's difficult to overeat minimally processed sources of protein, fat, and fiber, so it's hard to eat enough to stretch the stomach in this way. However, processed foods are easy to overeat quickly, making it easy to overly fill the stomach and cause you to feel bloated. On the same note, bacteria can quickly ferment processed foods, leading to a buildup of gas in the GI tract that makes you feel puffy, bloated, and overly stuffed.

- **Your pants suddenly feel tighter in the waistband.** This isn't from instant weight gain, but from bloating and expansion of the belly.

- **Your energy levels are variable.** Processed foods can cause more variable blood sugar levels, which means you might experience a sudden high and then a crash in energy.

- **You feel sleepy shortly after the meal.** This is due to that blood sugar crash.

- **You feel a little shaky a few hours after the meal.** Again, this is due to the blood sugar crash and your body experiencing low blood sugar.

- **You experience mood swings.** Low blood sugar can also cause feelings of irritability. Pair that with hunger, and you have the classic "hanger."

- **Even though you feel "full" and possibly bloated, you experience the urge to eat or snack within one to three hours after the meal.** This is due to low satiety hormones causing your appetite to go up while your body still feels physically "full" from the amount of processed foods you just ate. It is also quite common after eating a lot of pasta or pizza, both of which are high in processed carbs and low in protein.

If you've eaten a lot of processed foods, your gut reaction (no pun intended) might be to try to restrict your intake at your next meal, fast for a long time, or over-exercise. Although I understand the sentiment, these are not good choices. All of them will simply cause you to feel even hungrier and be even more likely to fall into binge eating behavior. Instead, when you start to feel hungry again, immediately go back to a satiating meal rich in protein, fat, and fiber. This will stop the blood sugar roller coaster and help bring you back to more stable levels. By eating a meal that supports satiety, you can get back on track much faster and bypass those tricky cravings that often result from eating processed foods.

FOODS THAT ARE HARD TO STOP EATING

There are two main categories of foods that bypass satiety and make it hard to stop eating. They are addictive foods and trigger foods.

ADDICTIVE FOODS

Addictive foods are usually hyperpalatable and have gone through numerous processing steps to make them hit various pleasure centers on your taste buds and in your brain. They are usually high in a combination of carbs, fat, and salt while being low in protein.

As we know, protein is required to boost satiety and prevent cravings, so we're off to a bad start. But studies have found that ultra-processed carbs and fats have addictive-like properties that are on par with alcohol and certain drugs. Similar to other types of addiction, those who suffer from some degree of food addiction experience symptoms such as excessive intake, loss of control once they've started, continued use despite negative consequences, and withdrawal symptoms when they stop. The study specifically highlights that this behavior isn't from *all* foods, but only ultra-processed carbs and fats.[6] This is why the nutrition ideology that you can eat "everything in moderation" doesn't work. You can't "moderate" an addiction. Snack food companies are well aware of this. Anyone remember this classic slogan for a popular chip company: "Once you pop, you can't stop"? At least they were honest!

Common foods that have addictive-like qualities are chips, crackers, cookies, ice cream, soda, cereal, packaged baked goods, and candy, although this is not an exhaustive list. Some people seem to be more susceptible to the addictive-like qualities of these foods, just like some people are more likely to become addicted to other substances. However, generally speaking, these foods appear to make it incredibly difficult to stop eating or to tune in to satiety cues.

It's not to say that you can never have these items, but they certainly shouldn't be daily foods, especially if you want to feel your best and achieve a weight-loss or wellness goal. Occasionally having chips with guacamole when you're out to dinner likely won't cause you to spiral (as long as you're also eating protein and fiber at that meal). But notice that many of the ultra-processed foods I listed are habitual foods. This means they are intended to be eaten on a daily basis. For example, when you buy cereal, you don't buy a single-serve packet; you buy a box that's supposed to last you a week. Same goes for a box of crackers, a bag of chips, or a case of soda. Also notice that most of these foods are considered "snack foods." While following a protein, fat, and fiber three-meal approach, you'll automatically remove the need for these snacks and greatly reduce your intake of ultra-processed foods.

Takeaway: Some foods provide zero nutritional value while triggering addictive-like behaviors. These foods should be greatly reduced or removed entirely if you believe you have a food addiction. However, if you are focusing on protein, fat, and fiber and you choose to have some of these more processed foods on the weekend as a treat, make sure to opt for a single-serve package; *don't* buy a larger multiple-serving package. Go for a scoop of ice cream at the local ice cream shop instead of a pint from the grocery store.

TRIGGER FOODS

The other category is "trigger foods." These foods aren't necessarily unhealthy but are difficult for *you* to stop eating once you start. For many people, peanut butter is a trigger food. My husband is one of those people. If he comes home hungry and reaches for a "tablespoon" of peanut butter, he ends up going through half the jar before he realizes what's happened.

There's nothing inherently wrong with peanut butter. In fact, it can be a great source of fat to add to a meal. But for my husband (and many others), it's one that he has to be careful with.

NOT LOSING WEIGHT?

If you find that you aren't losing weight, you might be making one or more of these common mistakes:

- **Gauging your progress on body weight alone.** A traditional scale won't tell you if you've lost muscle or body fat. You can lose fat while also gaining muscle. This results in a lower body fat percentage and better body recomposition but can look like a net zero loss on the scale. I recommend taking measurements with a tape measure to better track fat loss. Great areas to monitor include the hips, waist, arms, and neck. Check for inches going down rather than the scale moving. My other favorite tool is the InBody scan, which measures body fat and muscle mass and can let you know if you've lost fat or muscle since your last scan. This equipment can often be found at local gyms.

- **Eating too much fat and not enough protein.** My husband made the mistake for a long time of eating too much fat and not enough protein. This caused him to not make the fat-loss progress he was looking for. Once we reorganized his meals to focus on protein, then fiber, then fat, he started to gain muscle and lose body fat. With the rise of the keto diet, this is a common mistake that I've seen with many of my clients and community members as well. Check out the section "Building Your Plate" beginning on page 49 for how to properly form your meals.

- **Not watching your glycemic load.** You might be eating too high of a glycemic load for your carb tolerance. Try sticking to the low-GL fruits and veggies. (See page 35.)

- **Having too many sugary drinks.** Sugary drinks are really sneaky. Look out for sweetened coffees, energy drinks, teas, fruit juices, and sodas.

- **Eating too many sweet foods.** Although natural zero-sugar sweeteners such as stevia, monk fruit, and erythritol shouldn't negatively impact weight loss, they can alter your preferences to sweeter foods if you are in the habit of eating them often. Try a seven-day sugar detox to help reset your taste buds. My 7 Day Detox is a great resource. You can find it at autumnellenutrition.shop.

- **Neglecting strength training.** Strength training two to four days a week helps the body become more metabolically flexible and makes it easier to burn fat as fuel. It also helps prevent a slowing metabolism during weight loss.

Other common trigger foods are almonds, pistachios, sunflower seeds, popcorn, chocolate, and dried fruit.

Trigger foods don't usually have to be avoided entirely. Instead, it's important to eat it with a meal and not snack on it. When it's part of a meal, it can contribute to satiety and prevent hunger before you accidentally overeat the individual triggering ingredient. So, rather than snacking on a spoonful of peanut butter, you can add it to a smoothie, Greek yogurt bowl, or cottage cheese bowl as a topping. If you find that you didn't eat enough at your last meal and need a little something to hold you over, opt for a high-protein snack that doesn't include your trigger foods. The sidebar on pages 44 and 45 lists some great options.

It's important to identify which foods are your trigger foods so you can make sure to pair them with a meal and not snack on them.

ON-THE-GO, VACATION, AND TREAT MEALS

There will be times in life when you can't maintain your usual routine: when you're traveling, you're on vacation, or you want to have a treat. But this doesn't mean you need to go totally off the rails. You can enjoy your vacation and have the occasional treat meal while still feeling great and making progress toward your weight-loss or wellness goals. And if you travel a lot for work, I have some simple tips you can follow to optimize your meals.

TRAVEL AND ON-THE-GO TIPS

When traveling, whether it be by car, train, or plane, it's important to stick to protein, fat, and fiber as much as possible. Here are my top travel tips:

- **Bring proteins and veggies that are easy to travel with.**

  - Depending on your mode of travel, some proteins are easier to travel with than others.

  - When flying, opt for meat sticks, jerky, string cheese, hard-boiled eggs, bagged tuna (but I recommend eating it in the terminal rather than on the plane!), or deli meats with hard cheese. Depending on the protein you choose, you might want to pack it with a little bit of ice. Pair your protein with sliced veggies like cucumber, carrots, bell pepper, or cauliflower florets. Don't forget to add a fat! If you keep it to less than 3.4 ounces, you can bring a Greek yogurt–based sauce for dipping (like my Tzatziki on page 156). You can also bring sliced avocado or whole olives to cover your fat needs. Just don't mash that avocado into guacamole! Then you're subject to the 3.4-ounce rule. But feel free to mash the avocado once you're on the flight. Airport security rules are a bit bonkers like that.

- If you'll be on a long drive and you know you won't have time to stop, it's important to have a meal on hand that you can easily eat on-the-go. My protein-packed smoothies (see pages 88 and 89) are excellent options to sip on a full meal without much fuss. Just blend it in the morning and pack it in a thermos to keep it cool until you're ready to drink it. Give it a bit of a shake, and you're good to go!

- If you travel by train, you have a lot more flexibility with what you can bring. As you'll be sharing a space with other commuters, you might want to choose options that aren't very "smelly." Greek yogurt bowls (see pages 90 and 240) and cottage cheese bowls are excellent options. You can also pack a protein smoothie (see pages 88 and 89) for something fast and easy.

- **Know your airport terminal foods.**

  - If you're stuck in a terminal for a meal or two, it's important to make the best of the situation. Most terminals have a restaurant that offers burgers or salads. If that's the case, simply order a burger without a bun or a salad with extra protein. If the terminal only has one of those convenience store options, look for a meat and cheese pack in the fridge section. You can often find a salami, cheese, and cracker combination that will at least provide some protein and fat. Just ditch the crackers and focus on the salami and cheese. If you can also find an apple or a small refrigerated salad for some fiber, even better. It's okay if one or two meals aren't perfect. Just do your best!

What about when you've arrived at your vacation destination? Here are my top tips:

- **Start your day with protein.** Never skip protein at breakfast! It's easy to do while on vacation, but it can set you up for failure the rest of the day. If you at least get protein at breakfast, you know you're starting your day on the right foot. Eggs are likely your best bet. Try an omelet, scrambled eggs, or something more fun, like huevos rancheros, to get a boost of satiating protein.

- **Always eat your protein first.** You might want to have more frequent treats while on vacation. That choice is up to you and perhaps dependent on where you're traveling. For example, if you're vacationing in Italy, you probably want to try all of the pasta dishes and the gelato! If that's the case, just make sure to start off every single meal with some sort of protein, and *then* have your treat.

- **Explore by walking.** You can help your body absorb excess blood sugar and balance out some of the spikes from the treats by getting your steps in. I also love that you get to experience more of the place you're visiting when you're on foot.

- **Get back to your usual routine once home.** Don't try to "compensate" after the vacation by fasting for a long time or restricting your intake. This can lead to a binge-and-restrict habit and won't help you get back on track (or feel any better) faster. Instead, go straight back to your usual protein, fat, and fiber–rich meals. It can be helpful to plan the first few days of post-vacation meals before you leave so that you aren't needing to make decisions while traveling.

HOW TO HANDLE TREAT MEALS

First, let's define a treat. A treat is not a "cheat." It's a food that probably spikes your blood sugar and very likely has some addictive properties, but is part of a celebration or your heritage or simply is something you love the taste of. Treats are part of life. It's the cake at a wedding or the ice cream at a birthday party. It can also be something savory, like a cheesy homemade pizza or your grandma's famous lasagna. In short, you shouldn't think of it as cheating when you occasionally eat a treat. Instead, you just want to make sure you properly balance the treat with foods that support health, wellness, and stable blood sugar levels.

Whether the treat is a savory main dish or a sweet dessert, it is considered a "treat meal." So having Grandma's famous lasagna for dinner and birthday cake right after for dessert would be considered *two* treat meals.

I have found that most people do best with one or two treat meals per week while working toward a weight-loss or body recomposition goal. Any more than two, and those "treat meals" start to become more of a habit. And when I say "treat meal," I mean *meal*, not *day*. If you view a full day as a treat or "cheat day," it can lead to very unstable blood sugar levels that spike cravings throughout the rest of the week.

When including treat meals, I encourage you to follow a four-step process:

1. **Schedule it.** When you plan for a treat rather than give in to an urge that pops up during the day, you're less likely to fall into a habitual cycle. This way, you can make it an exciting event. Perhaps you'll do a weekend movie and popcorn night or try that homemade pasta recipe you've been eyeing. This approach keeps the treat fun and makes it less likely that you'll start leaning on treats to cope with stressful days or habitually saying yes to random acts of candy at the office.

2. **Keep it to later in the day.** Starting the day with a treat, such as pancakes with syrup, sets you off with unstable blood sugar levels. These unstable levels can cause a multitude of crashes throughout the day, making you feel low in energy and more likely to reach for something sugary to lift you up. I've found

the best times to schedule a treat are either with dinner or after dinner (as a dessert). That way, you've already stabilized your blood sugar levels all day and have fewer opportunities to experience sugar cravings after your treat. If you're able to go for a five-minute walk after eating the treat, you can also help your muscles absorb the excess carbs and sugar before bed and further prevent next-day cravings.

3. **Eat protein first.** If you go into the treat feeling hungry, you're much more likely to overindulge. However, if you start with a serving of protein, then you're going to feel satisfied with eating less of the treat. For example, if your treat is pizza, order an appetizer of meatballs or chicken wings to eat first. Or, if you're planning on having a dessert, have a protein-rich dinner before you eat the dessert. That way, you can quite literally have your cake and eat it too!

4. **Immediately go back to your regularly scheduled meals.** Many people feel that they need to compensate for a treat by eating less the next day or fasting longer. Neither of these strategies is a good idea. It's important to restabilize your blood sugar levels as soon as possible after the treat to help prevent further cravings. Instead of trying to eat less to account for the "extra calories," just go back to your protein, fat, and fiber–rich meals.

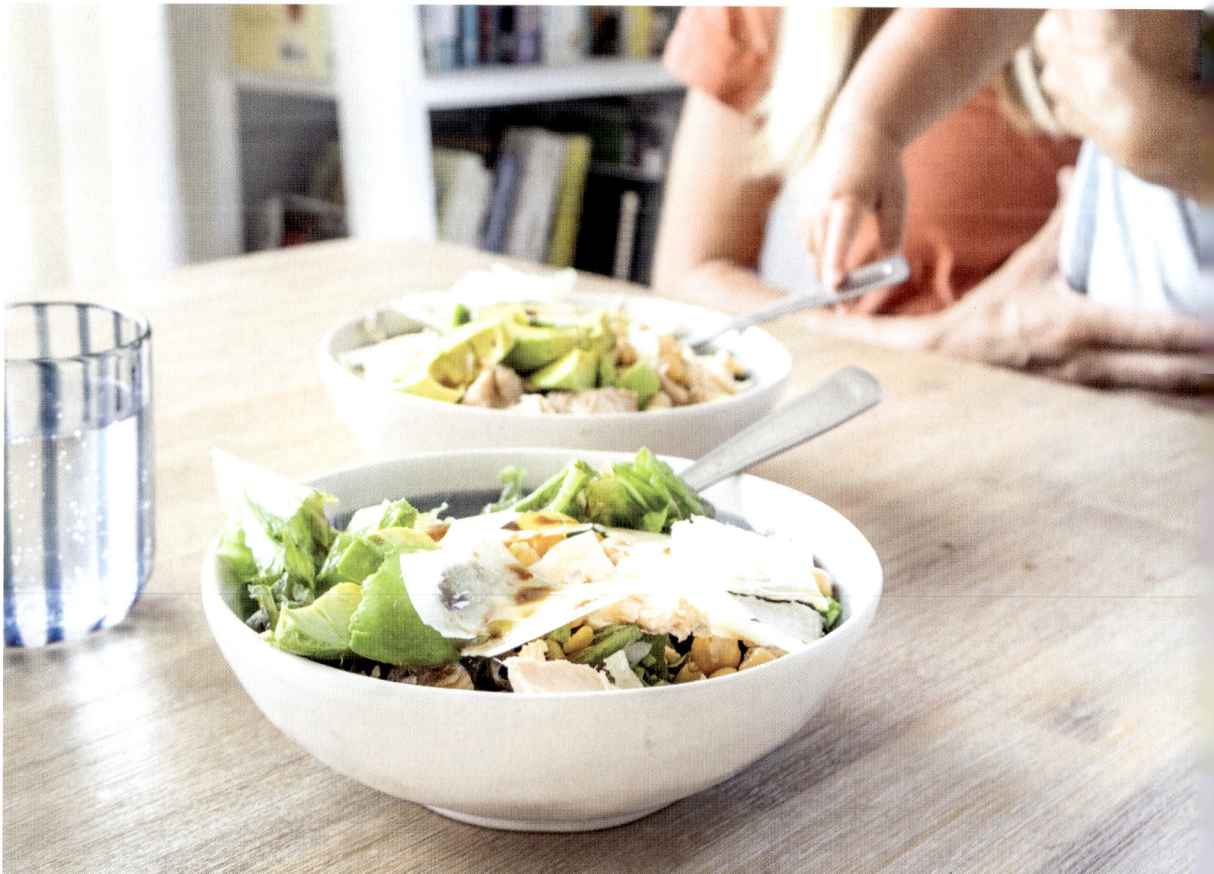

REFERENCES

[1] Leidy, Heather J. et al. "The Effects of Consuming Frequent, Higher Protein Meals on Appetite and Satiety During Weight Loss in Overweight/Obese Men." *Obesity* (Silver Spring, Md.) 19, no. 4 (2011): 818–824. doi:10.1038/oby.2010.203

[2] Southey, Flora. "The European 'Snackers': Who Is Snacking on What, Where?" *Food Navigator Europe,* June 9, 2022.

[3] "Obesity Rates by Country 2025." World Population Review. https://worldpopulationreview.com/country-rankings/obesity-rates-by-country, accessed July 14, 2025.

[4] Aleman, Ricardo Santos et al. "Leaky Gut and the Ingredients That Help Treat It: A Review." *Molecules* (Basel, Switzerland) 28, no. 2 (2023): 619. doi:10.3390/molecules28020619

[5] Bali, Atul, and Roopa Naik. "The Impact of a Vegan Diet on Many Aspects of Health: The Overlooked Side of Veganism." *Cureus* 15, no. 2 (2023): e35148. doi:10.7759/cureus.35148

[6] Gearhardt, Ashley N. et al. "Social, Clinical, and Policy Implications of Ultra-Processed Food Addiction." *BMJ (Clinical Research Ed.)* 383 (2023): e075354. doi:10.1136/bmj-2023-075354

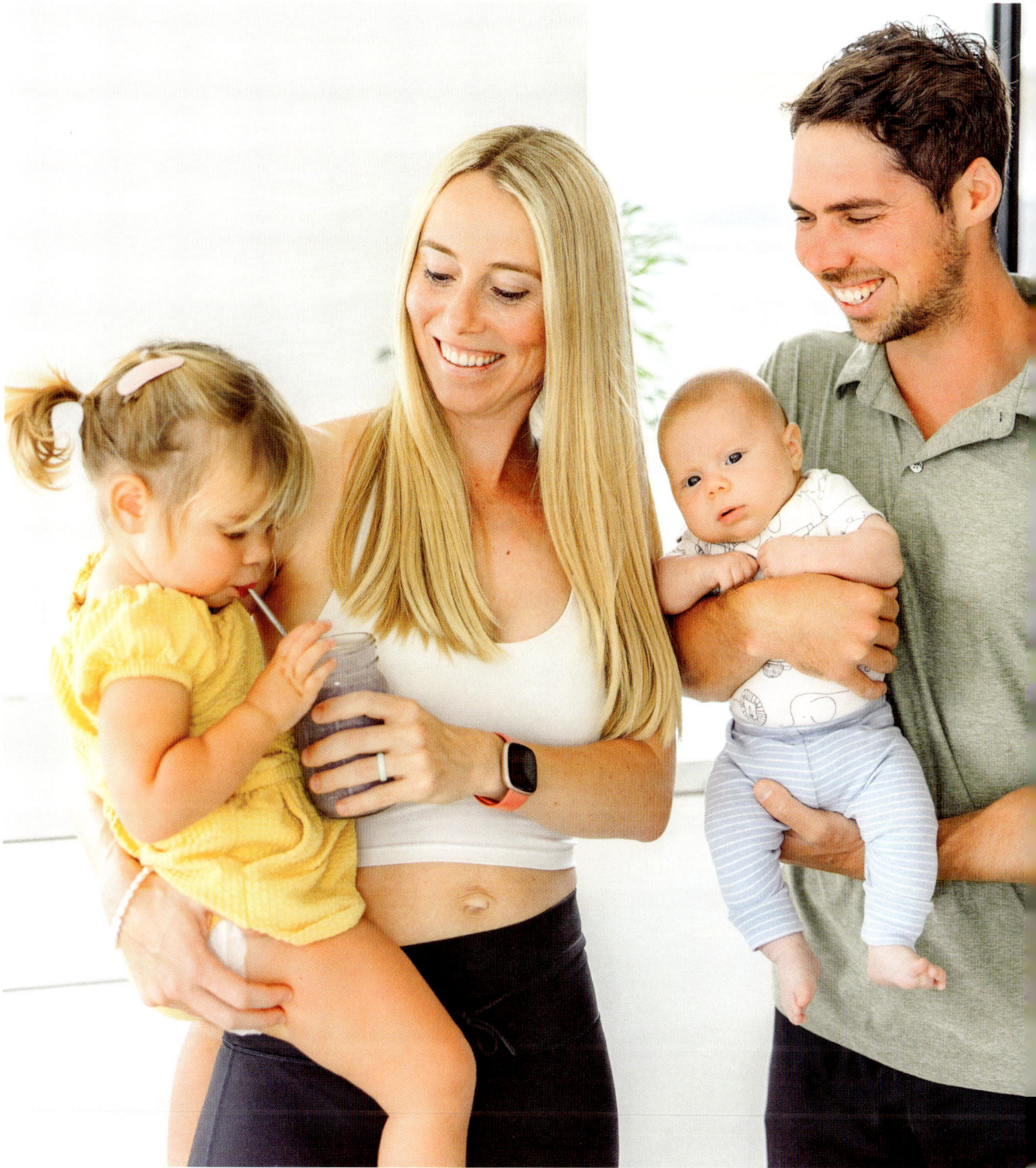

RECIPES

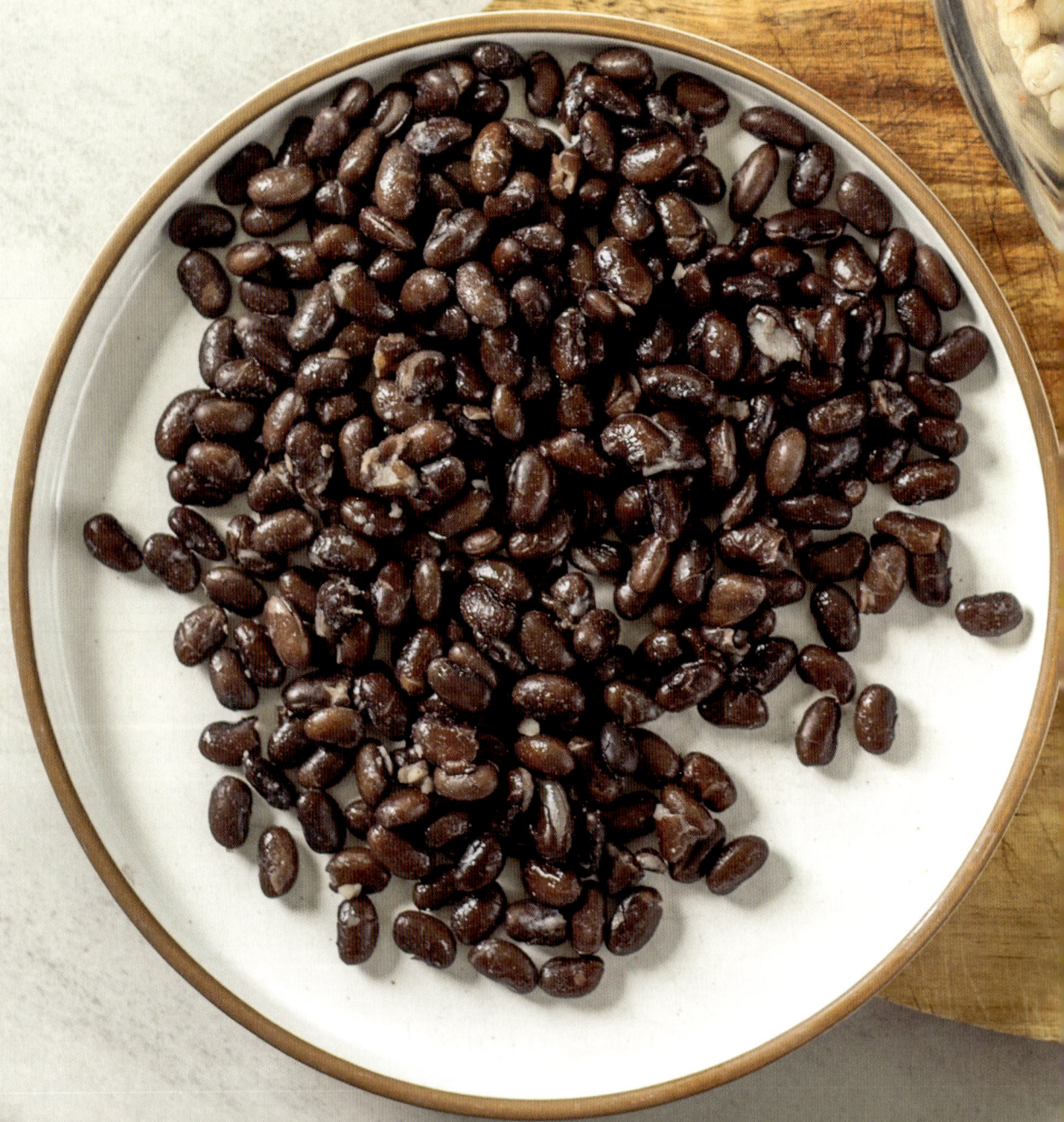

BASICS

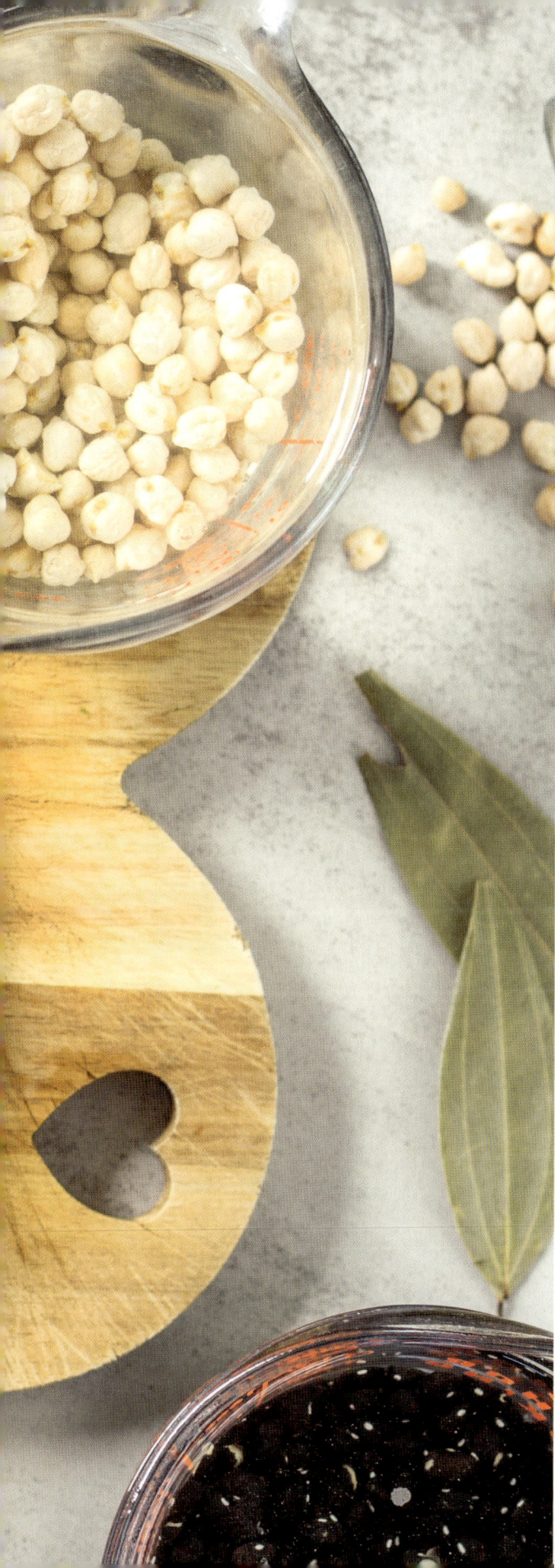

RED ENCHILADA SAUCE

MAKES 2½ cups

PREP TIME 5 minutes

COOK TIME 20 minutes

I use enchilada sauce to flavor meat for tacos and to make my enchilada pies (see pages 140 and 164). This recipe is great to prepare in large batches and store extra in the freezer to use whenever you need it. If you have trouble finding dried ancho chiles at your local grocery store, you can always find them at Mexican markets or on Amazon or Thrive Market. I like to buy them in bulk to keep in my pantry.

2 cups water

2 dried ancho chiles, stems and seeds removed

1 tablespoon olive oil

½ medium yellow onion, diced

4 cloves garlic, chopped

Salt

2 cups chicken or vegetable broth

2 tablespoons tomato paste

1 tablespoon dried oregano leaves

½ teaspoon ground cumin

Juice of ½ lime (about 1 tablespoon)

¼ to ½ teaspoon red pepper flakes, according to taste

1. In a medium-sized saucepan, bring the water and ancho chiles to a boil, then lower the heat to a simmer and cook for 5 minutes. Remove the pan from the heat and carefully pour 1 cup of the cooking liquid and the softened chiles into a blender. Set aside without blending.

2. Heat the olive oil in a large skillet over medium heat, then add the onion, garlic, and a heavy pinch of salt. Sauté for 5 minutes, or until the onion has softened. Stir in the broth, tomato paste, oregano, and cumin. Lower the heat to a simmer. Continue to cook for 10 minutes, then slide the pan off the heat and allow to cool for 5 to 10 minutes.

3. Pour the broth mixture into the blender with the chiles and cooking liquid. Add the lime juice and red pepper flakes. Slowly bring the blender up to medium-high speed and blend until smooth.

4. Use immediately or store in the fridge for up to 5 days or in the freezer for up to 6 months.

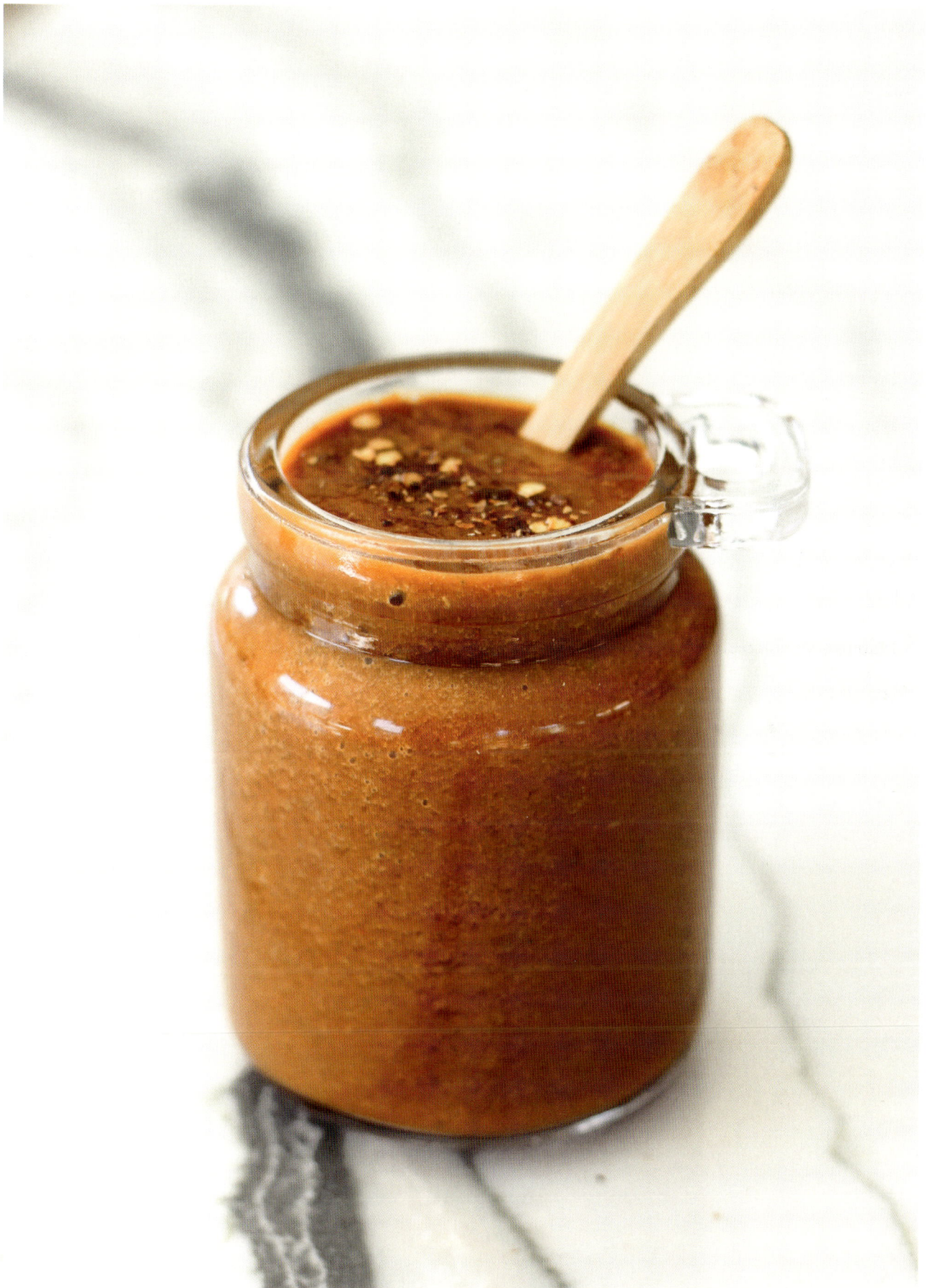

Note If you don't have a tortilla press, a rolling pin works fine, although if you plan on making tortillas frequently, a press is well worth the investment. When looking for a tortilla press, I recommend one made of cast iron or a similar heavy material, which will help flatten your tortillas more efficiently. You can also purchase tortilla press liners, which make the tortillas easier to remove from the press, but you don't have to. I use parchment paper with great results.

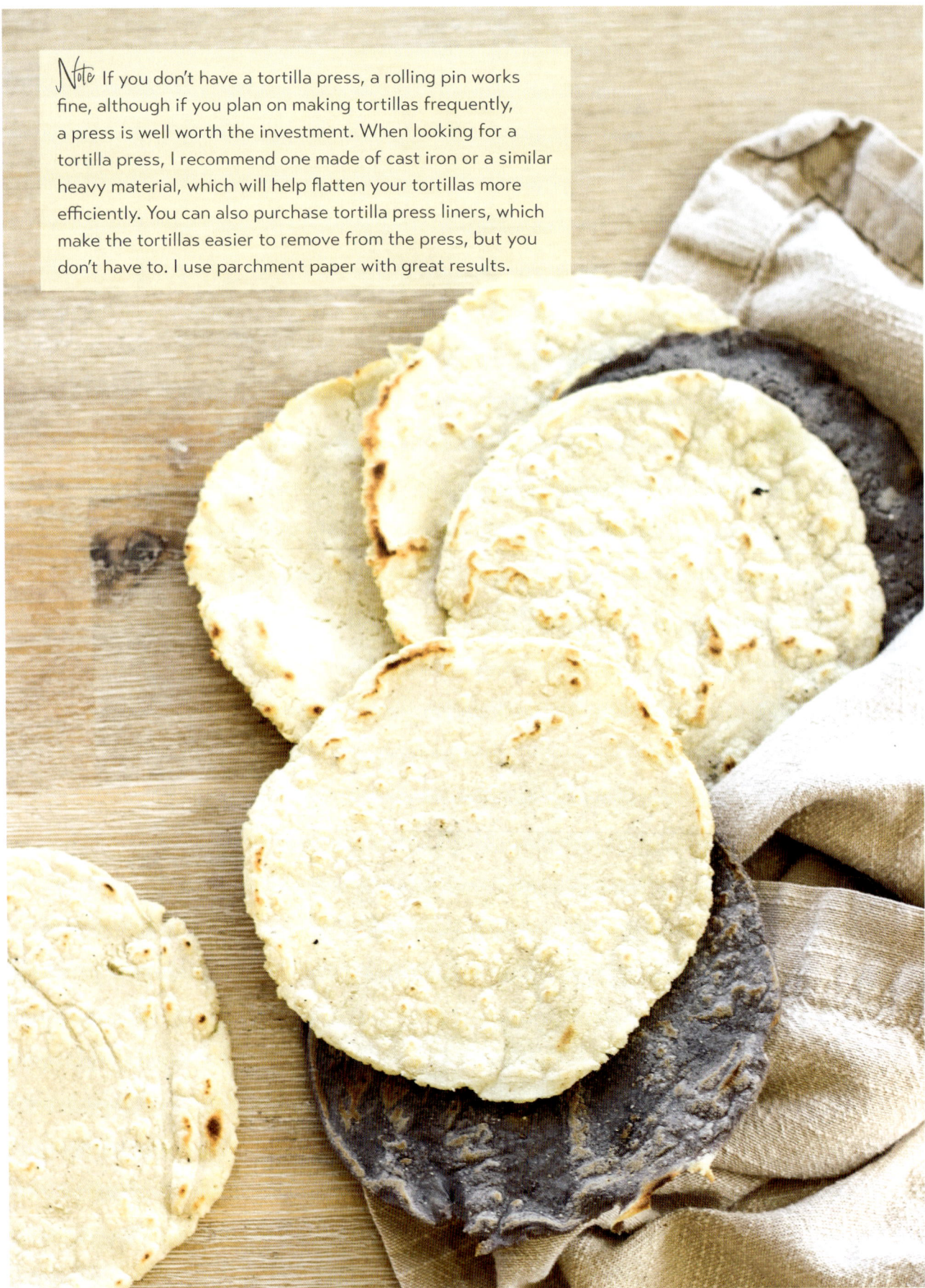

CORN TORTILLAS

MAKES ten 6-inch tortillas

PREP TIME 10 minutes

COOK TIME 10 to 20 minutes, depending on size of griddle/skillet

Corn tortillas have a fairly high glycemic load, so I recommend eating them only if you're physically active and not working toward a weight-loss goal. If you do choose to have them, it's well worth making your own. Homemade tortillas are easy to prepare and so much tastier than store-bought varieties. Plus, you need only two ingredients: masa harina and water. Masa harina is a "nixtamalized" corn flour, which means the nutrients have been made more bioavailable, and therefore it is a more nutrient-dense option than regular corn flour. It can be made from a variety of types of corn, such as blue, white, or yellow. The type you use will dictate the color of your tortillas, but they all taste similar, so feel free to experiment! My favorite brand is Masienda.

1 cup masa harina

1 cup warm water

Special equipment: 8-inch (or larger) tortilla press (optional)

1. In a medium-sized mixing bowl, mix the masa harina and warm water with a fork until you have a smooth, uniform dough that can easily be rolled into a ball. If it sticks to your hands, add a bit more masa harina. If it's too dry and can't hold a ball shape, add a bit more water. You might need to knead the dough with your hand a bit to evenly combine the ingredients.

2. Heat a griddle or large skillet over medium-high heat.

3. Scoop up about 3 tablespoons of the dough and roll into a ball. Repeat with the rest of the dough to make a total of ten balls.

4. Take a piece of parchment paper and fold it in half so that it covers both sides of the tortilla press. Place a dough ball on the paper and press down on the tortilla press to flatten. If you don't have a press, working on a sheet of parchment, use a rolling pin to evenly flatten each ball of dough to about $\frac{1}{16}$ inch thick.

5. Lay the tortilla on the hot pan (don't add any oil). Sear for 30 seconds, then flip and sear the other side for 30 seconds. Flip the tortilla back to the original side and cook until it puffs. This should take another 1 to 2 minutes. Repeat the process for the remaining tortillas.

6. Wrap the cooked tortillas in a clean dish towel until ready to eat. This helps them soften. The tortillas are best eaten the same day, but leftovers can be stored in a plastic bag in the freezer. To reheat, sear the tortillas on a hot griddle or skillet for about 30 seconds on each side.

CHIA JAM, TWO WAYS

Chia jam is a staple in my house. I like to have it on hand as a topping for Greek yogurt parfaits, cottage cheese bowls, protein pancakes, and protein waffles. My recipe uses chia seeds as the binder instead of sugar, making it less sweet than store-bought jam while adding healthy fiber. Don't be tempted to go for pricey fresh berries for this recipe! Frozen fruit is less expensive and creates a juicier jam.

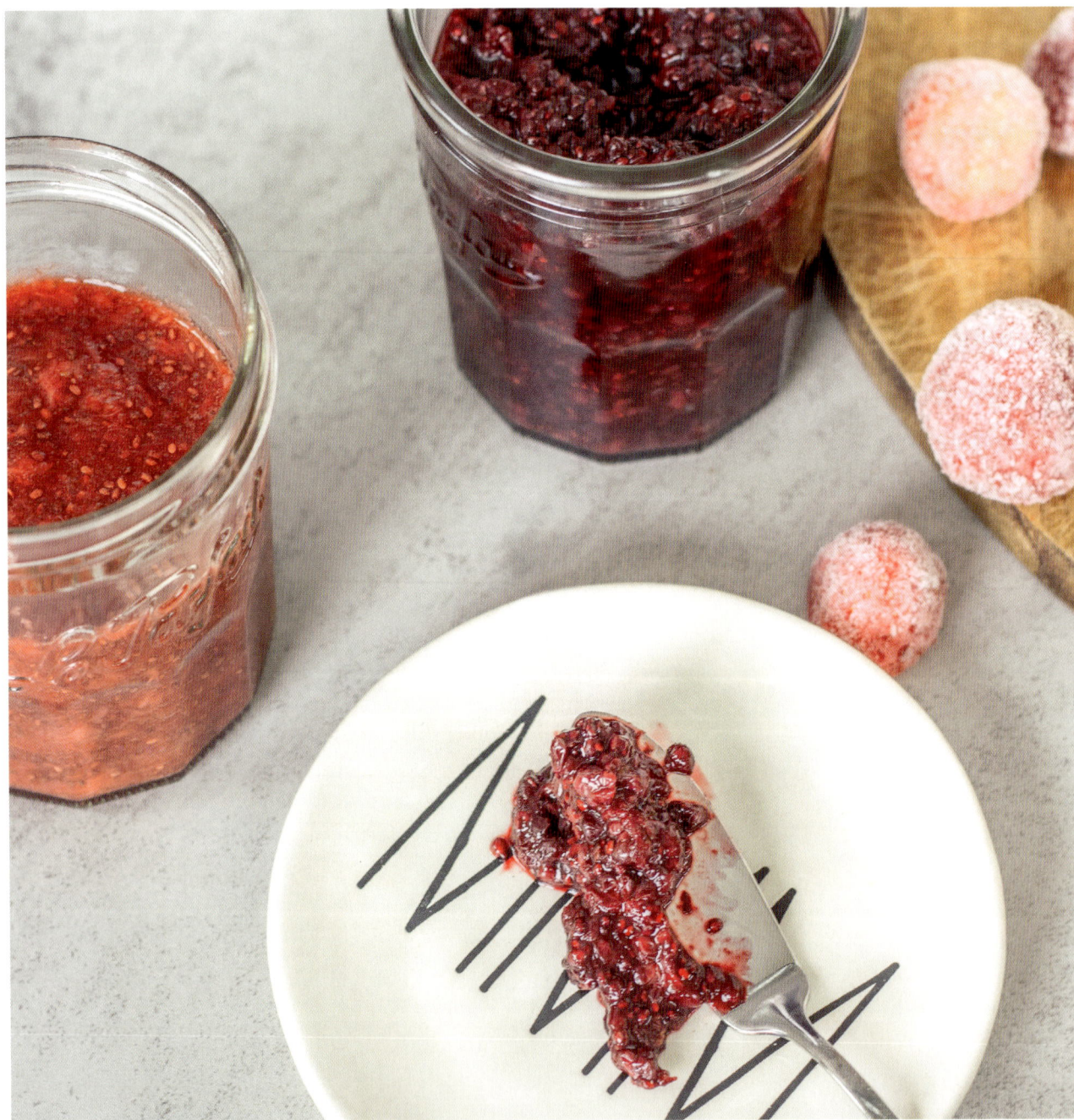

BLACKBERRY CHIA JAM

MAKES about 1 cup

PREP TIME 1 minute

COOK TIME 7 minutes

2 cups frozen blackberries

1 teaspoon grated lemon zest

1 tablespoon chia seeds

1. In a medium-sized saucepan over medium heat, cook the blackberries and lemon zest, stirring occasionally, for 5 to 7 minutes, until the berries are soft and squishy.

2. Remove the pan from the heat and mash the berries with a fork or potato masher until liquefied.

3. Stir in the chia seeds and transfer to an 8-ounce glass jar. Use immediately if you prefer a softer jam. For a firmer texture, allow to set up in the fridge for 30 minutes before using. Store in the fridge for up to 5 days.

STRAWBERRY LEMON CHIA JAM

MAKES about 1 cup

PREP TIME 1 minute

COOK TIME 7 minutes

2 cups frozen strawberries

Grated zest and juice of 1 lemon (2 to 3 tablespoons)

1 teaspoon vanilla extract

1 tablespoon chia seeds

1. In a medium-sized saucepan over medium heat, cook the strawberries, lemon zest and juice, and vanilla extract, stirring occasionally, for 5 to 7 minutes, until the berries are soft and squishy.

2. Remove the pan from the heat and mash the berries with a fork or potato masher until liquefied.

3. Stir in the chia seeds and transfer to an 8-ounce glass jar. Use immediately if you prefer a softer jam. For a firmer texture, allow to set up in the fridge for 30 minutes before using. Store in the fridge for up to 5 days.

EASY POACHED CHICKEN

MAKES about 1½ pounds shredded chicken (6 servings)

PREP TIME 1 minute

COOK TIME 20 minutes

Poaching is a hassle-free way to prepare a lot of chicken for use in so many different recipes. I like to shred this chicken for my Mini Chicken Enchilada Pies (page 164). You can also use poached chicken as a simple way to add protein to a salad.

2 pounds boneless, skinless chicken breasts

1 bay leaf

1 teaspoon salt

1. Put the chicken in a large pot and fill with enough water to cover the chicken. Add the bay leaf and salt.

2. Bring to a boil, then reduce to a simmer. Cook for 20 minutes, or until the internal temperature of the chicken is 165°F. Drain and allow to cool for 5 minutes.

3. If shredding the chicken, use two forks to pull it apart. Store in a sealed container in the fridge for up to 4 days.

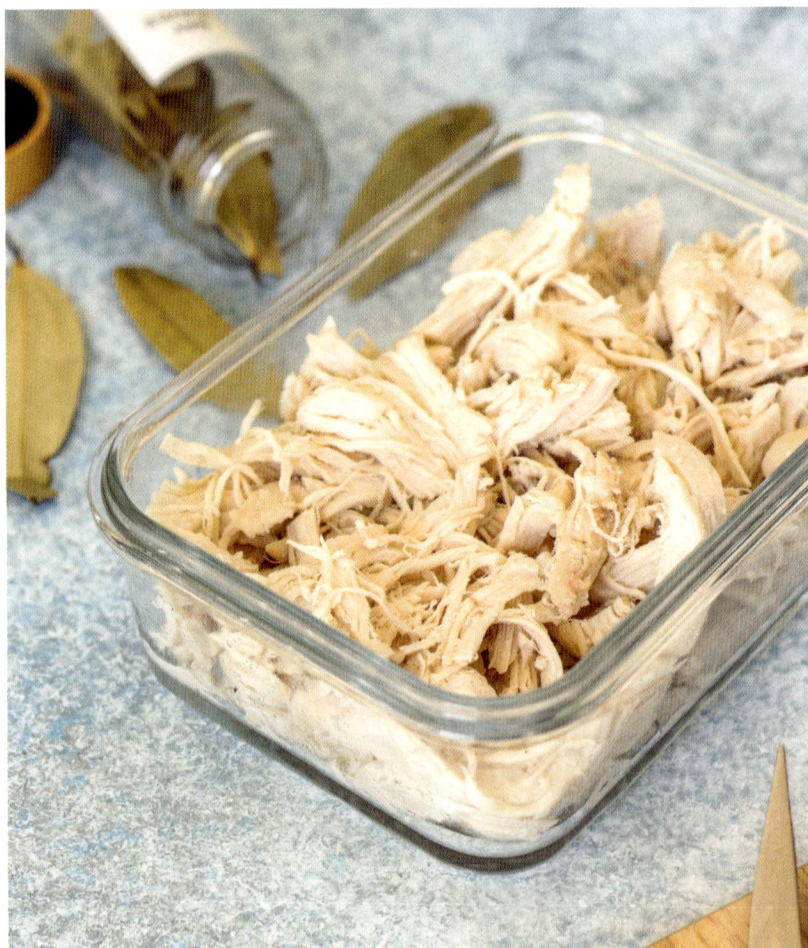

GREEK YOGURT, TWO WAYS

When I reintroduced dairy into my diet, Greek yogurt was one of the first things I added. It's very high in protein (about 30 grams per 1½ cups), rich in calcium and vitamin K2, and so versatile. I use it in place of mayonnaise in recipes to bump up the protein content of my meals. I also use it in smoothies, parfaits, and sauces and as a topping. But yogurt can be pricey when you eat it often. Plus, some stores don't carry full-fat Greek yogurt, which is important for satiety and nutrient density. So, to reduce my family's grocery bill while ensuring the quality of my yogurt, I started making it myself from scratch. It is a super fun and fairly simple process that saves us about $450 per year. I learned how to make it by using a tool I already had on hand: a slow cooker. This method worked well for years, but as I got more serious about yogurt making, I decided to upgrade to a yogurt maker. I've shared both methods here so you can start with what you have. If you have an Instant Pot, then you can use the yogurt maker method, as the directions are nearly identical. If you're brand-new to making yogurt, I recommend starting with the slow cooker option, as it's a very simple process. Regardless of which method you use, after the straining step you'll be left with Greek yogurt and a greenish-yellow liquid called whey water. You can keep this liquid and use it in place of water or broth in soups. If you have chickens, you can feed it to them as well. Mine love whey water!

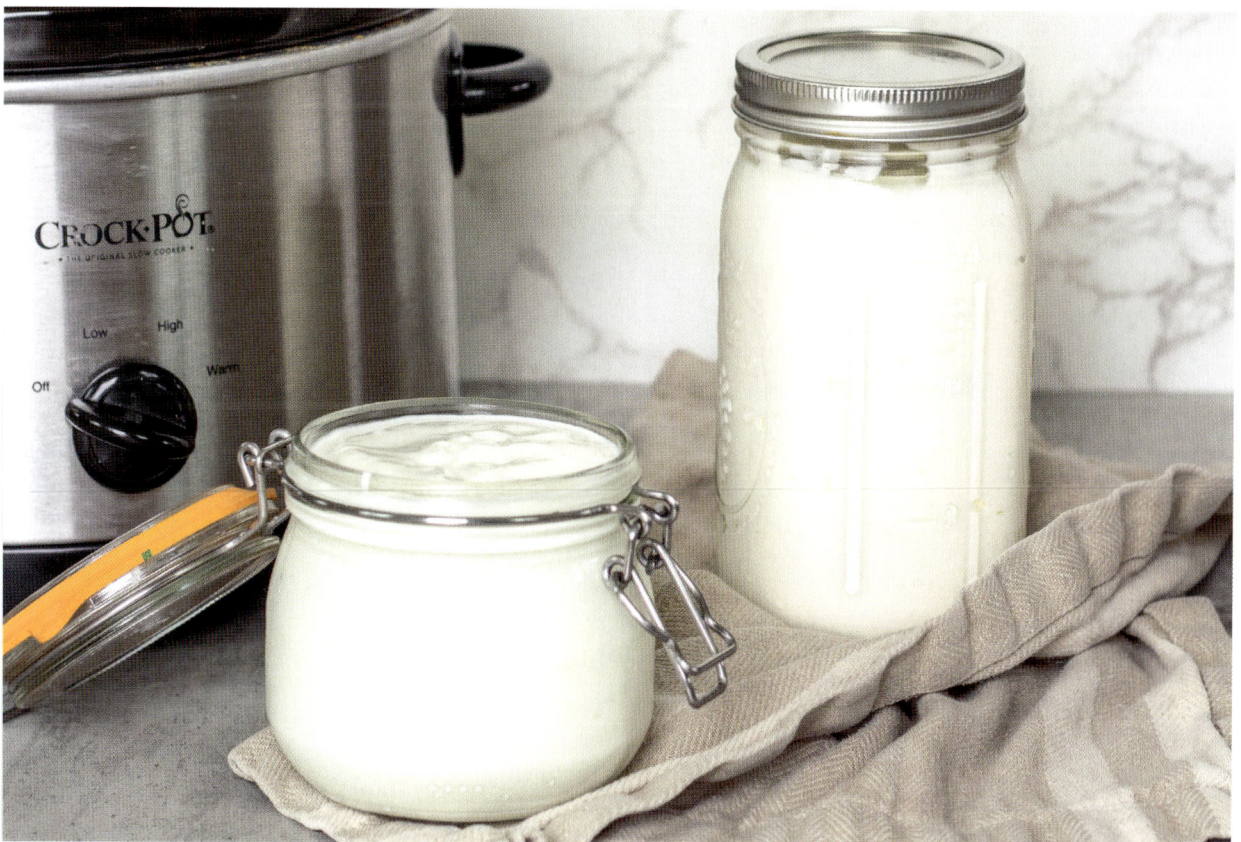

GREEK YOGURT IN A SLOW COOKER

MAKES about 6 cups

PREP TIME 5 minutes, plus 15 to 21 hours to cool and ferment and 8 hours to strain

COOK TIME 2½ hours

This is the original method I used when starting to make Greek yogurt. The only difference between Greek and regular yogurt is that Greek yogurt has been strained to remove excess lactose and whey. I prefer Greek yogurt because it contains about triple the amount of protein. If you already have a slow cooker, then all you need to get started is a yogurt strainer. Mine is from the brand Euro Cuisine.

I recommend starting this recipe 5 to 6 hours before your usual bedtime. The longer the yogurt ferments, the lower the lactose content will be, making it better for those who are lactose intolerant. However, the longer fermentation time also makes it more sour, so if you prefer it less sour, then you can ferment it for 12 hours.

½ gallon whole milk (see note)

¼ cup plain whole milk Greek yogurt with live active cultures

Special equipment: 5- to 7-quart slow cooker and 2-quart yogurt strainer (or a colander lined with butter muslin)

1. Pour the milk into the slow cooker and cover. Turn to the low setting and set a timer for 2½ hours.

2. When the timer goes off, turn the slow cooker off and unplug it. Set a timer for 3 hours.

3. When the second timer goes off, stir the yogurt into the milk with a fork or whisk until it is fully broken up and incorporated into the milk. Cover the slow cooker and wrap with a towel. If possible, keep it in a warm, draft-free area of your kitchen. Let the yogurt ferment for 12 to 18 hours.

4. After the fermentation time, you officially have yogurt! But to make it Greek yogurt, it needs to be strained. Pour the yogurt into a yogurt strainer or a colander lined with butter muslin. Cover and put in the fridge to strain for 8 hours.

5. Transfer the strained yogurt to a couple of large mason jars. Store in the fridge for up to 2 weeks.

Note This recipe can only be made with cow milk (either vat or ultra pasteurized). Dairy-free alternatives will not work.

GREEK YOGURT IN A YOGURT MAKER

MAKES about 3 cups

PREP TIME 5 minutes, plus 10 hours to ferment and 6 hours to strain

COOK TIME 10 minutes

A yogurt maker provides more reliable results by keeping the temperature of the yogurt constant. I like the brand called Bear. Other yogurt makers use multiple small jars for the fermentation process, which just creates extra cleanup time. You can speed up the cooling process by pouring the heated milk into a separate bowl.

4 cups whole milk (see note)

2 tablespoons plain whole milk Greek yogurt with live active cultures

Special equipment: yogurt maker, candy thermometer, and yogurt strainer (or a colander lined with butter muslin)

1. Pour the milk into a medium-sized pot. Bring to medium heat and stir every couple of minutes until the temperature reaches 160°F. Remove the pot from the heat and let cool until the temperature reaches 110°F, stirring every few minutes.

2. Plug in the yogurt maker and pour the yogurt into it. Add the cooled milk and stir to combine. Cover and turn the yogurt maker to the yogurt setting. Allow to ferment for 10 hours.

3. After fermentation, you have yogurt! To make Greek yogurt, you'll need to strain it. Pour the yogurt into the yogurt strainer or a colander lined with butter muslin. Cover and place in the fridge to strain for 6 hours.

4. Transfer the strained yogurt to a large mason jar. Store in the fridge for up to 2 weeks.

Note This recipe can only be made with cow milk (either vat or ultra pasteurized). Dairy-free alternatives will not work.

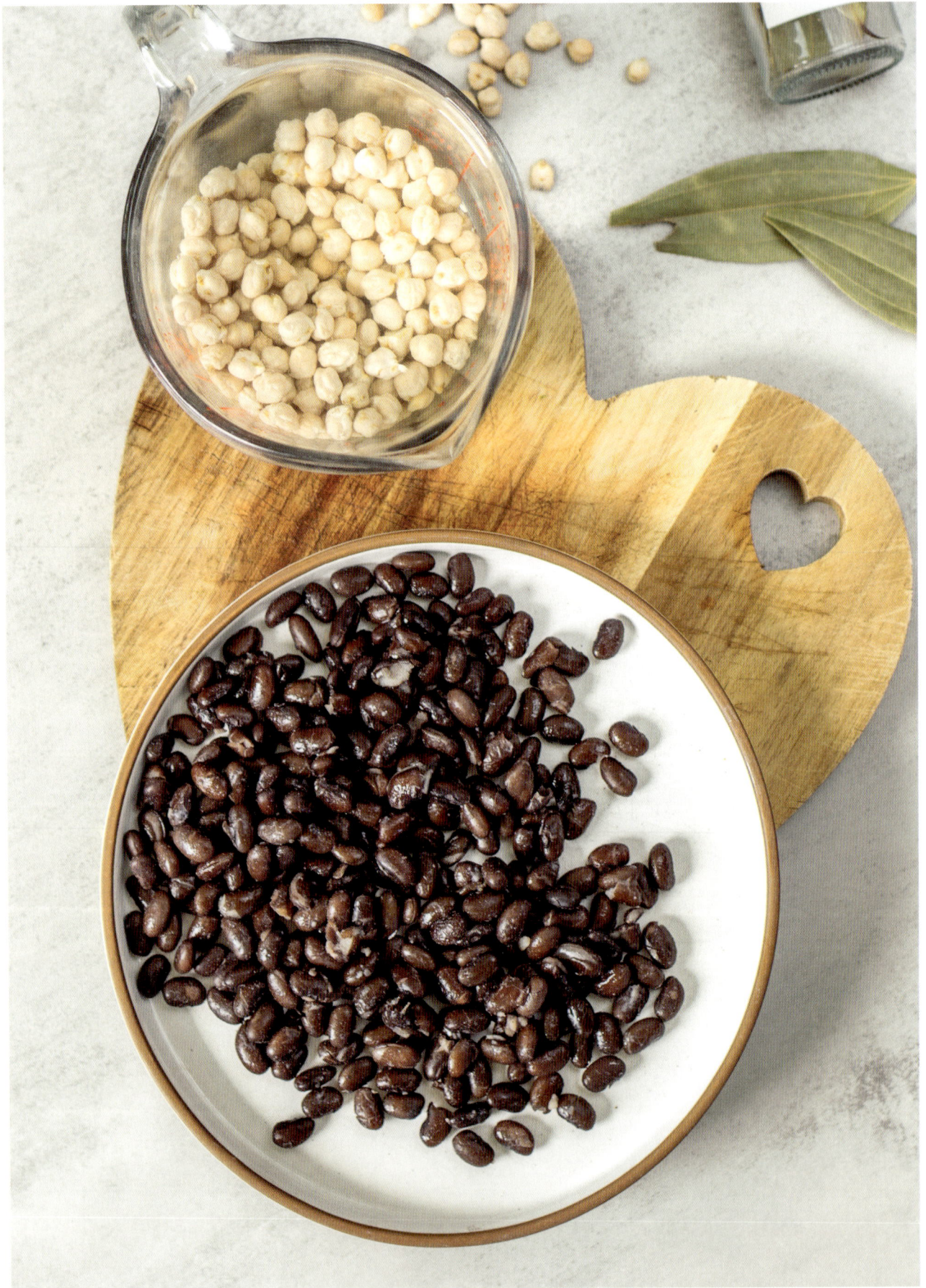

HOMEMADE BEANS

MAKES about 2 cups

PREP TIME 1 minute, plus 12 to 24 hours to soak

COOK TIME 30 minutes to 2 hours, depending on type of beans

I've been making beans from scratch since I learned the method in college. I found that when I soaked and cooked beans at home, it drastically reduced the bloating often associated with canned beans. This is because the antinutrients in the beans are broken down during the soaking process, making the end product more nourishing and gut health friendly. This recipe can be used for any type of bean. Some of my favorites are black beans, kidney beans, pinto beans, and chickpeas. But the cook time will vary greatly depending on the type. For example, chickpeas tend to cook quite quickly, in 25 to 30 minutes. On the flip side, kidney beans can take a lot longer. Just check every now and then and test a bean the same way you would test pasta. You're looking for it to be soft but still maintain its shape. You can also double or triple this recipe and store extras in the freezer for later. These can be used in any recipe that calls for beans, such as Cowboy Chili (page 126) and Spiced Chicken and Chickpeas with Quick Pickled Carrots (page 170).

1 cup dry beans or chickpeas

1 teaspoon baking soda

2 cups water

1 bay leaf

Salt

1. Pour the dry beans or chickpeas, baking soda, and water into a medium-sized bowl. Give it a quick stir and cover with a clean dish towel. Let sit at room temperature for 12 to 24 hours.

2. Drain the beans, give them a quick rinse, and then drain again. Pour the beans into a medium-sized pot and fill with enough water to cover the beans by at least 2 inches. Add the bay leaf and a heavy pinch of salt. Bring to a boil, then reduce to a simmer. Cook for 30 minutes to 2 hours, until the beans are soft. You might need to add extra water if the cook time is on the longer side; make sure that the beans remain fully submerged.

3. Drain the beans and remove the bay leaf. Use immediately or store in the fridge for up to 5 days or in the freezer for up to 6 months.

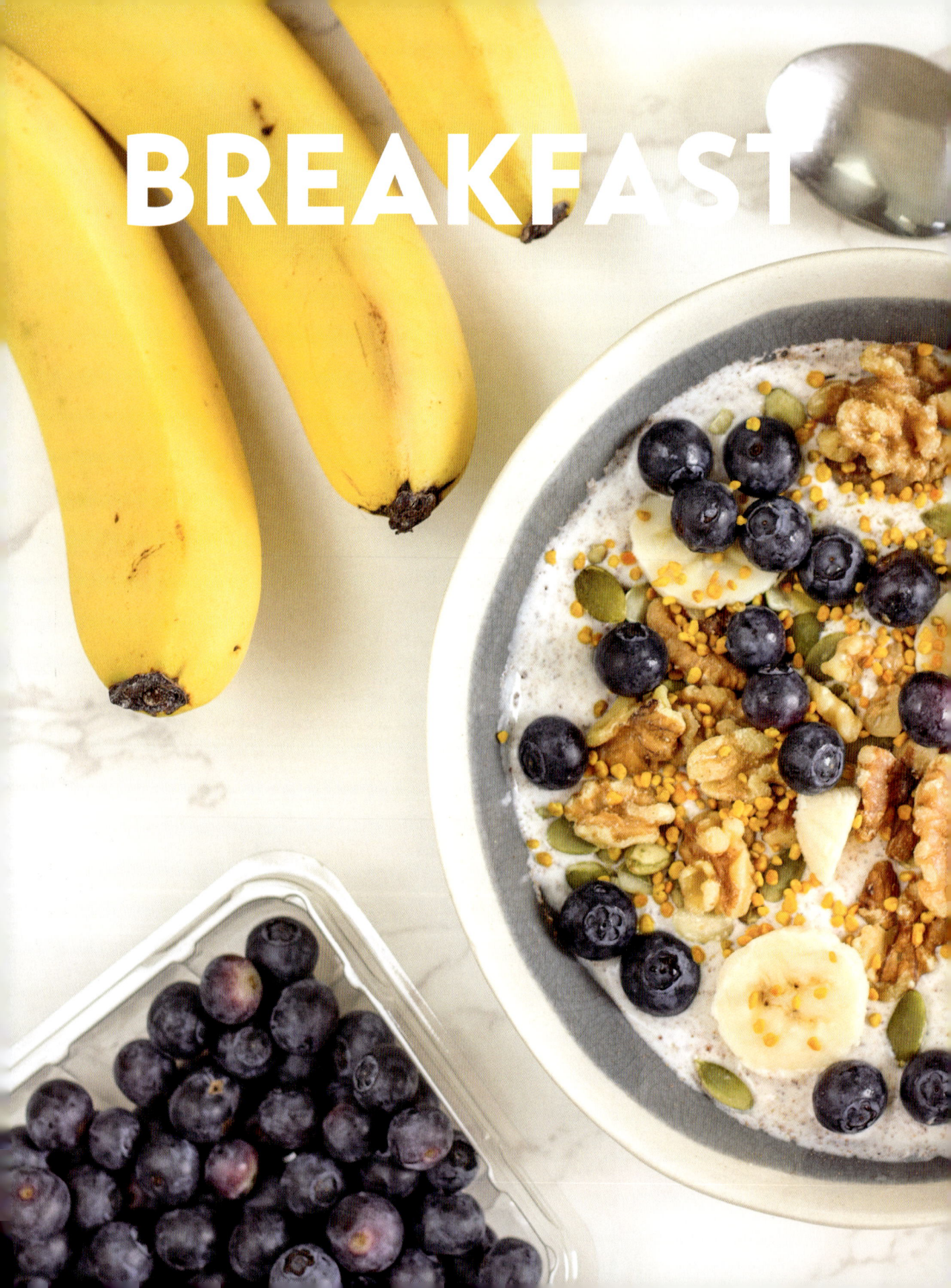

BREAKFAST

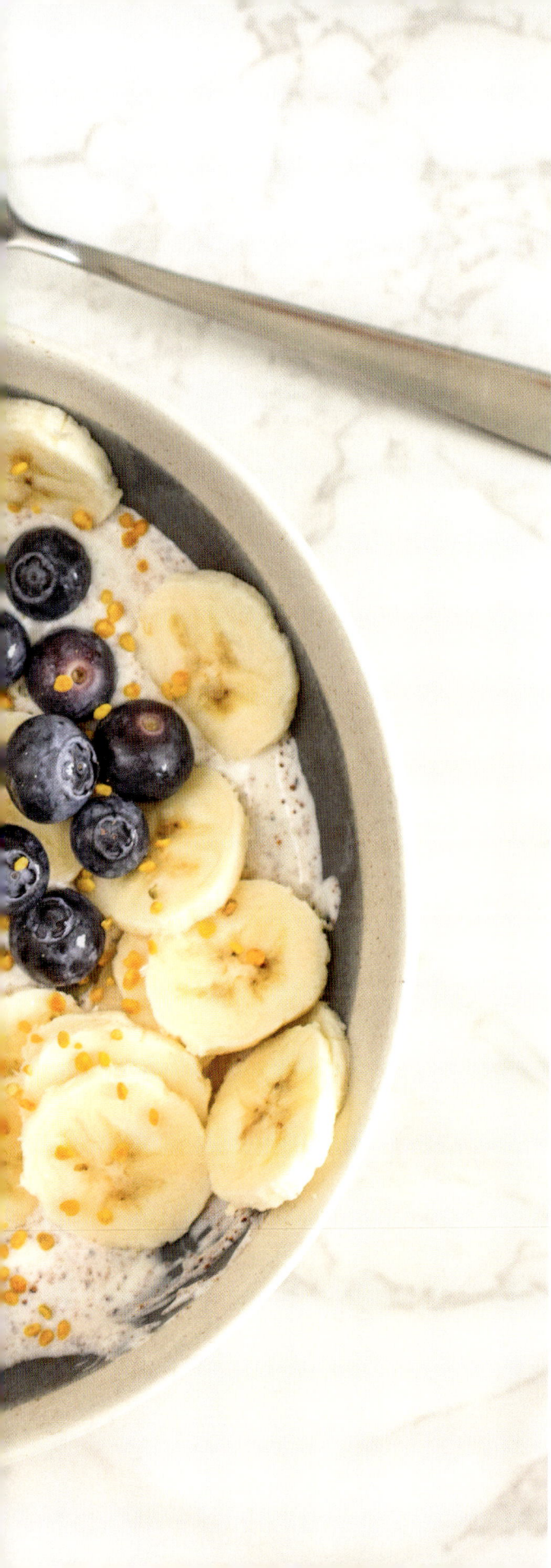

BLUEBERRY CHOCOLATE KEFIR SMOOTHIE

SERVES 1

PREP TIME 5 minutes

Kefir is a fermented dairy product that's rich, creamy, and naturally packed with probiotics. It's very thick, so I like to cut it with some water so that the smoothie isn't gloopy. This smoothie recipe sneaks in an unconventional source of fiber: cacao nibs. Cacao nibs are the raw form of chocolate and are very high in antioxidants and fiber. You can often find them at health food stores or online. This smoothie was designed to be a complete meal with 30 grams of protein and high-quality sources of fat and fiber. If you find that you're still hungry after drinking it, you can try bumping up the hemp seeds to 2 tablespoons for a boost of satiating healthy fat.

⅔ cup unsweetened kefir

½ cup water

½ cup frozen blueberries

2 scoops chocolate protein powder (or 1 serving that equates to 20 grams of protein)

1 tablespoon cacao nibs

1 tablespoon hulled hemp seeds

2 Brazil nuts

1 teaspoon bee pollen, for topping (optional)

Put all of the ingredients except the bee pollen in a blender. Blend until smooth. If desired, top with the bee pollen.

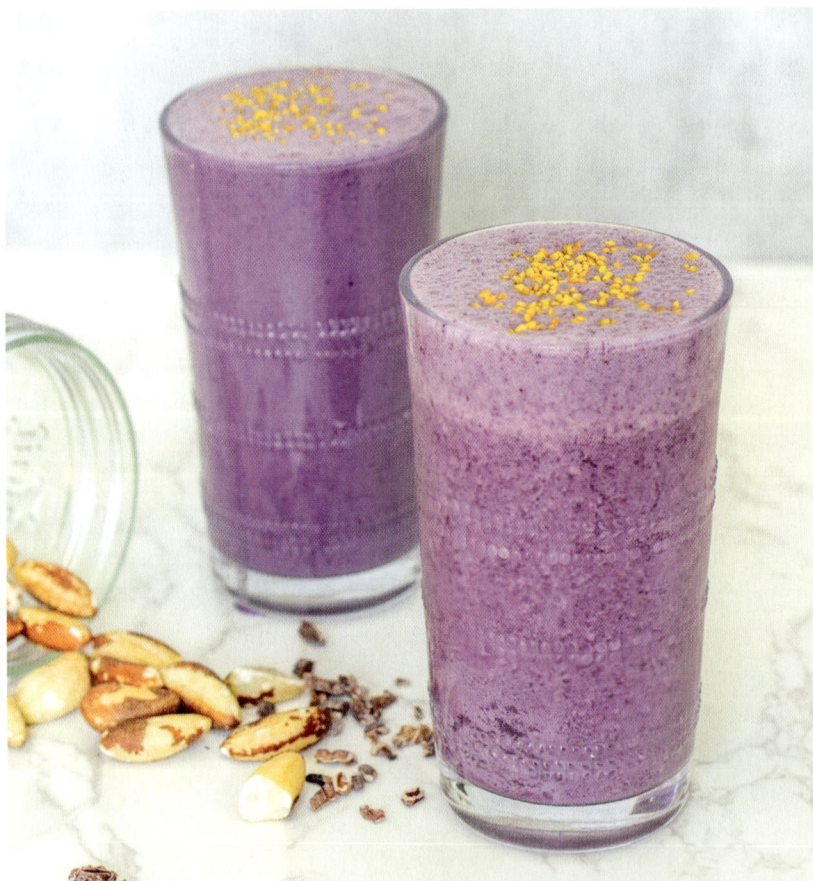

GREEN MINT SMOOTHIE

SERVES 1

PREP TIME 5 minutes

Did you ever let your ice cream melt into the bowl as a kid so that it would turn into "soup"? I used to. This smoothie tastes like melted mint chip ice cream. I like to use peppermint extract, which can be found in the grocery store spice aisle, but you can also use fresh mint leaves, which will give the smoothie a bit more of an "herby" mint flavor. I also prefer frozen kale for this recipe because it's precooked before freezing. Cooking helps reduce the antinutrients that are typically present in raw kale and make it more digestible.

1 cup water

½ cup plain whole milk Greek yogurt, store-bought or homemade (page 81)

½ frozen banana

½ cup frozen kale

2 scoops vanilla protein powder (or 1 serving that equates to 20 grams of protein)

3 tablespoons unsweetened coconut flakes

1 tablespoon cacao nibs

3 drops peppermint extract, or ¼ cup fresh mint leaves

Put all of the ingredients in a blender and blend until smooth.

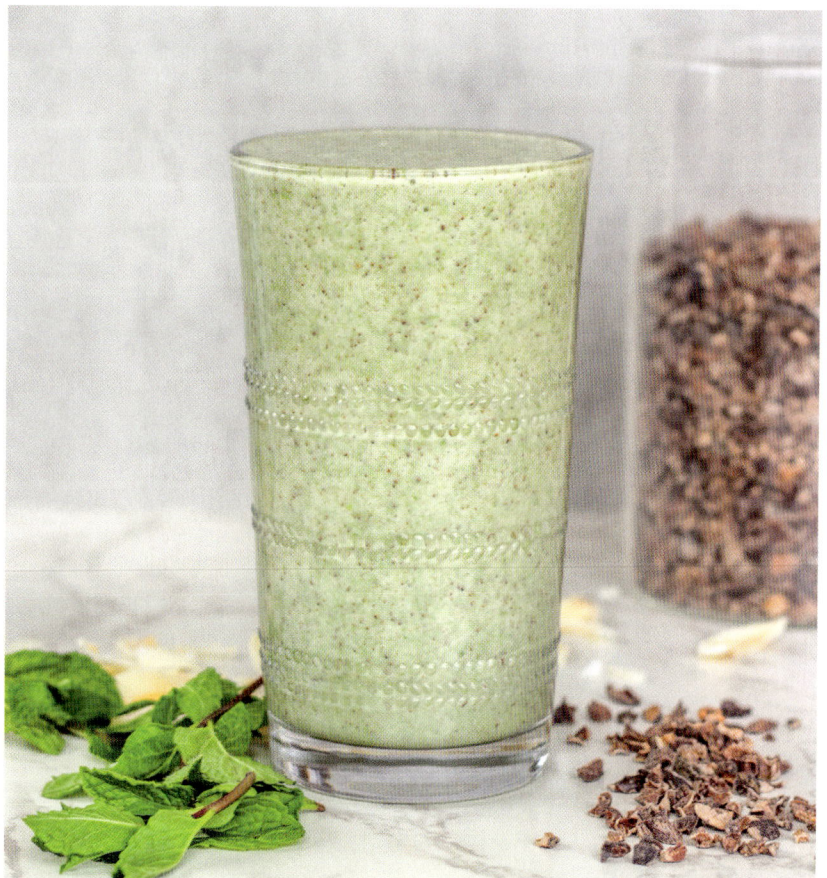

PEACH COBBLER BREKKY BOWL

SERVES 1

PREP TIME 5 minutes

Getting enough protein from yogurt alone can be tricky. Regular yogurt has only 5 to 7 grams of protein per cup, so it's important to opt for high-protein yogurts like Greek or skyr, both of which have about 20 grams per cup. I like to bring the protein up even further and add a hint of vanilla sweetness by stirring in vanilla protein powder. Not all protein powder will blend in well. From my experience, plant-based proteins tend to make the mixture chalky. I use my zero-sugar vanilla protein powder, which blends in very nicely while adding a hint of sweetness. If you aren't in the States and can't get your hands on my protein powder, try a 100 percent whey protein isolate that's low in sugar and local to you. I also add collagen to this bowl because it promotes even higher levels of satiety when combined with other proteins like protein powder and yogurt. If peaches aren't in season, you can opt for frozen peaches and lightly sauté them in a bit of oil before adding the fruit to your brekky bowl.

1 cup plain whole milk Greek yogurt, store-bought or homemade (page 81)

1 scoop vanilla protein powder (or ½ serving that equates to 10 grams of protein)

1 scoop unflavored collagen powder (optional)

1 medium peach, sliced

2 tablespoons chopped walnuts

1 tablespoon almond butter

Ground cinnamon, for sprinkling

Ground nutmeg, for sprinkling

1. Put the yogurt, protein powder, and collagen (if using) in a bowl and stir to combine.

2. Top the yogurt mixture with the peach slices, walnuts, almond butter, a sprinkle of cinnamon, and a sprinkle of nutmeg.

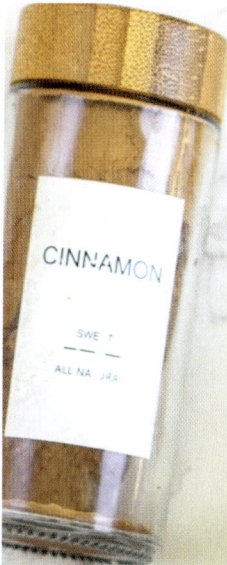

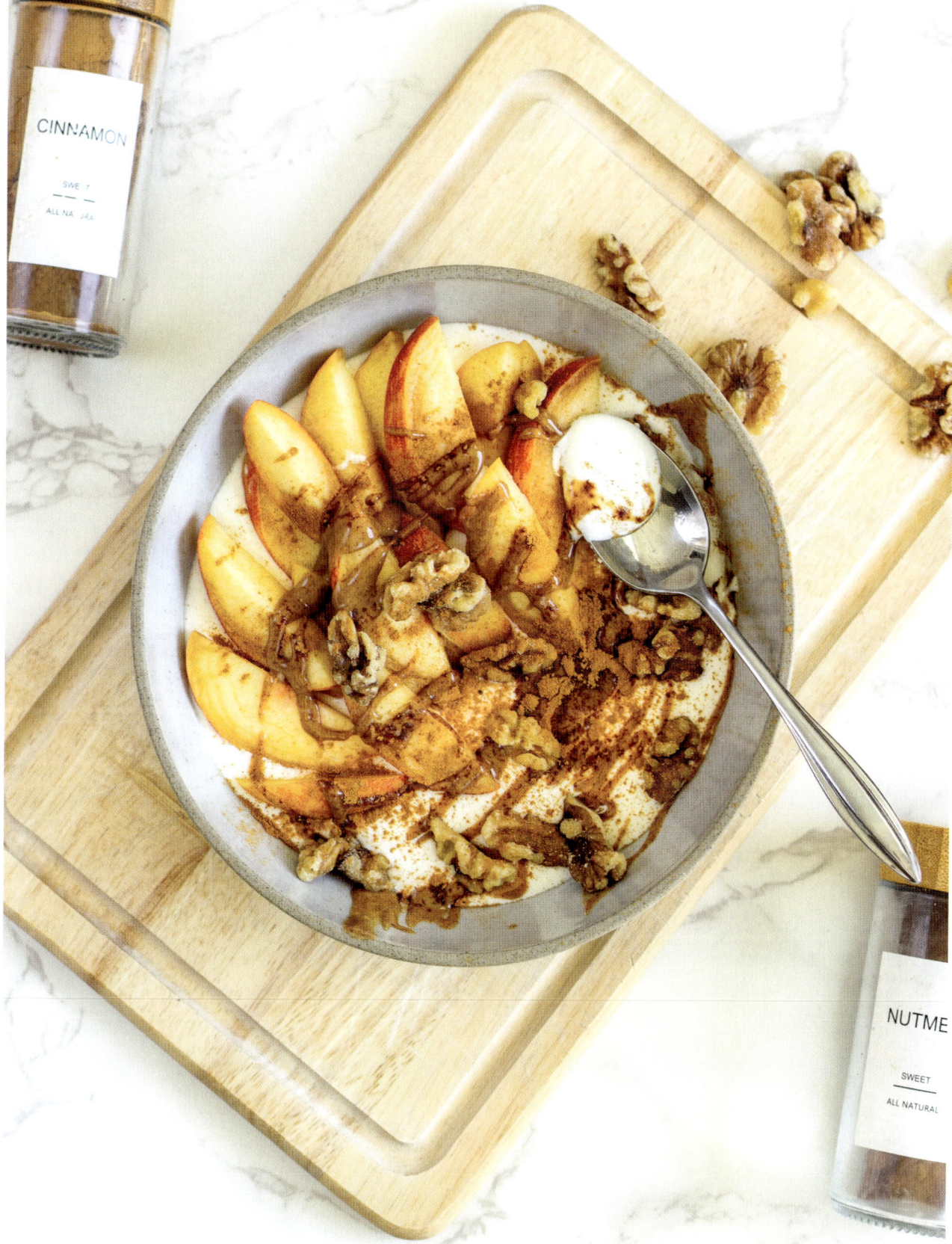

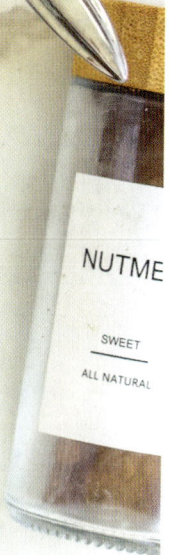

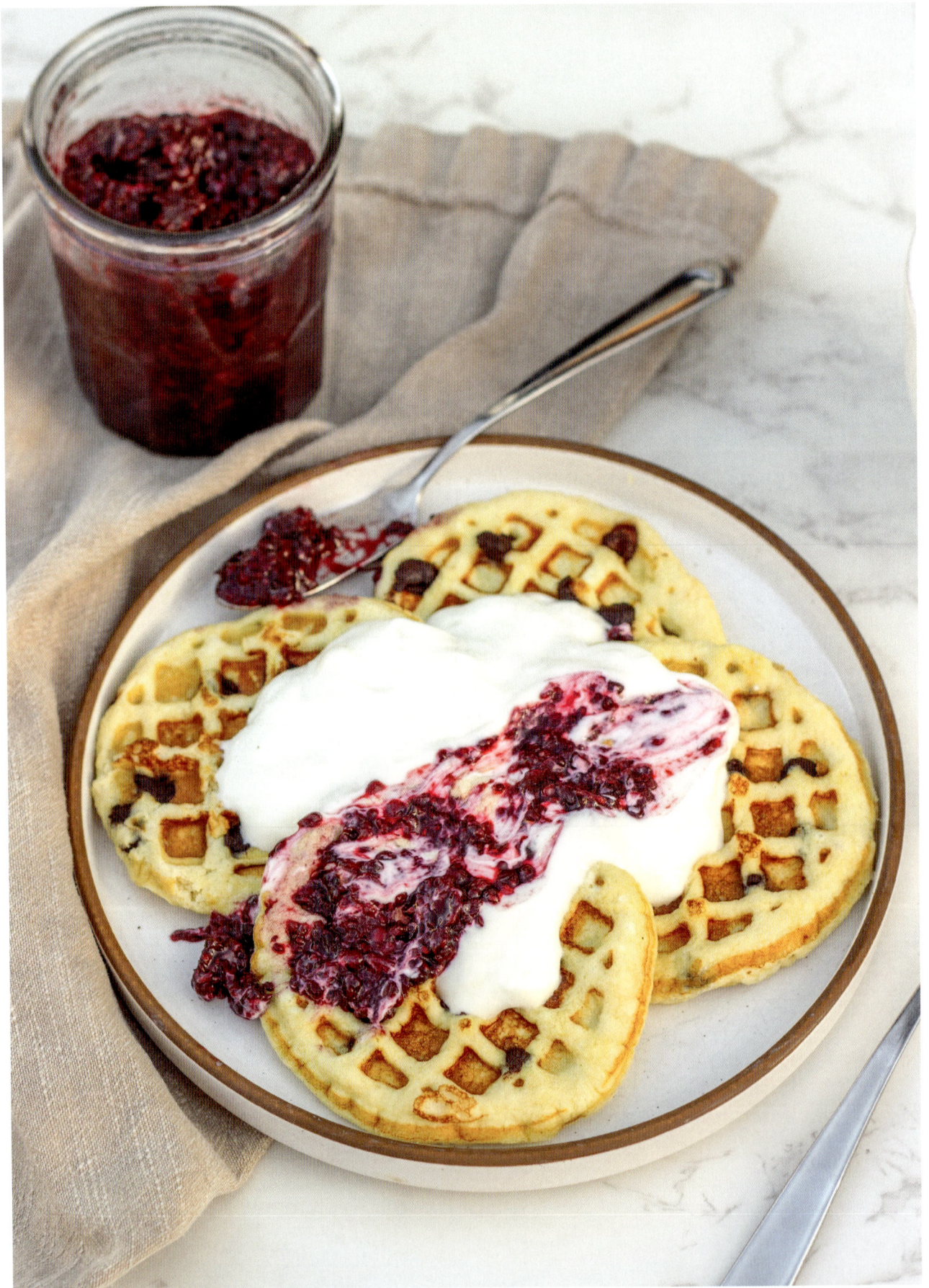

BLACKBERRY CHOCOLATE CHIP PROTEIN WAFFLES

MAKES 2 waffles (1 serving)

PREP TIME 5 minutes (not including time to make jam)

COOK TIME about 5 minutes (varies depending on waffle iron)

Throughout my postpartum weight-loss journey, I lived on these waffles. Unlike typical waffles, they are packed with 26 grams of protein per serving. I bump up the protein content even further by topping them with Greek yogurt instead of maple syrup. I like to triple or quadruple this recipe on the weekend to make a big batch of waffles for the week. Once cooled, store the waffles in a plastic bag in the freezer for up to 6 months. Then just pop a couple in the toaster for a fast and easy breakfast! If you're not a fan of banana or if you're very carb sensitive, you can swap the banana for ¼ cup of cottage cheese or canned pumpkin puree.

WAFFLES

2 scoops vanilla protein powder (or 1 serving that equates to 20 grams of protein)

1 large egg

½ medium banana, mashed

½ teaspoon vanilla extract

1 tablespoon zero-sugar chocolate chips

Avocado oil spray

TOPPINGS

½ cup plain whole milk Greek yogurt, store-bought or homemade (page 81)

¼ cup Blackberry Chia Jam (page 78)

1 tablespoon almond butter

Special equipment: waffle iron (preferably 4-inch)

1. Preheat the waffle iron.

2. Combine the protein powder, egg, banana, and vanilla extract in a medium-sized mixing bowl. Fold in the chocolate chips.

3. Spray the waffle iron with avocado oil spray to prevent sticking. Pour half of the batter onto the waffle iron and cook according to the manufacturer's instructions (see notes if not using a mini waffle iron). Repeat with the remaining batter.

4. Top the waffles with the yogurt, jam, and almond butter.

Notes

• If you are using a standard-sized waffle iron that makes four waffles at a time, consider doubling this recipe so you have enough batter to completely fill the iron. Otherwise, you'll end up with very thin waffles.

• Not all protein powders are created for baked recipes. Some can make the end result dry or artificial tasting. I only use my zero-sugar pasture-raised protein powder, which I specifically designed to taste amazing in baked goods; scan the QR code for details. If you can't get your hands on my protein powder, look for a 100 percent whey protein isolate that's free of artificial flavors and sweeteners.

SCRAMBLED EGGS AND SAUERKRAUT

SERVES 1

PREP TIME 5 minutes

COOK TIME 13 minutes

Eggs are a great source of protein, but it can be tricky to eat enough eggs in one sitting to hit 30 grams of complete protein. To put this in perspective, you would need to eat five to six scrambled eggs to get enough protein. To boost the protein in the meal while also adding some cheesy goodness, I like to combine eggs with cottage cheese before cooking them. This brings the total protein up to 30 grams without going through a half dozen eggs. The cottage cheese also makes the eggs extra light and fluffy. I love serving eggs with sauerkraut for an added boost of probiotics and fiber as well. Feel free to use even more sauerkraut than the recipe recommends. If you find that you need a little extra food with this meal to feel fully satisfied, try adding one-half to one avocado per serving.

2 teaspoons olive oil

½ Roma tomato, diced

¼ cup diced red onions

Salt

3 large eggs

½ cup cottage cheese

½ teaspoon dried basil leaves

¼ cup sauerkraut, for serving

Fresh parsley, for garnish

1. Heat the olive oil in a medium-sized skillet over medium-high heat. Add the tomato, onions, and a heavy pinch of salt. Sauté for 5 minutes, or until the tomato is softened.

2. In a medium-sized mixing bowl, whisk the eggs, cottage cheese, and basil. Pour the egg mixture into the pan with the tomato mixture and cook for 5 to 8 minutes, stirring with a rubber spatula or spoon every few minutes, until the scrambled eggs are firm and not runny. (However, they won't brown as much as regular scrambled eggs.)

3. Remove the pan from the heat and serve the eggs with the sauerkraut, garnished with parsley.

> Note Cottage cheese adds moisture to the eggs, which causes the cooking time to be a few minutes longer than for standard scrambled eggs.

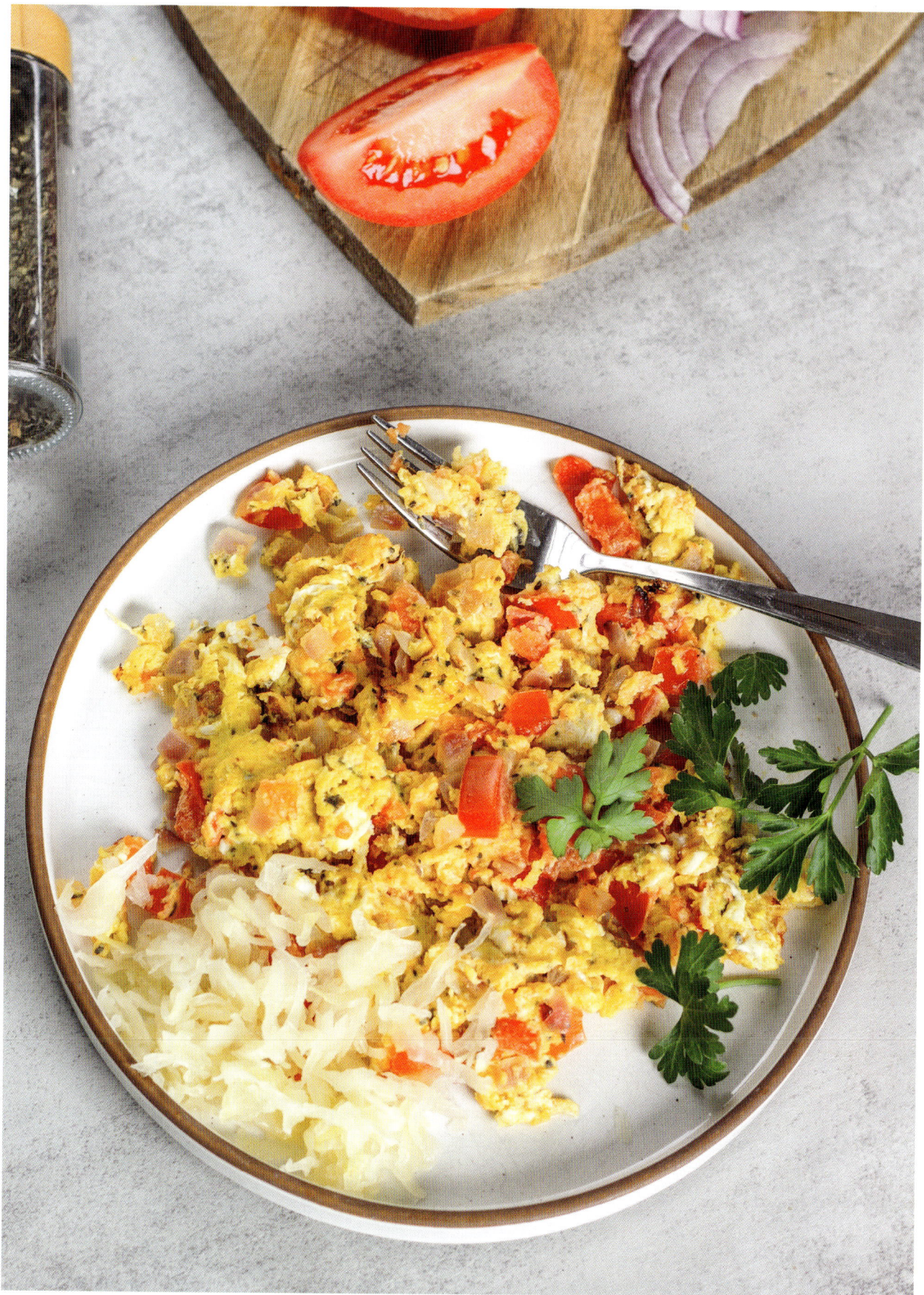

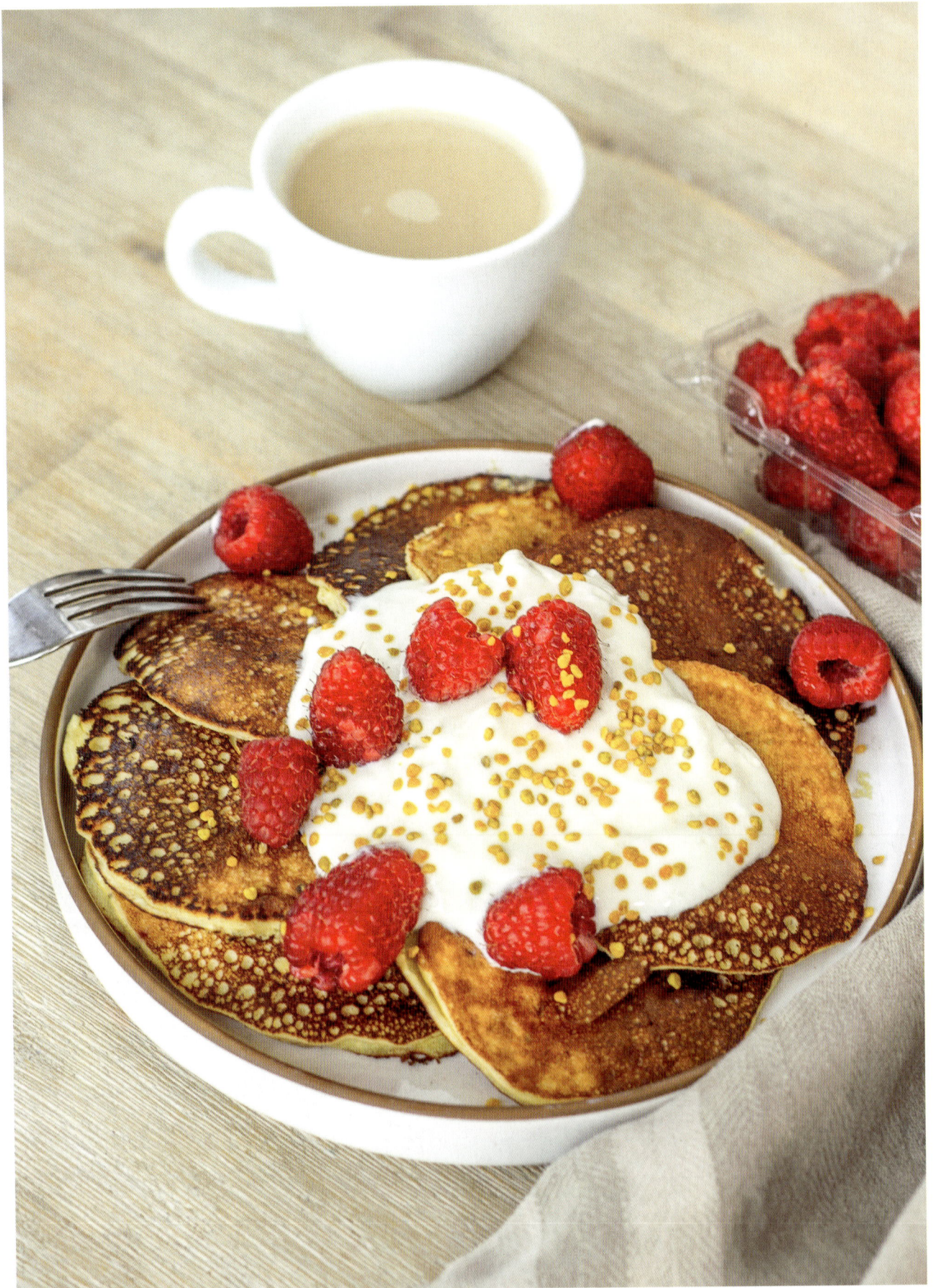

RASPBERRY LEMON PROTEIN PANCAKES

SERVES 1

PREP TIME 5 minutes

COOK TIME 6 minutes

When I have a little extra time to cook a fresh, warm breakfast, I like to make protein pancakes. The batter is identical to my protein waffles, but I've found that it's much easier to add a variety of fun mix-ins to pancakes without them sticking and falling apart. The combination of raspberries and lemon zest in this recipe makes it light and refreshing while still satiating enough to be considered a full meal. But just like with the waffles, the type of protein powder you use really matters (see notes, page 93).

PANCAKES

2 scoops vanilla protein powder (or 1 serving that equates to 20 grams of protein)

1 large egg

½ medium banana, mashed

½ teaspoon grated lemon zest

¼ cup frozen or fresh raspberries, roughly chopped

Coconut oil or avocado oil spray, for greasing

TOPPINGS

½ cup plain whole milk Greek yogurt, store-bought or homemade (page 81)

1 teaspoon bee pollen

¼ cup fresh raspberries

1. Combine the protein powder, egg, banana, and lemon zest in a medium-sized mixing bowl. Once well mixed and smooth, stir in the raspberries.

2. Preheat a griddle and grease it with oil or spray. Use a ladle to pour about one-quarter of the batter onto the hot griddle. Cook for 2 to 3 minutes, until the pancake is lightly browned on the bottom. Then flip and cook for another 2 to 3 minutes, until lightly browned on the other side. Repeat with the remaining batter; you should get three or four pancakes.

3. Top the pancakes with the yogurt, bee pollen, and fresh raspberries.

TREVOR'S YOGURT PARFAIT

SERVES 1

PREP TIME 5 minutes

I was just finishing writing the first chapter of this book when my husband, Trevor, came into my office saying, "You need to try this." He had taken a "kitchen sink" approach to his breakfast, and the results were surprisingly delicious. We use our zero-sugar vanilla protein powder for this recipe, and it dissolves perfectly. The protein powder helps bring the total protein in the meal up to a whopping 40 grams while cutting through the sourness of the Greek yogurt. We designed our powder to be used in recipes (like this!) and complement other ingredients rather than overpower them. If you are located outside of the US and unable to get your hands on our protein powder, then you'll want to stick with an unflavored whey protein isolate for this recipe.

2 teaspoons cacao nibs

1 cup plain whole milk Greek yogurt, store-bought or homemade (page 81)

2 scoops vanilla protein powder (or 1 serving that equates to 20 grams of protein)

¼ medium banana, sliced

¼ cup blueberries

1 tablespoon pumpkin seeds

1 tablespoon raw walnuts

¼ teaspoon bee pollen

1. Pour the cacao nibs into a coffee or spice grinder. Pulse until it forms a fine powder (aka cacao powder).

2. Scoop the yogurt into a bowl. Stir the cacao powder and protein powder into the yogurt until dissolved.

3. Top the yogurt mixture with the banana, blueberries, pumpkin seeds, walnuts, and bee pollen before serving.

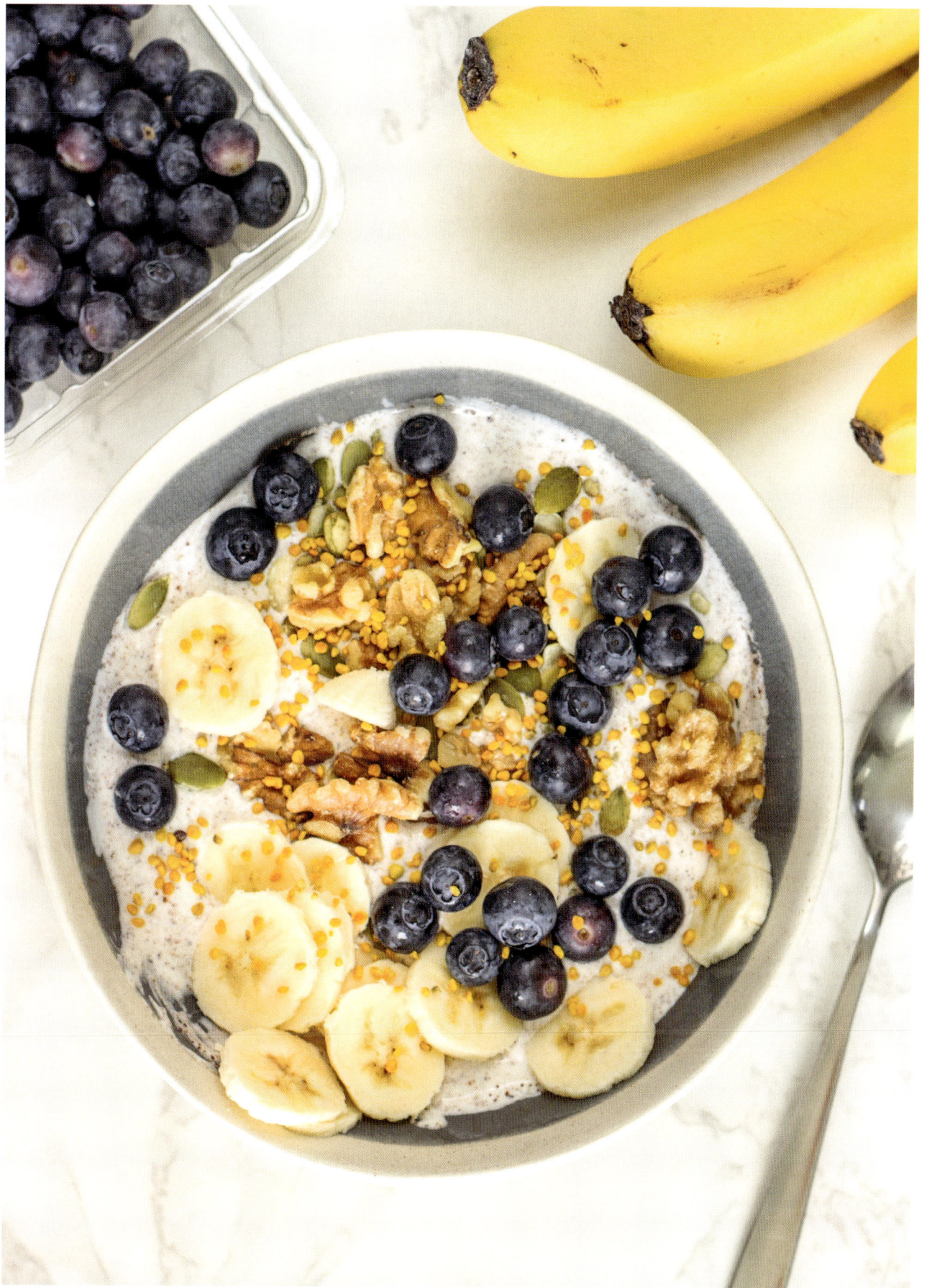

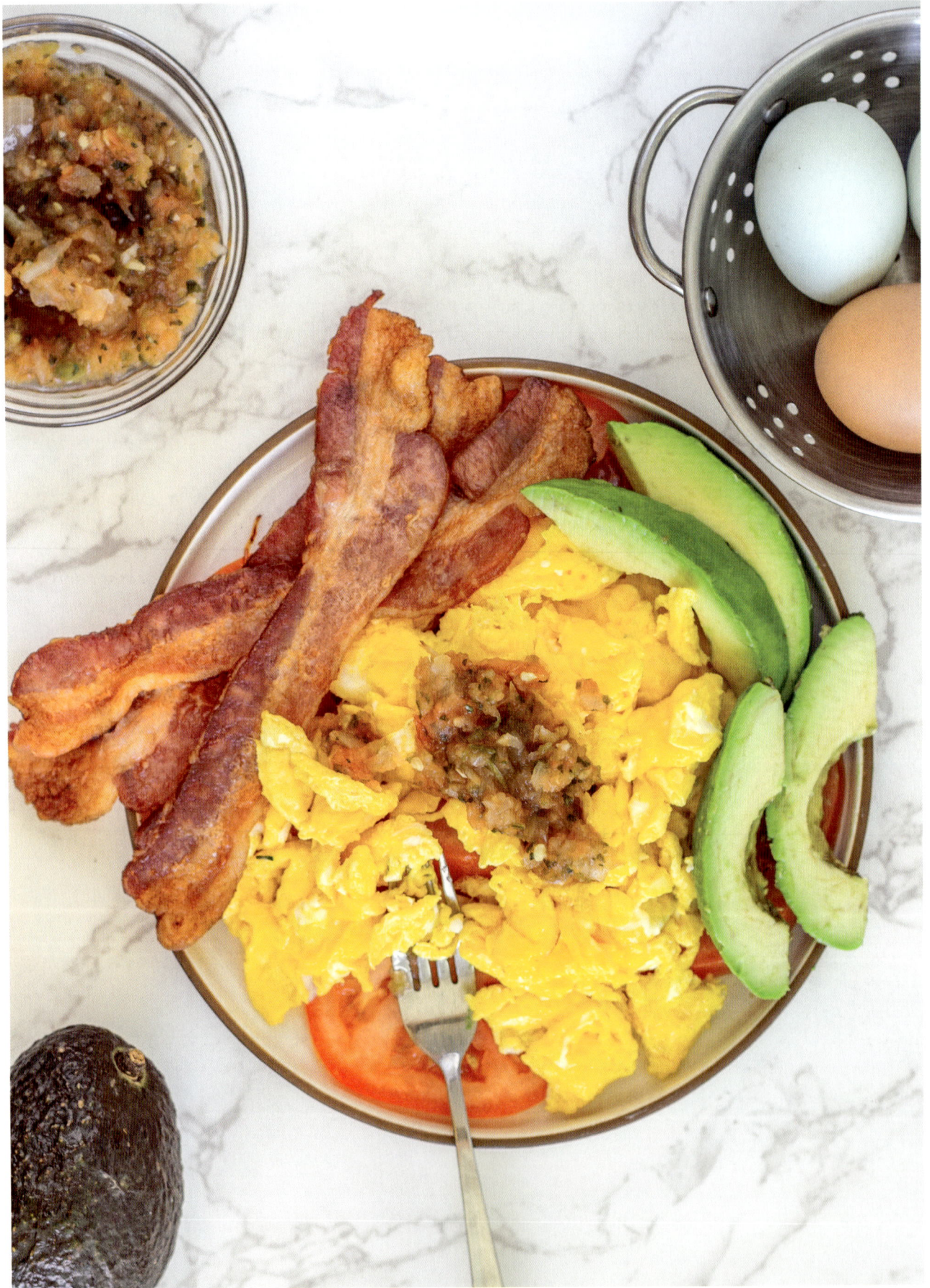

BREKKY BURRITO BOWL

SERVES 1

PREP TIME 5 minutes

COOK TIME 30 minutes
(18 minutes if the
salsa is already
prepped)

Growing up in southern California, I ate a lot of breakfast burritos.
Salsa, eggs, cheese, bacon, and avocado—all you need is a warm, sunny
beach, and you're describing a typical summer day of mine in high school.
Here, I took my well-loved breakfast burrito and turned it into a bowl
to maximize the protein, fat, and fiber while minimizing the processed
grains. Even though this meal doesn't have many obvious signs of fiber,
it's packed with over 7 grams of fiber, mostly from the avocado. If you
don't have time to make homemade salsa, your favorite store-bought
salsa will do. And feel free to spice this dish up even further by drizzling
hot sauce on top!

ROASTED SALSA

(makes about 2 cups)

5 medium tomatoes

½ medium yellow onion,
chopped

5 jalapeño peppers, chopped
(remove membranes and
seeds if you prefer less heat)

3 cloves garlic

½ cup chopped fresh cilantro

Juice of 1 lime (about
2 tablespoons)

1 teaspoon salt

BURRITO BOWL

3 slices bacon

3 large eggs

2 tablespoons whole milk

2 tablespoons Mexican-style
shredded cheese

1 medium tomato (preferably
heirloom), sliced

½ avocado, sliced

Special equipment: food
processor

For the salsa:

1. Set the oven to broil. Spread the tomatoes, onion, and jalapeños
    on a sheet pan. Broil for 7 to 10 minutes, until the veggies are a
    bit blackened.

2. Carefully transfer the broiled veggies to a food processor and
    add the garlic, cilantro, lime juice, and salt. Pulse until the salsa
    is mostly pureed but still slightly chunky.

3. Store in a glass container in the fridge for up to 4 days.

For the brekky bowl:

4. In a medium-sized skillet over medium-high heat, cook the bacon
    for 5 minutes on each side, or until crispy. Remove the bacon to
    a plate but leave the rendered fat in the pan.

5. Crack the eggs into a small bowl, add the milk, and whisk to
    combine. Pour the egg mixture into the skillet. Cook for 3 to
    5 minutes, stirring with a rubber spatula or spoon every few
    minutes, until scrambled to the desired doneness.

6. Put the scrambled eggs in a serving bowl and top with the
    cheese. Serve with the bacon, tomato, avocado, and some salsa.

Note This recipe makes much more salsa than you'll need for
one brekky bowl. Make a batch and use it on your eggs and
tacos for the week!

LEBANESE-STYLE BREKKY BOWL

SERVES 1

PREP TIME 5 minutes (not including time to make tabbouleh)

COOK TIME 5 minutes

Tabbouleh originates from Lebanon and is one of my favorite refreshing veggie-packed side dishes to add to a meal. I like making a big batch of Cauliflower Avocado Tabbouleh for the week so that I can whip up protein-packed breakfasts or lunches in a matter of minutes. To hit the goal of 30 grams of protein, this recipe pairs four eggs with feta cheese. Both are high-quality and nutrient-dense protein sources packed with a combination of calcium, vitamin K2, vitamin A, and B12. This meal makes a delicious breakfast or lunch.

1 teaspoon salted butter

4 large eggs

2 tablespoons whole milk

¼ batch Cauliflower Avocado Tabbouleh (page 234)

3 tablespoons crumbled feta cheese

½ avocado, sliced

Salt

1. Melt the butter in a medium-sized skillet over medium-high heat. In a small bowl, whisk the eggs and milk. Pour the egg mixture into the skillet and cook for 3 to 5 minutes, stirring with a rubber spatula or spoon every few minutes, until scrambled to your desired doneness.

2. Place the tabbouleh and scrambled eggs in a serving bowl. Sprinkle on the feta and sliced avocado before serving. Season with salt to taste.

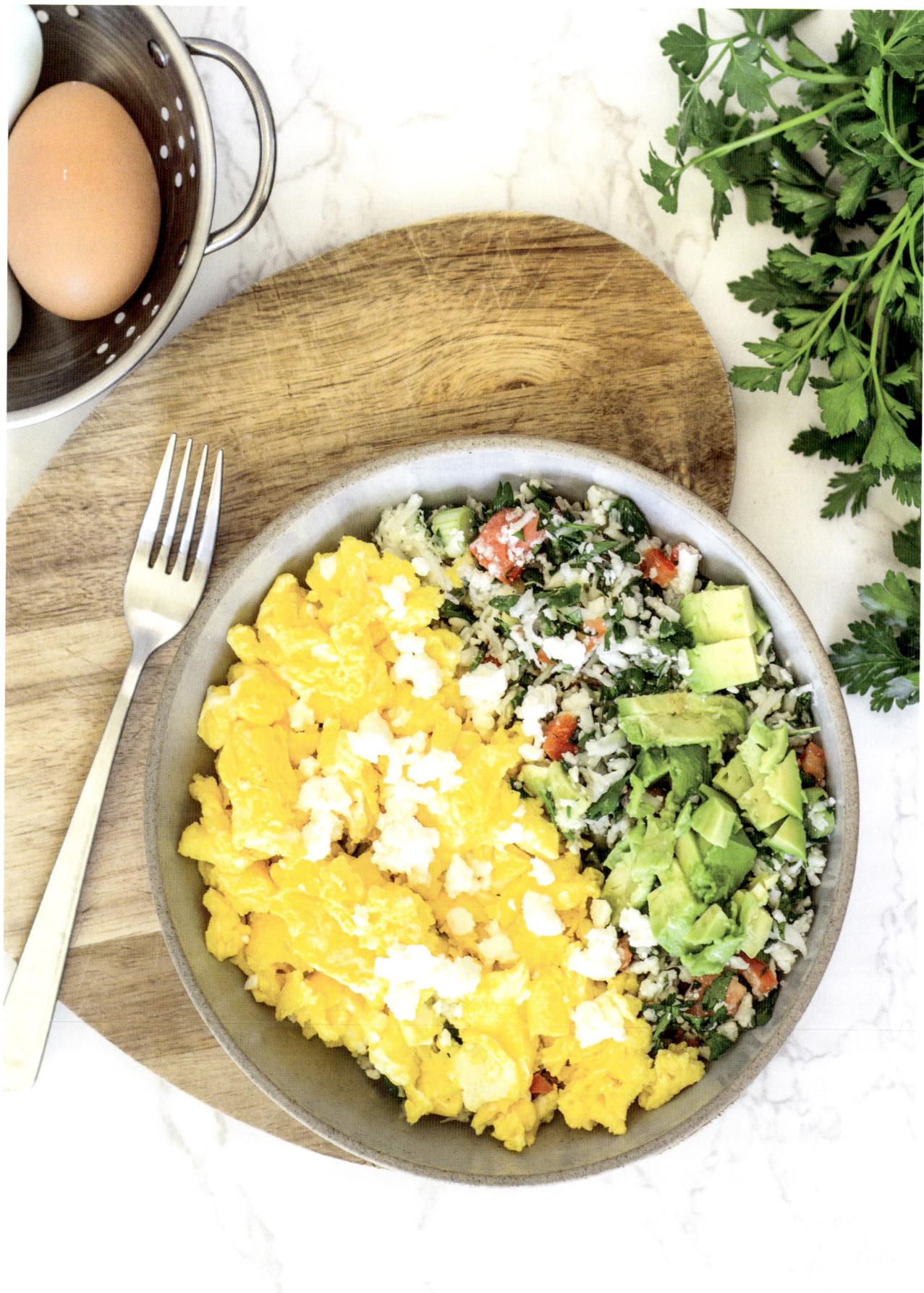

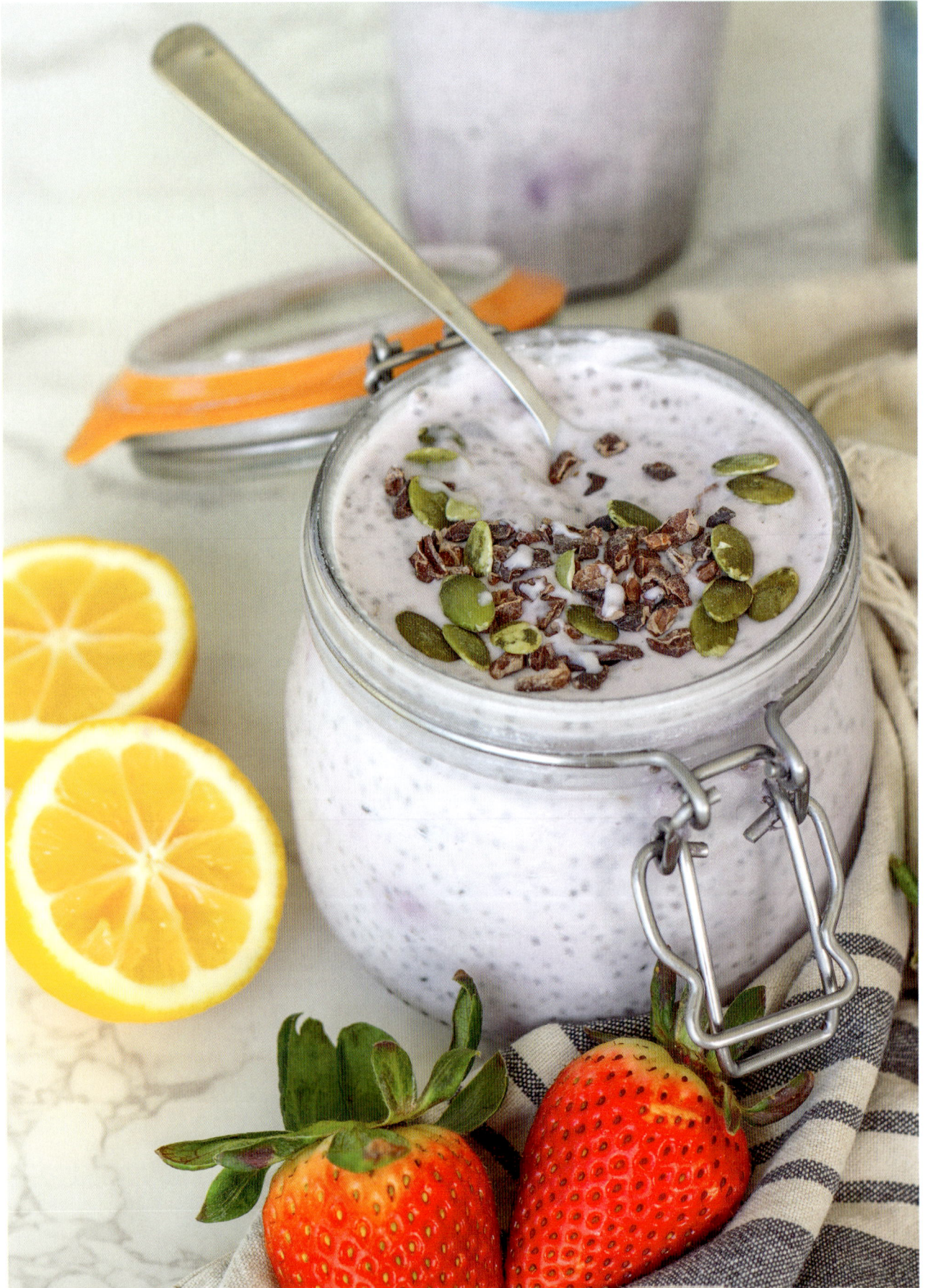

BLUEBERRY LEMON CHIA PUDDING

SERVES 3

PREP TIME 10 minutes, plus at least 30 minutes to soak chia seeds

COOK TIME 5 minutes

Chia pudding is a staple for my community because you can easily whip up a whole workweek's worth of breakfasts or lunches in a matter of minutes, making this one of the simplest foods to meal prep. When done right, chia pudding is loaded with protein, fat, and fiber to boost satiety and prevent cravings. My chia pudding recipes always focus on adding extra flavor and crunch with toppings and mix-ins. This version uses a combination of blueberries and lemon juice for a slightly sweet base, plus pumpkin seeds, cacao nibs, and strawberries on top for some low-sugar crunch and texture.

CHIA PUDDING

1 cup frozen blueberries

Grated zest and juice of 1 lemon (2 to 3 tablespoons)

⅓ cup chia seeds

3 tablespoons hulled hemp seeds

1½ cups plain whole milk Greek yogurt, store-bought or homemade (page 81)

1½ cups unsweetened almond or coconut milk

4 scoops vanilla protein powder (or 2 servings that equate to 40 grams of protein)

Pinch of salt

TOPPINGS PER SERVING

1 tablespoon cacao nibs

1 tablespoon pumpkin seeds

1 cup sliced fresh strawberries

1. In a small skillet over medium heat, combine the blueberries and lemon zest and juice. Sauté for about 5 minutes, until the blueberries start to release their juices. Remove from the heat and set aside.

2. Put the chia seeds, hemp seeds, yogurt, milk, protein powder, and salt in a mixing bowl. Use a fork to mix until the ingredients are evenly distributed.

3. Pour the blueberry mixture into the bowl with the pudding and stir until the entire mixture turns a light purple color. Cover with plastic wrap and refrigerate for at least 30 minutes or overnight to allow the chia seeds to bloom and the pudding to develop a thick consistency. If it hasn't, refrigerate it for a little longer.

4. Divide the pudding into three equal servings and store in the fridge for up to 5 days. Add the toppings just before eating.

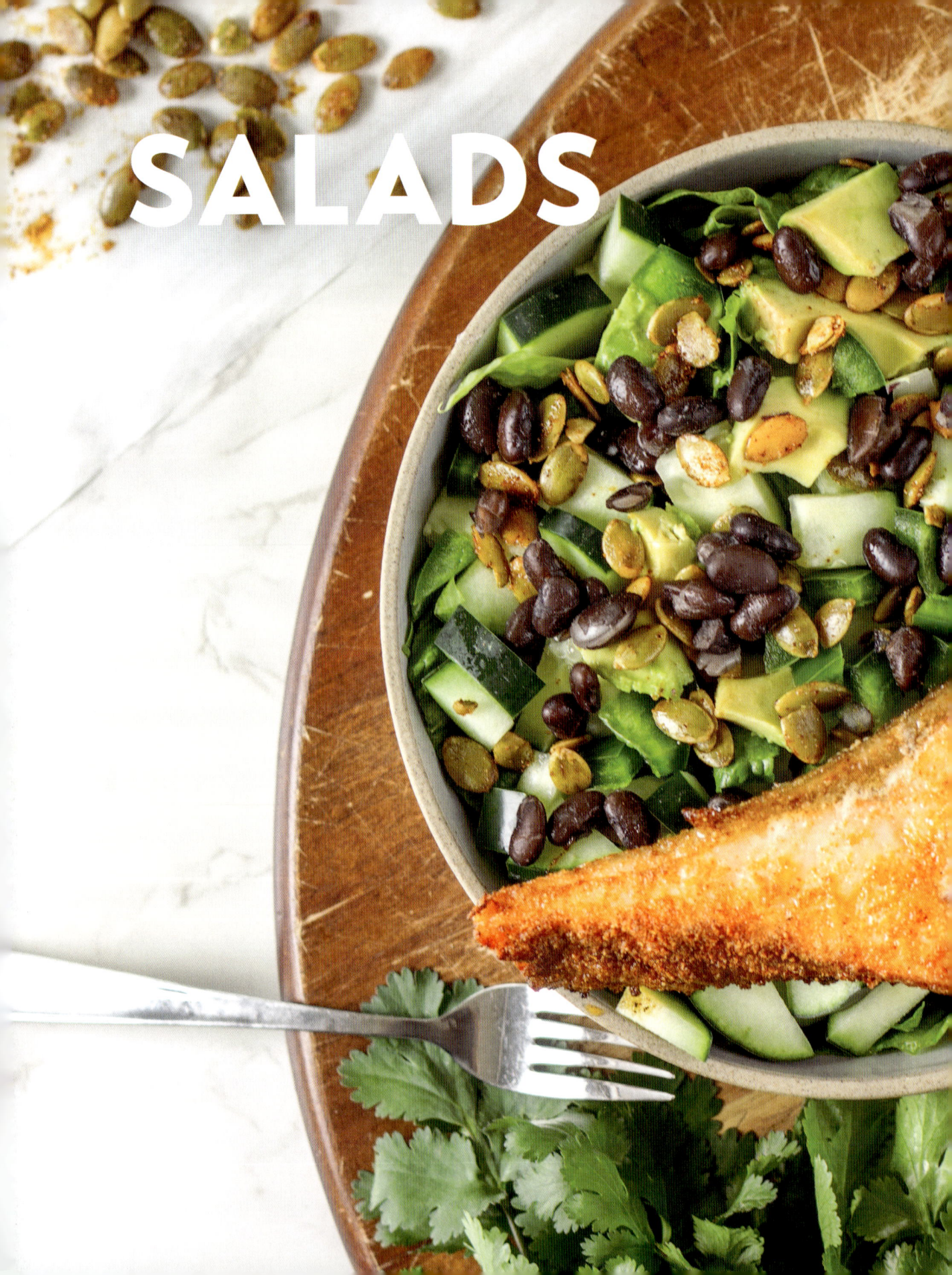

SALADS

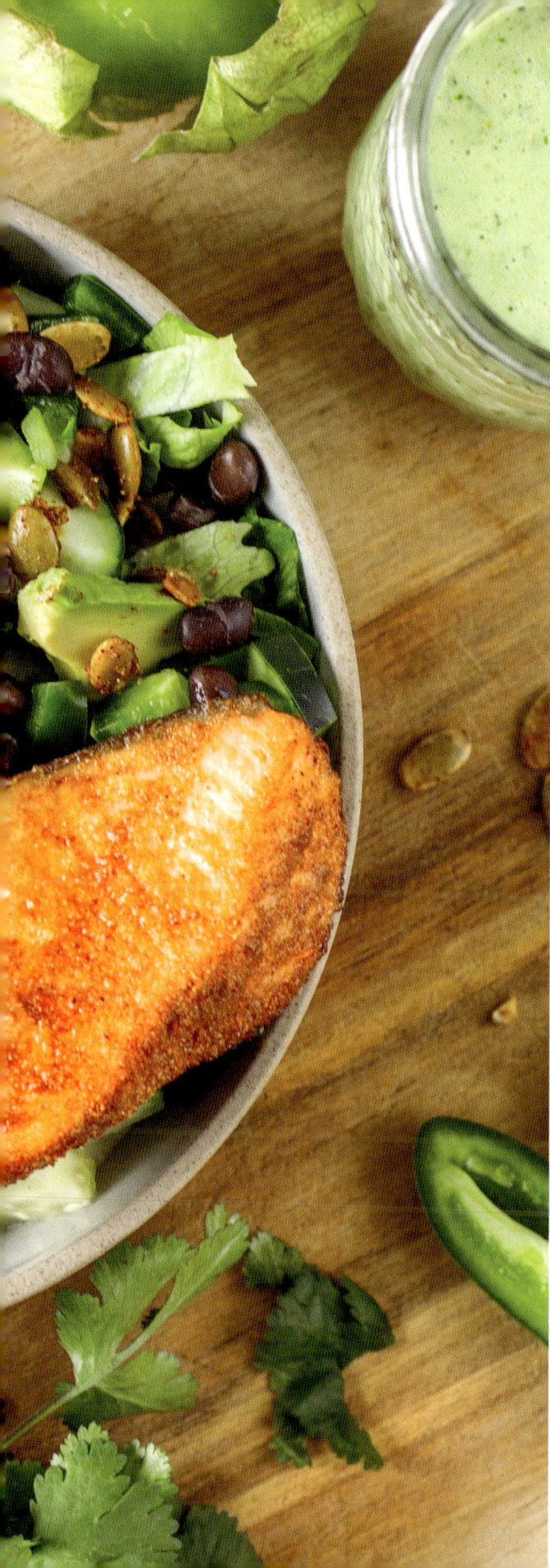

KALE PECORINO SALAD

SERVES 1

PREP TIME 10 minutes (not including time to cook buckwheat groats)

This salad can be served as either a side dish or a main meal. If you choose to have it as a main meal, make sure to pair it with 4 to 5 ounces of complete protein per serving. I love it with my Balsamic Grilled Chicken (page 168) when eating it for lunch. This recipe also uses buckwheat, which is a pseudograin like quinoa. In the quantity called for in this recipe, buckwheat's glycemic load is considered low. However, if you're particularly carb sensitive, you can leave it out of the salad.

¼ cup pumpkin seeds

1 large bunch curly kale, chopped

¼ cup olive oil

¼ cup balsamic vinegar

¼ teaspoon salt

4 radishes, sliced into half-moons

2 medium carrots, shredded

½ cup chopped red onions

½ cup shredded Pecorino Romano cheese

½ cup buckwheat groats, cooked according to package instructions and cooled

1. Toast the pumpkin seeds: Preheat a small skillet over medium-high heat. Pour in the pumpkin seeds and toast, shaking the pan every 20 seconds or so to prevent burning. When the seeds are lightly browned, transfer them to a small bowl to cool slightly.

2. Put the kale, olive oil, balsamic vinegar, and salt in a large salad bowl. Massage the kale by gently squeezing the ingredients together with your hands for 1 to 2 minutes. Add the remaining ingredients and toss to combine. Taste and add more salt if needed.

3. Leftovers can be stored in the fridge for up to 5 days.

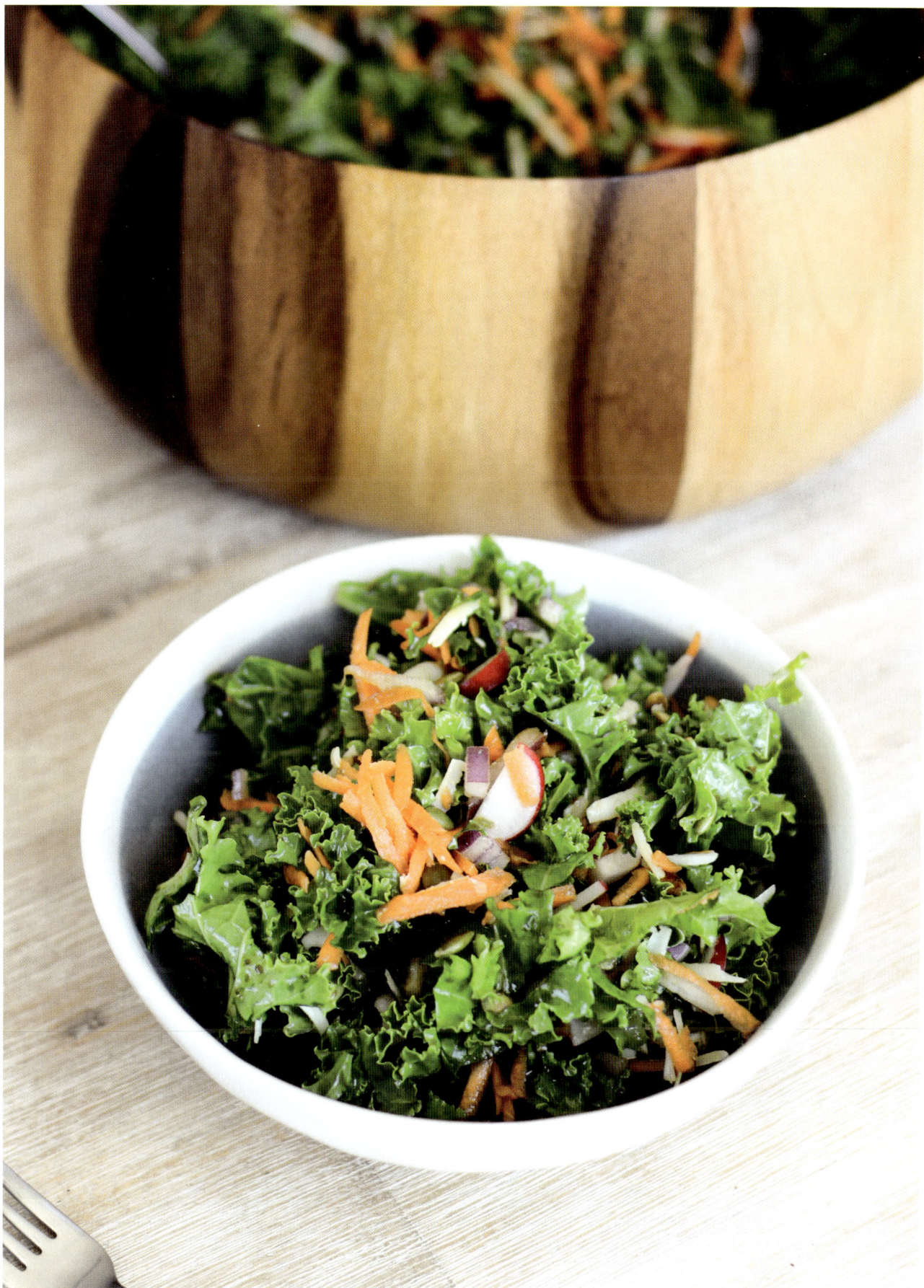

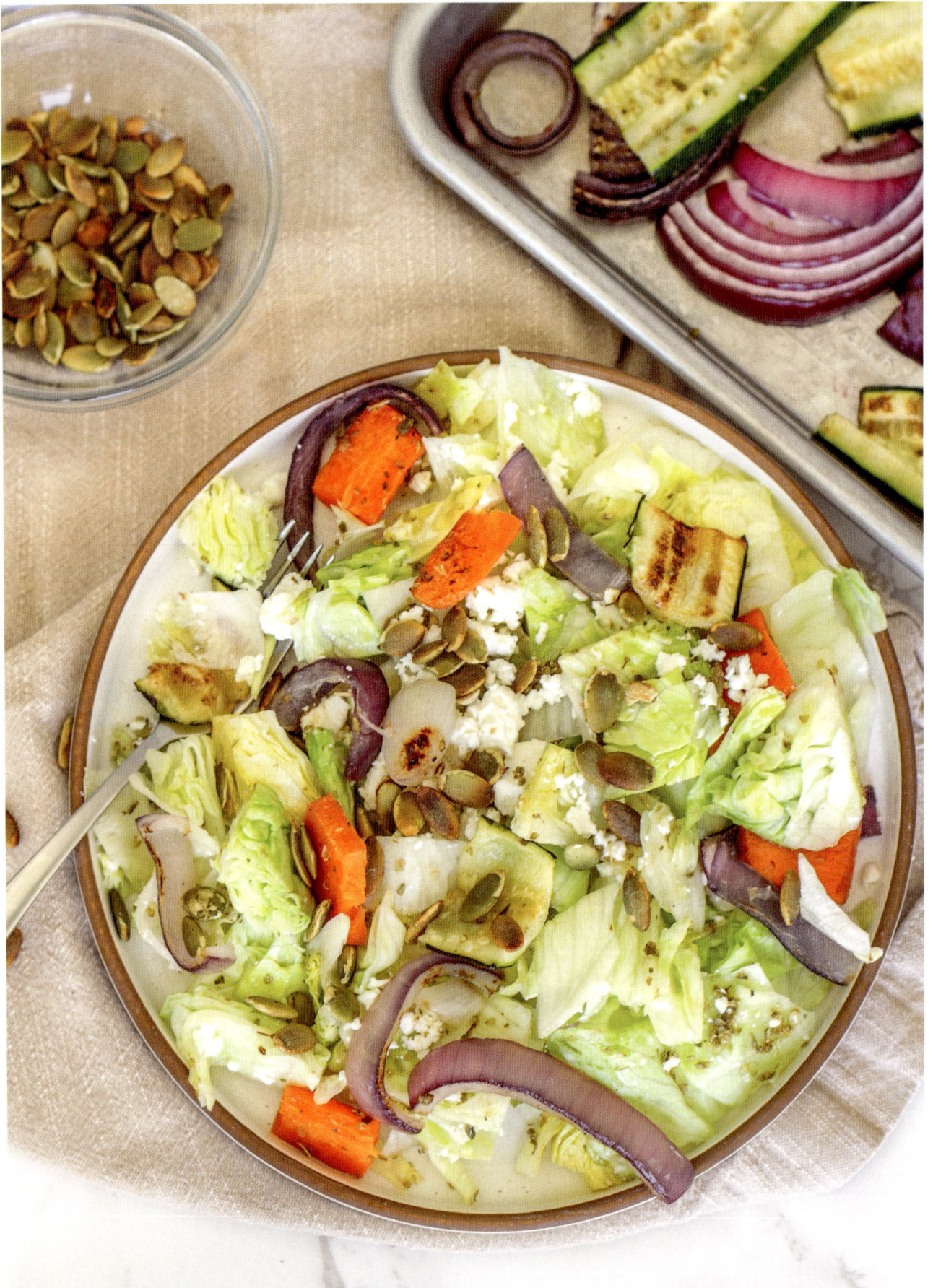

GRILLED VEGGIE SALAD

SERVES 4

PREP TIME 10 minutes

COOK TIME 20 minutes

Iceberg lettuce isn't going to win any nutrient density awards, but what it lacks in nutrition, it makes up for with crunch. This recipe also uses nutrient-dense ingredients like carrots, pumpkin seeds, and feta cheese to help round out the salad. The result is a crunchy, light, and flavorful side that pairs perfectly with meals that are heavier on spice, like my Cowboy Chili (page 126). It's also a great way to use up leftover iceberg lettuce from making lettuce buns, such as for my Swiss Smash Burgers (page 144). If you choose to serve this salad as a main meal, make sure to pair it with 4 to 5 ounces of complete protein per person.

2 medium zucchini, cut into ¼- to ½-inch planks

2 medium carrots, cut into ¼- to ½-inch planks

1 medium red onion, cut into 1-inch rounds

3 tablespoons olive oil, divided

2 teaspoons dried oregano leaves, divided

Salt

1 head iceberg lettuce, chopped

2 tablespoons rice vinegar

¼ cup crumbled feta cheese

¼ cup pumpkin seeds, toasted (see page 108)

1. Preheat a grill to medium-high heat (425°F to 450°F).

2. Prepare the veggies: Lay the zucchini, carrots, and red onion on a sheet pan. Drizzle with 1 tablespoon of the olive oil and sprinkle with 1 teaspoon of the oregano and a heavy pinch of salt, then toss to coat.

3. Grill for 12 minutes, then flip over and cook for an additional 8 minutes, or until the veggies are tender and have grill marks. Remove from the grill and allow to cool for at least 5 minutes.

4. Assemble the salad: Using a knife or kitchen scissors, roughly chop the grilled veggies into bite-sized pieces. Put the lettuce in a large salad bowl, then add the grilled veggies, rice vinegar, remaining 2 tablespoons of olive oil, remaining teaspoon of oregano, feta, toasted pumpkin seeds, and another heavy pinch of salt. Toss to combine.

MEXICAN-STYLE SALMON SALAD

SERVES 4

PREP TIME 15 minutes

COOK TIME 15 minutes

My husband and I like to have this salad for dinner and save the extra two servings for lunches later in the week. If you plan on storing leftovers, toss only the portion you are going to eat with dressing; otherwise, the leftovers will be soggy and lose their refreshing crunch. Instead, store leftovers in individual glass containers with the dressing in its own glass jar. Once you're ready to eat, you can toss the salad with the dressing.

SALMON

1 tablespoon olive oil

1 teaspoon paprika

½ teaspoon garlic powder

½ teaspoon onion powder

½ teaspoon ground cumin

Salt

1 (1¼-pound) skin-on salmon fillet

SPICED PEPITAS

¼ cup pumpkin seeds

½ teaspoon paprika

¼ teaspoon garlic powder

⅛ teaspoon cayenne pepper

Salt

1 teaspoon olive oil

CILANTRO-LIME DRESSING

2 tomatillos, chopped

½ packed cup fresh cilantro

1 jalapeño pepper, diced (remove membranes and seeds if you prefer less heat)

2 cloves garlic, minced

1 cup plain whole milk Greek yogurt, store-bought or homemade (page 81)

Juice of 1 lime (about 2 tablespoons)

½ teaspoon onion powder

¼ teaspoon paprika

Salt

SALAD

1 large head romaine lettuce, thinly sliced

1 (15-ounce) can black beans, or 1¾ cups homemade black beans (page 85)

1 medium cucumber, diced

1 red bell pepper, diced

½ medium red onion, diced

1 avocado, cubed

1. Cook the salmon: Preheat the oven to 425°F and line two sheet pans with parchment paper. In a small bowl, stir together the olive oil, paprika, garlic powder, onion powder, cumin, and a heavy pinch of salt. Place the salmon on one of the prepared pans, skin side down. Brush the oil mixture over the fish. Bake for 11 to 15 minutes, until the internal temperature reaches 145°F. The thicker the fillet, the longer the cook time. Once done, remove from the oven and allow to cool for about 5 minutes before slicing into four equal portions.

2. Prepare the pepitas: Spread the pumpkin seeds on the second parchment-lined pan. Sprinkle the paprika, garlic, cayenne, and a heavy pinch of salt over the seeds. Drizzle the olive oil on top. Toss to combine and put in the oven with the salmon. Bake for 4 minutes, or until the seeds are lightly browned. Remove from the oven and pour into a bowl to stop the cooking.

3. Make the dressing: Put all of the ingredients in a blender and blend until smooth.

4. Assemble the salad: Put the lettuce, black beans, cucumber, bell pepper, red onion, and avocado in a large bowl. Top with the spiced pepitas and toss to combine. Split among four serving bowls. Allow each person to add dressing according to their preference. Toss the salads before topping with the salmon.

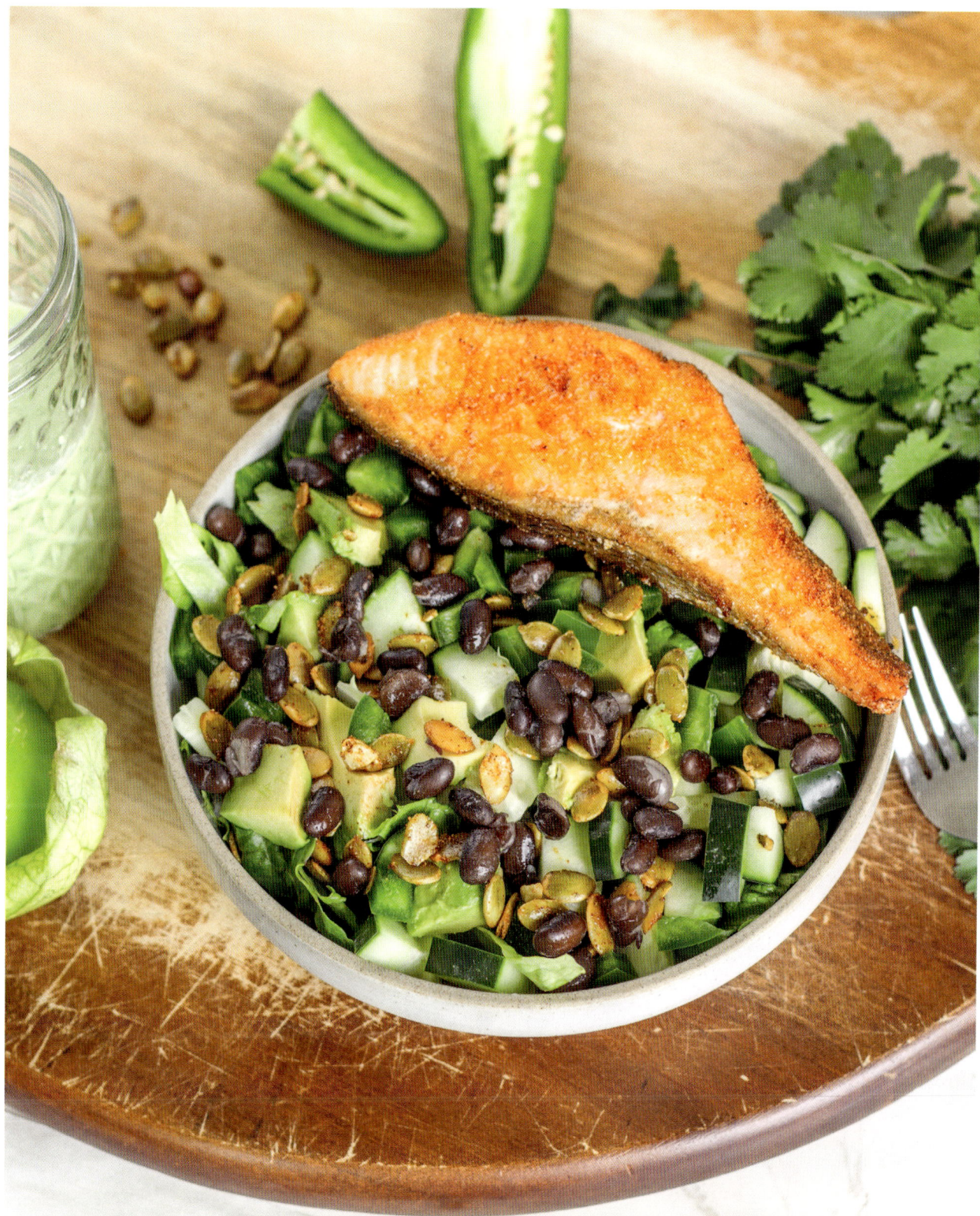

Note This recipe makes more dressing than you will need for four salads. Store the extra dressing in a glass container in the fridge for up to 5 days.

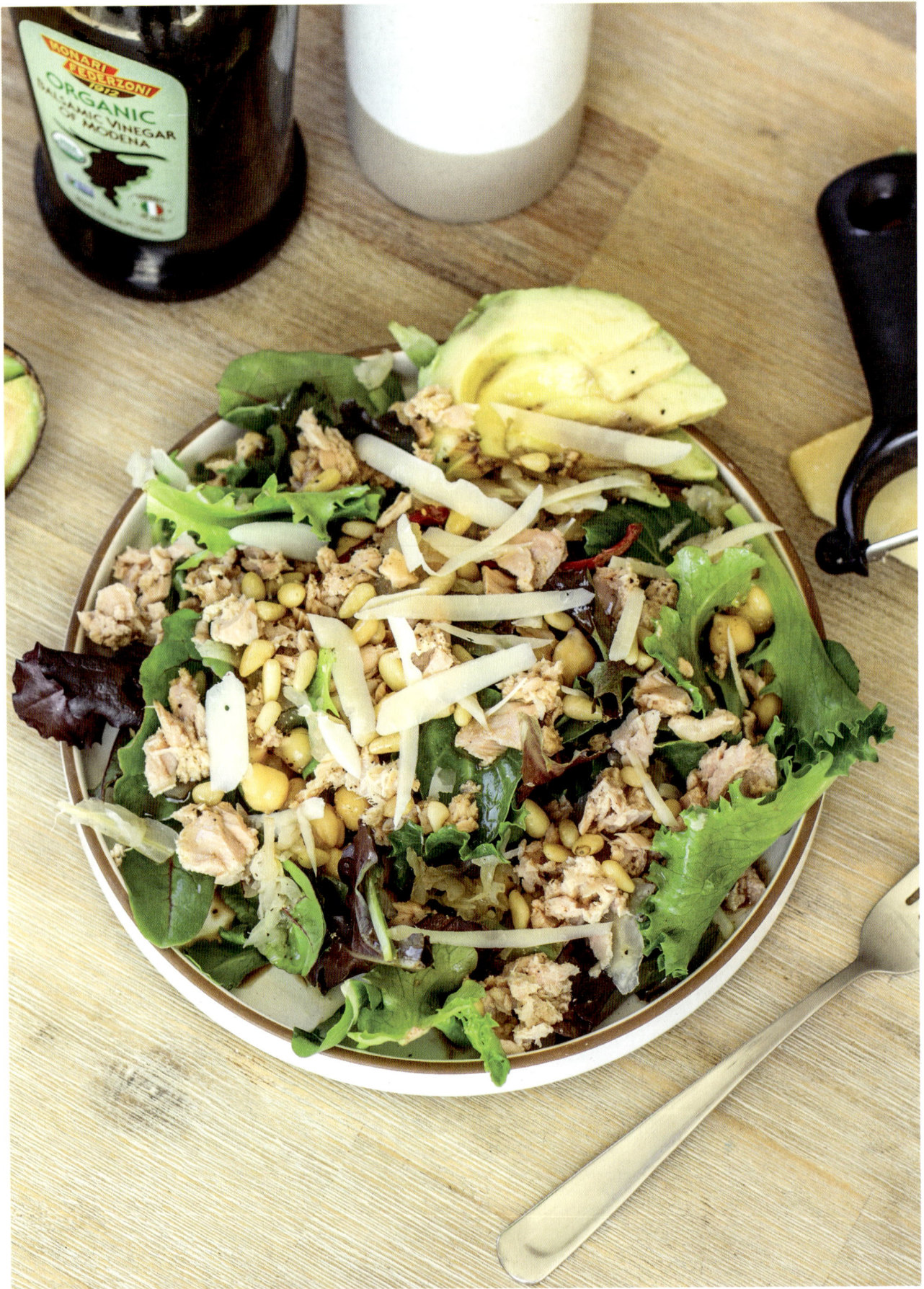

QUICKIE LOADED SALAD

SERVES 1

PREP TIME 5 minutes

Protein, fat, and fiber: This salad couldn't be a better example of this combination. It's loaded with 10 grams of fiber and nearly 45 grams of protein. You also get a variety of satiating fats from the olive oil, pine nuts, Parmesan, avocado, and tuna. Plus, your gut gets a healthy boost of natural probiotics from the sauerkraut. And the best part? This meal can be made in a matter of minutes. As a super busy mom and full-time business owner, I make sure to always have these ingredients as pantry or fridge staples so that I can quickly throw together a nutrient-dense and satisfying lunch to keep me full for hours.

2 cups mixed greens

¼ cup sauerkraut

¼ cup cooked chickpeas, canned or homemade (page 85)

¼ avocado, sliced

1 tablespoon shredded Parmesan cheese

1 tablespoon pine nuts

1 tablespoon olive oil

1 teaspoon balsamic vinegar

1 (4-ounce) can tuna, drained

Salt and pepper

1. Put the mixed greens, sauerkraut, chickpeas, avocado, Parmesan, and pine nuts in a salad bowl. Drizzle with the olive oil and balsamic and toss to combine.

2. Top the salad with the canned tuna, breaking it up with a fork and tossing it into the salad. Sprinkle with a pinch of salt and pepper.

CHICKPEA, LENTIL, AND CUCUMBER SALAD

SERVES 4

PREP TIME 10 minutes (not including time to soak and cook chickpeas and lentils if making from scratch)

This salad reminds me of my time studying abroad in Italy and our various visits to seaside towns. It's hearty yet light and pairs perfectly with grilled salmon or any other type of seafood. On its own, this salad doesn't have much protein. Technically, the chickpeas, lentils, and feta provide about 12 grams, but this is quite shy of the 30 grams or more that most people need per meal. If you plan on having it for lunch, try pairing it with 3 to 4 ounces of grilled fish or halloumi (a grillable cheese that's high in protein). If you're plant based, you can add 4 ounces of tempeh instead.

SALAD

1 cucumber

1 cup cooked chickpeas, canned or homemade (page 85)

1 cup cooked green or brown lentils, canned or homemade (see note)

1 bell pepper (any color), diced

¼ cup diced red onions

¼ cup chopped fresh mint

¼ cup crumbled feta cheese

8 cups mixed greens

CITRUS DRESSING

3 tablespoons olive oil

Juice of 1 lemon (2 to 3 tablespoons)

Juice of ½ navel orange (about 2 tablespoons)

1 tablespoon Dijon mustard

Heavy pinch of salt

1. Cut the cucumber in half lengthwise and use a spoon to scrape out the seeds. Dice the scooped cucumber and place in a large salad bowl.

2. Add all of the remaining salad ingredients to the bowl. If you plan on making this meal for lunches for the week, leave out the mixed greens and only add when you're ready to eat it.

3. Put all of the dressing ingredients in a small bowl or measuring cup and whisk to combine. Pour the dressing over the salad and give it a toss before serving.

Note You can buy canned precooked lentils, but it's easy to make them from scratch. Just combine 1 cup of dry lentils in a saucepan with at least 3 cups of water or broth. This will make 2½ to 3 cups of cooked lentils—more than you'll need for this recipe. Bring to a boil and then reduce to a simmer. Depending on the type of lentils you use (French, green, etc.), they will take between 15 and 25 minutes to cook. You want them to be cooked through but not mushy. Drain off any excess liquid before using.

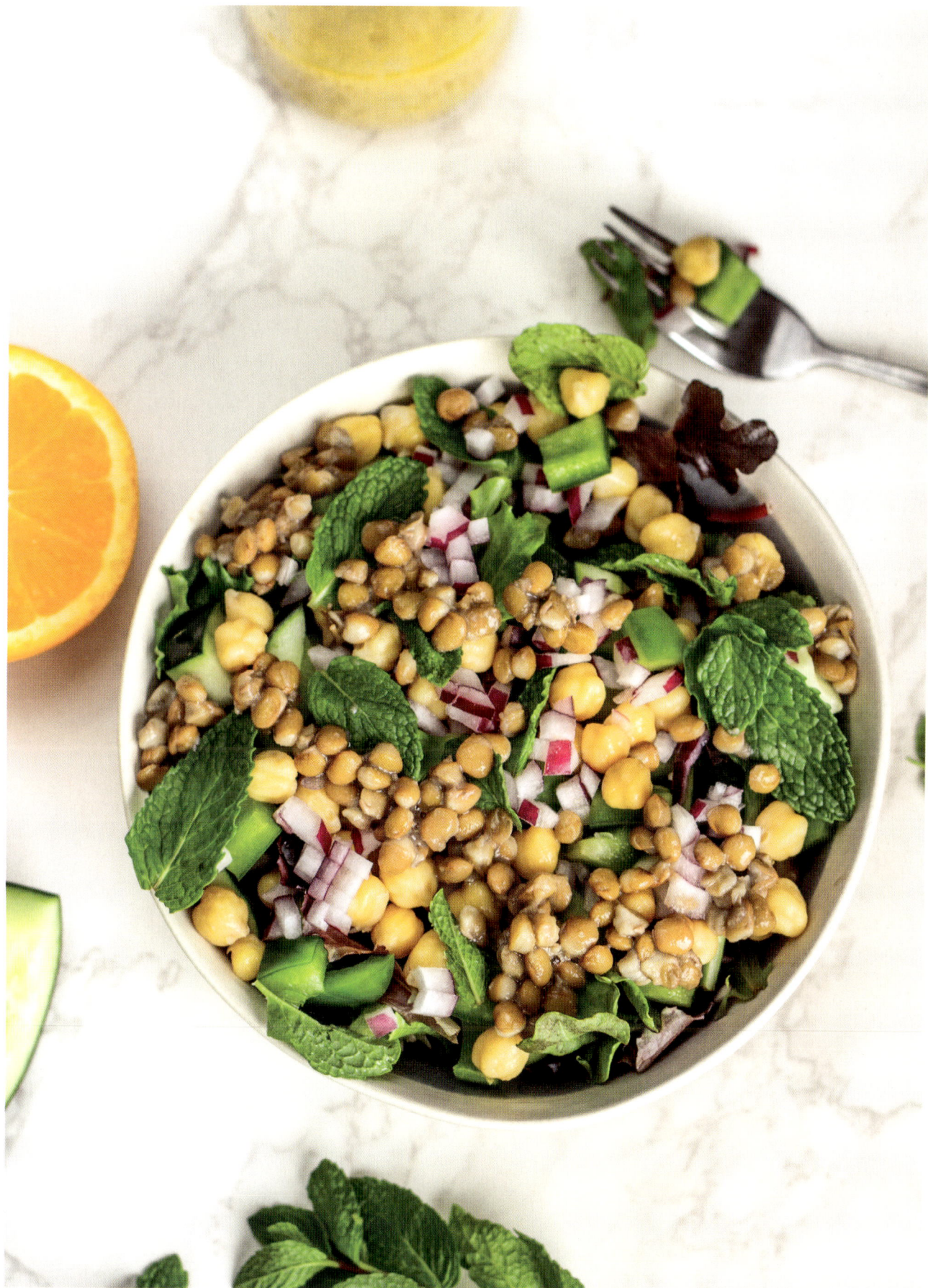

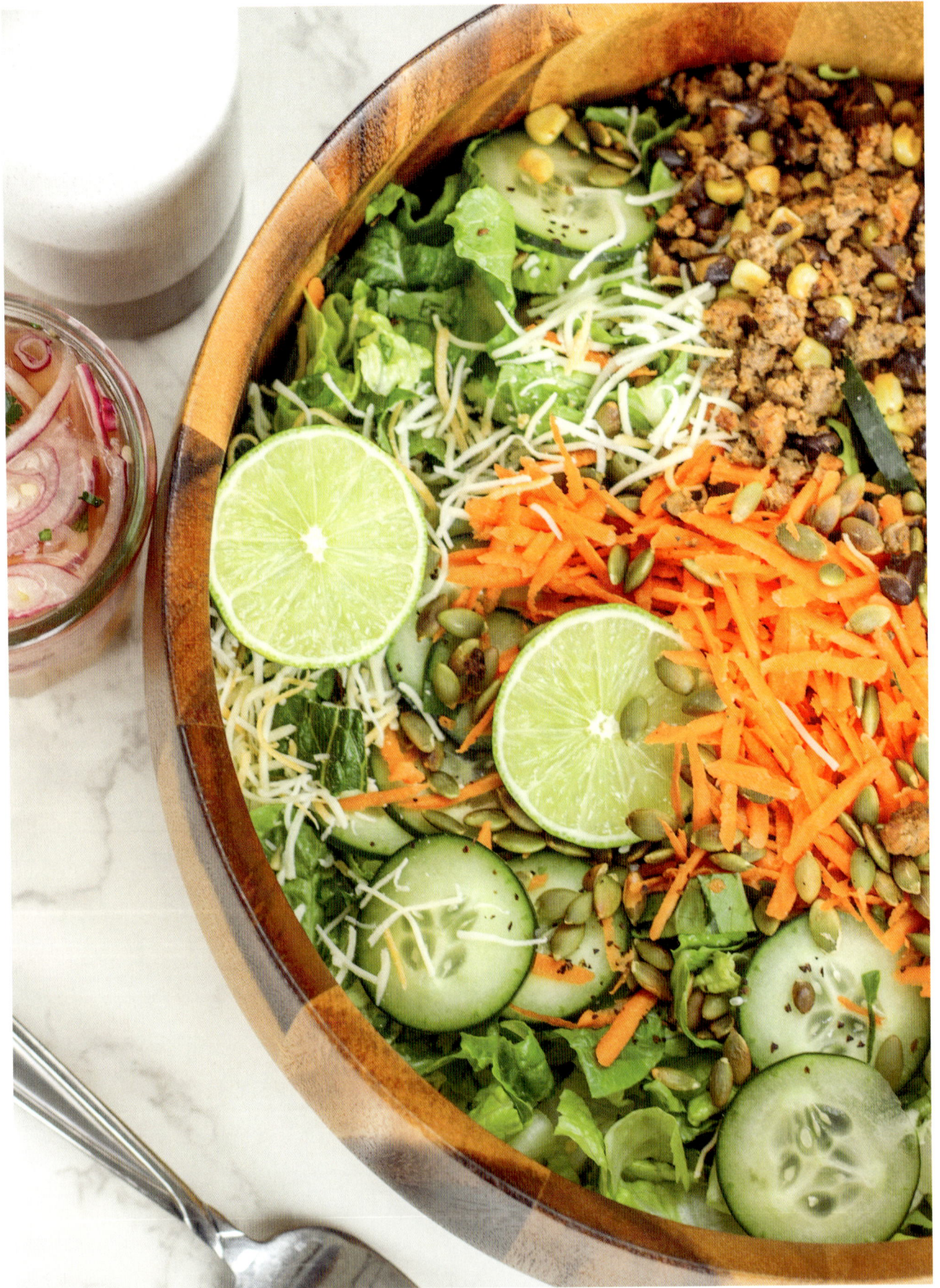

SPICY SAUSAGE SALAD

SERVES 2

PREP TIME 10 minutes

COOK TIME 12 minutes

This is a *very* satisfying and flavorful salad. Because chorizo has so much flavor on its own, you don't need to add a lot of dressing to this meal. The simple combo of olive oil and lime juice is the perfect refreshing hit to lighten up the chorizo and cheese. This recipe makes a very large salad, so if you choose to split it up between more than two people, just make sure to add more protein to compensate. For example, if you want to serve this to four people, increase the ground beef to 1 pound and the chorizo to two links.

1 raw chorizo sausage link, casing removed

8 ounces ground beef

½ cup cooked black beans, canned or homemade (page 85)

½ cup frozen corn (preferably fire roasted)

6 cups chopped romaine lettuce

1 cup chopped fresh cilantro

¼ cup chopped green onions

½ medium cucumber, thinly sliced

1 medium carrot, shredded

¼ cup Mexican-style shredded cheese

2 tablespoons pumpkin seeds, toasted (see page 108)

1 tablespoon olive oil

Juice of 1 lime (about 2 tablespoons)

Salt

1. Cook the chorizo in a medium-sized skillet over medium heat, using a rubber spatula to break it up as it cooks. Once the chorizo has started to brown and release its oil, add the ground beef. Sauté for another 8 minutes, or until both meats are fully cooked.

2. Add the beans and corn and sauté for 1 to 2 minutes, until warmed through. Remove the pan from the heat and set aside while you prepare the salad.

3. In a large salad bowl, toss the lettuce, cilantro, green onions, cucumber, carrot, cheese, toasted pumpkin seeds, olive oil, and lime juice. Add the cooked sausage mixture and toss again to combine. Season with salt to taste before serving.

MEDITERRANEAN CHICKPEA SALAD

SERVES 3

PREP TIME 5 minutes

Chickpeas are one of my favorite legumes because even though they aren't a complete protein, they are a decent source of amino acids. They're also hearty and make a great addition to any salad. The "dressing" here is extremely simple, but you won't miss out on flavor due to the fresh herbs, red onions, and olives. I often serve this salad as a side dish to grilled chicken or steak for bright, summery vibes.

1 cup cooked chickpeas, canned or homemade (page 85)

1 medium cucumber, diced

½ cup pitted Kalamata olives

½ cup finely chopped fresh mint

½ cup finely chopped fresh parsley

¼ cup finely chopped red onions

2 tablespoons crumbled feta cheese

2 tablespoons pine nuts

2 tablespoons olive oil

2 tablespoons red wine vinegar

Heavy pinch of salt

Put all of the ingredients in a large salad bowl and toss to combine. Feel free to add a little more salt, vinegar, or olive oil according to your taste preference.

Note If you want to make this salad a complete meal, add 4 ounces of your favorite cooked protein (like grilled chicken or steak) per serving.

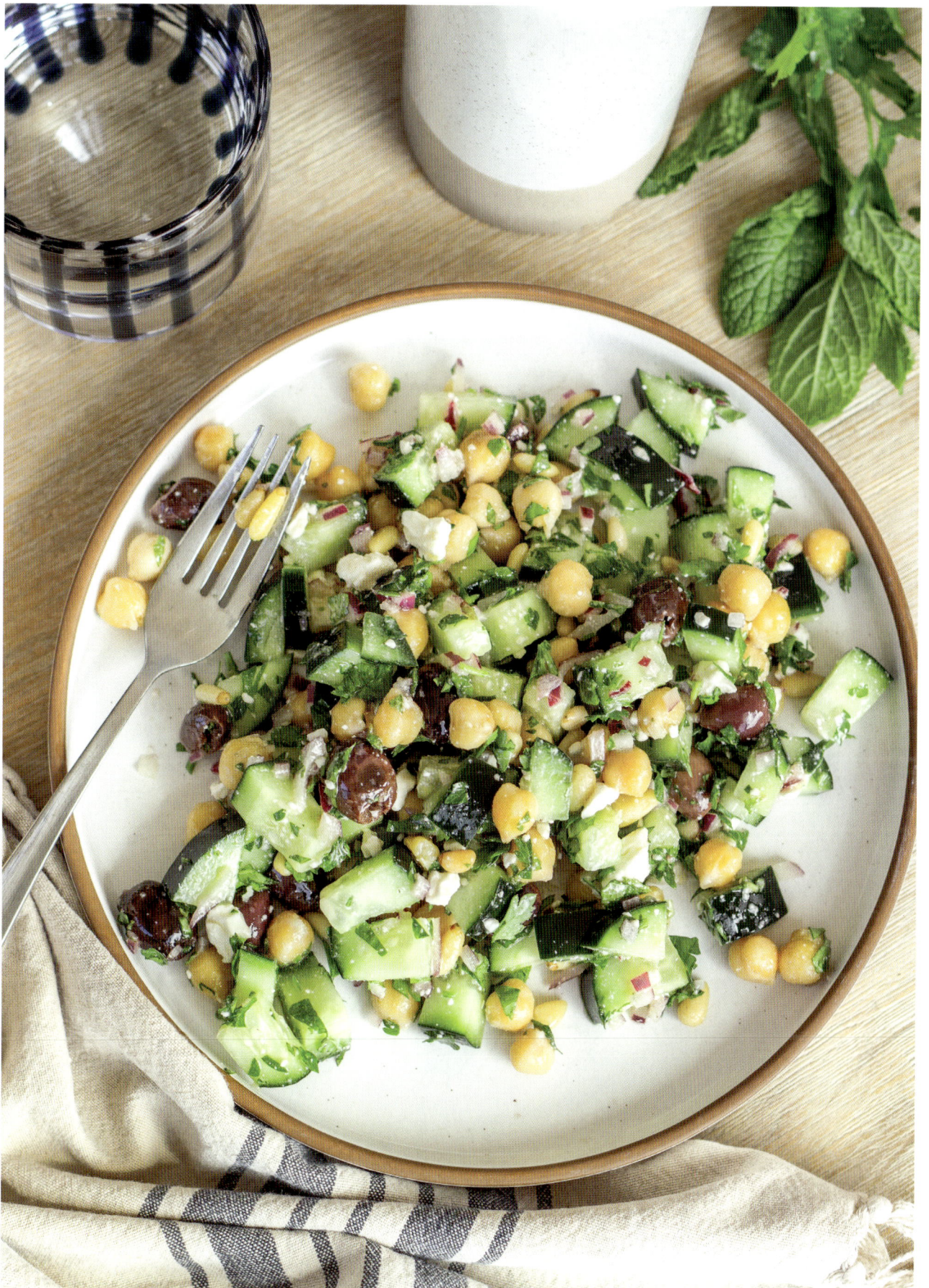

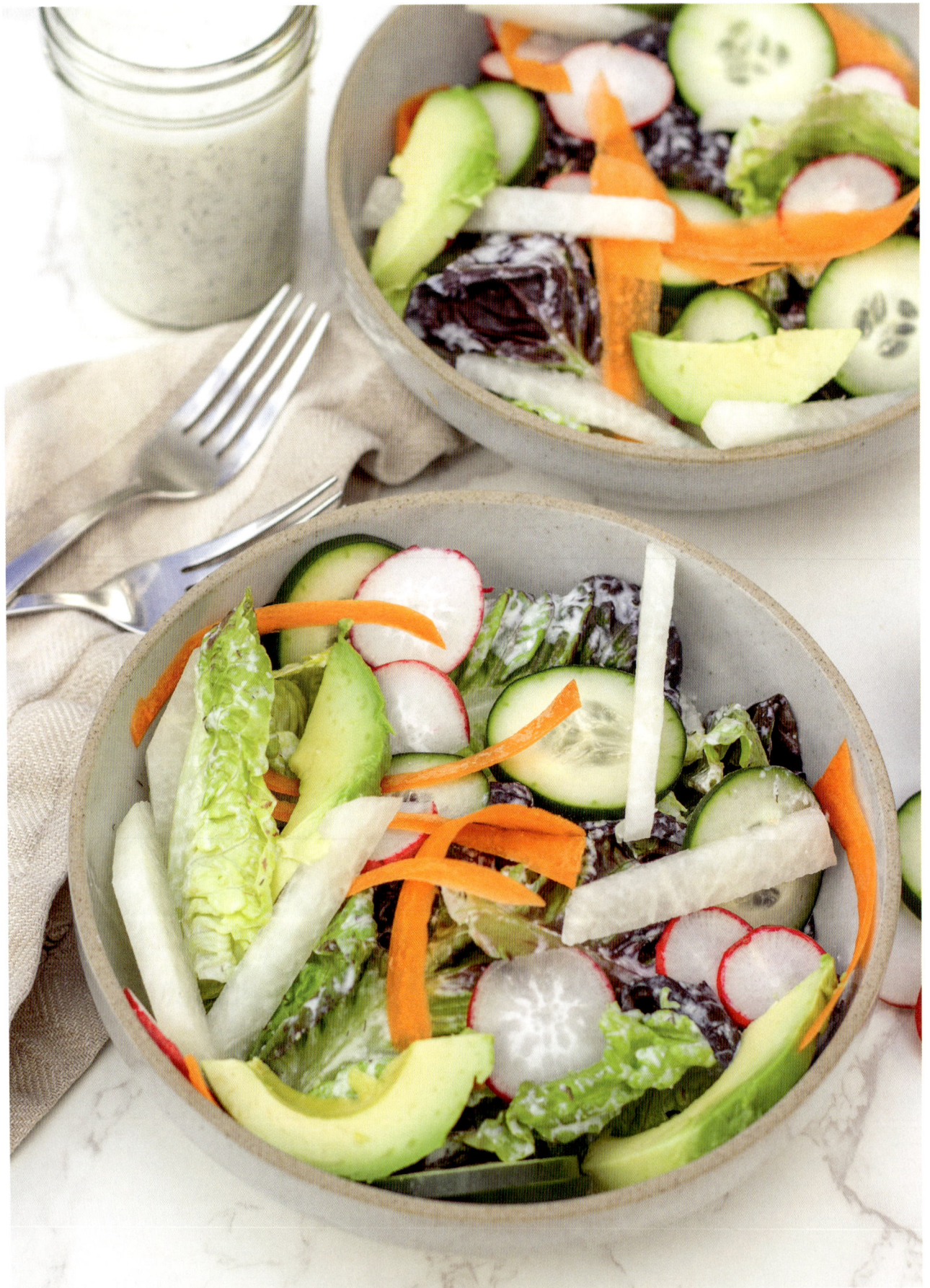

GARDEN HOUSE SALAD
WITH "BUTTERMILK" RANCH

SERVES 4

PREP TIME 10 minutes

Here in Santa Barbara, there's a great local burger spot that my husband and I like to go to on the weekends. Not only do they have an incredible smash burger, but they also have a simple yet tasty garden salad made with crunchy jicama and homemade buttermilk ranch dressing. I'm not usually one to order a simple house salad, but I *always* get this salad when I'm there. It's light, crunchy, and perfectly balanced, making it a refreshing side dish to any meal. I love it so much that I decided to re-create the recipe with higher protein and a healthier version of the classic buttermilk ranch dressing.

SALAD

8 cups little gem lettuce, leaves separated

4 radishes, thinly sliced

1 medium carrot, shaved

1 medium cucumber, cut into thin rounds

1 cup chopped jicama

1 avocado, sliced

"BUTTERMILK" RANCH DRESSING

¼ cup plain whole milk Greek yogurt, store-bought or homemade (page 81)

3 tablespoons whole milk

Juice of ½ lemon (1 to 1½ tablespoons)

1 teaspoon dried dill weed

½ teaspoon garlic powder

½ teaspoon onion powder

¼ teaspoon salt

1. Put all of the salad ingredients in a large salad bowl.

2. In a small bowl or jar, whisk together all of the dressing ingredients until smooth.

3. Pour half of the dressing over the salad and toss to combine. Leave the remaining dressing on the table in case anyone wants to add a little more.

SOUPS, STEWS, and CHILIS

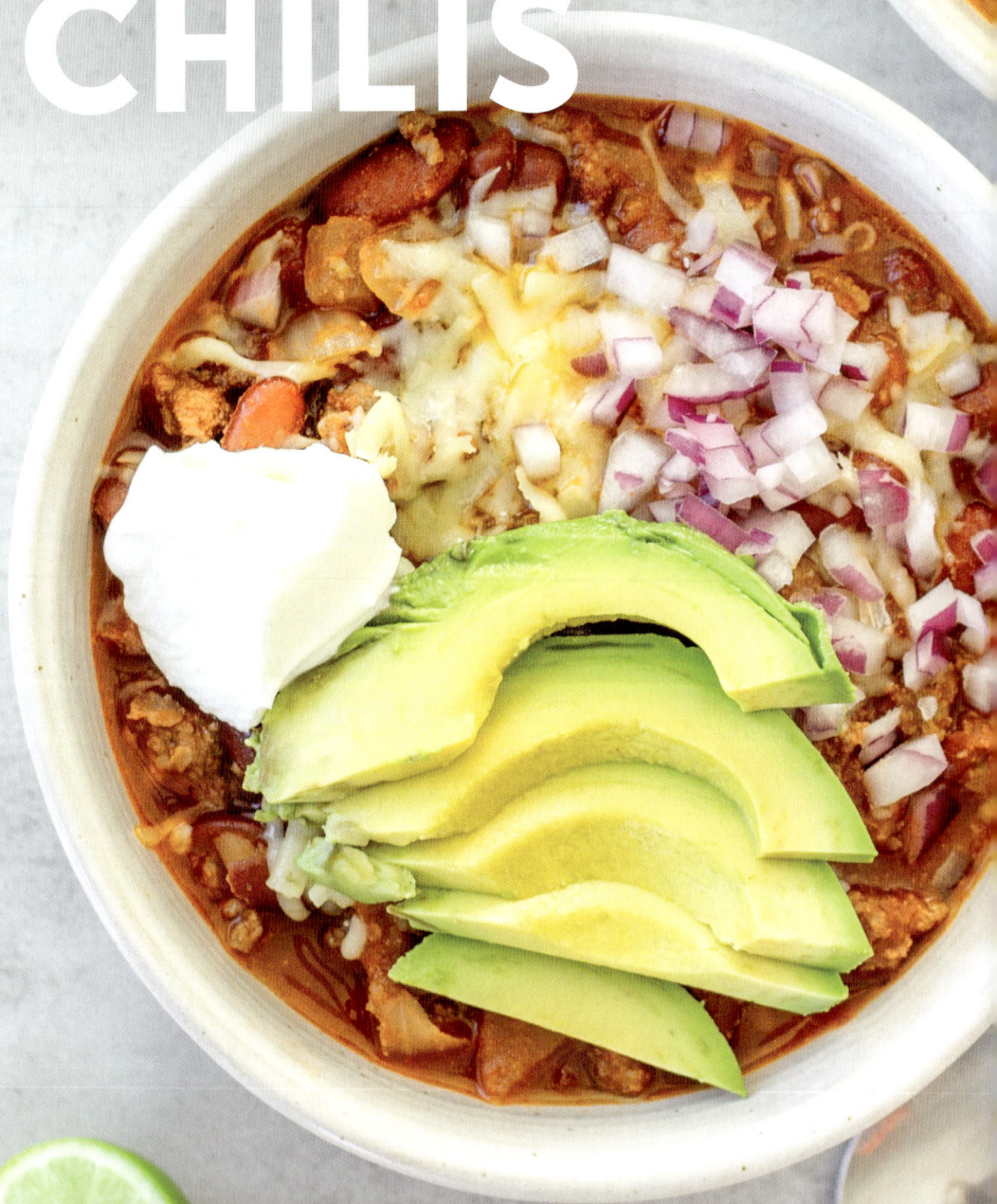

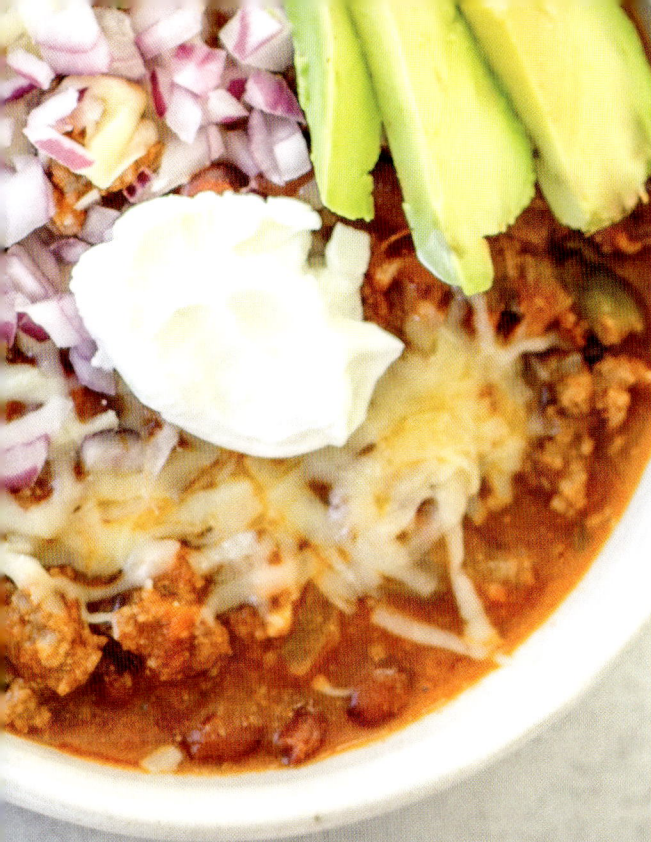

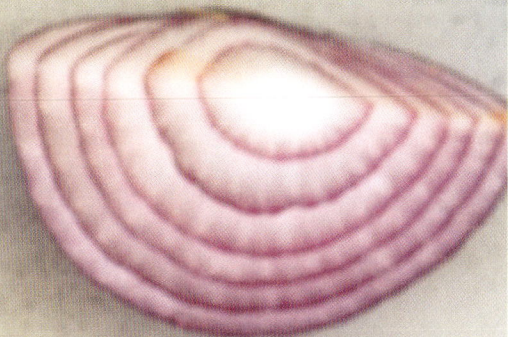

COWBOY CHILI

SERVES 10

PREP TIME 5 minutes

COOK TIME 3 hours
45 minutes

My Cowboy Chili is a hearty, satiating meal that emphasizes big chunks of slow-cooked meat that fall apart when you bite into them. This recipe calls for a mix of herbs and spices that might look odd if you haven't used them in this combination before (specifically the cocoa powder), but they infuse so much rich flavor into the meal. Don't be deceived by the long cook time! Most of it is hands-off, allowing you to do other things while your chili simmers. This recipe also serves a lot of people or leaves you with a good amount of leftovers that can be frozen for more days of delicious dinners. Try serving this with my Grilled Veggie Salad (page 111) for a light and crunchy pairing.

CHILI

1 tablespoon olive oil

Salt and pepper

3 pounds stewing beef or chuck roast, cut into 2-inch chunks

1 medium yellow onion, diced

10 cloves garlic, minced

2 jalapeño peppers, diced (remove membranes and seeds if you prefer less heat)

2 poblano peppers, diced

3 tablespoons ancho chili powder

2 tablespoons paprika

1 tablespoon ground cumin

1 tablespoon unsweetened cocoa powder

2 teaspoons ground coriander

2 teaspoons dried oregano leaves

1 (14-ounce) can fire-roasted tomatoes

4 cups beef or chicken bone broth

2½ (15-ounce) cans black beans, or 4 cups homemade black beans (page 85)

TOPPINGS PER SERVING

2 tablespoons plain whole milk Greek yogurt, store-bought or homemade (page 81)

¼ cup diced white or yellow onions

½ lime

1. In a 5- to 5½-quart Dutch oven or soup pot, heat the olive oil over medium-high heat. Sprinkle a heavy pinch of salt and pepper over the chunks of beef. Place the beef in the hot pot, leaving a little bit of space between pieces. You will likely need to cook it in three batches. Sear the beef until browned on all sides, flipping each piece after 4 to 5 minutes. Once all sides are browned, remove the beef from the pot and set aside on a plate. Repeat until all of the beef has been browned.

2. In the same hot pot, combine the onion, garlic, jalapeños, and poblanos. Sauté for 2 to 3 minutes, until the veggies are softened. Add the chili powder, paprika, cumin, cocoa powder, coriander, oregano, and a heavy pinch of salt. Sauté for 2 more minutes.

3. Return the beef to the pot and pour in the tomatoes (with juices) and broth. Bring the mixture to a boil, then reduce to a simmer. Cover and cook for 2 hours, stirring every 20 minutes or so.

4. After 2 hours, add the beans. Simmer, covered, for 1 more hour.

5. Serve the chili with the yogurt, raw onions, and lime half. Store leftovers in the fridge for up to 4 days or in the freezer for up to 6 months.

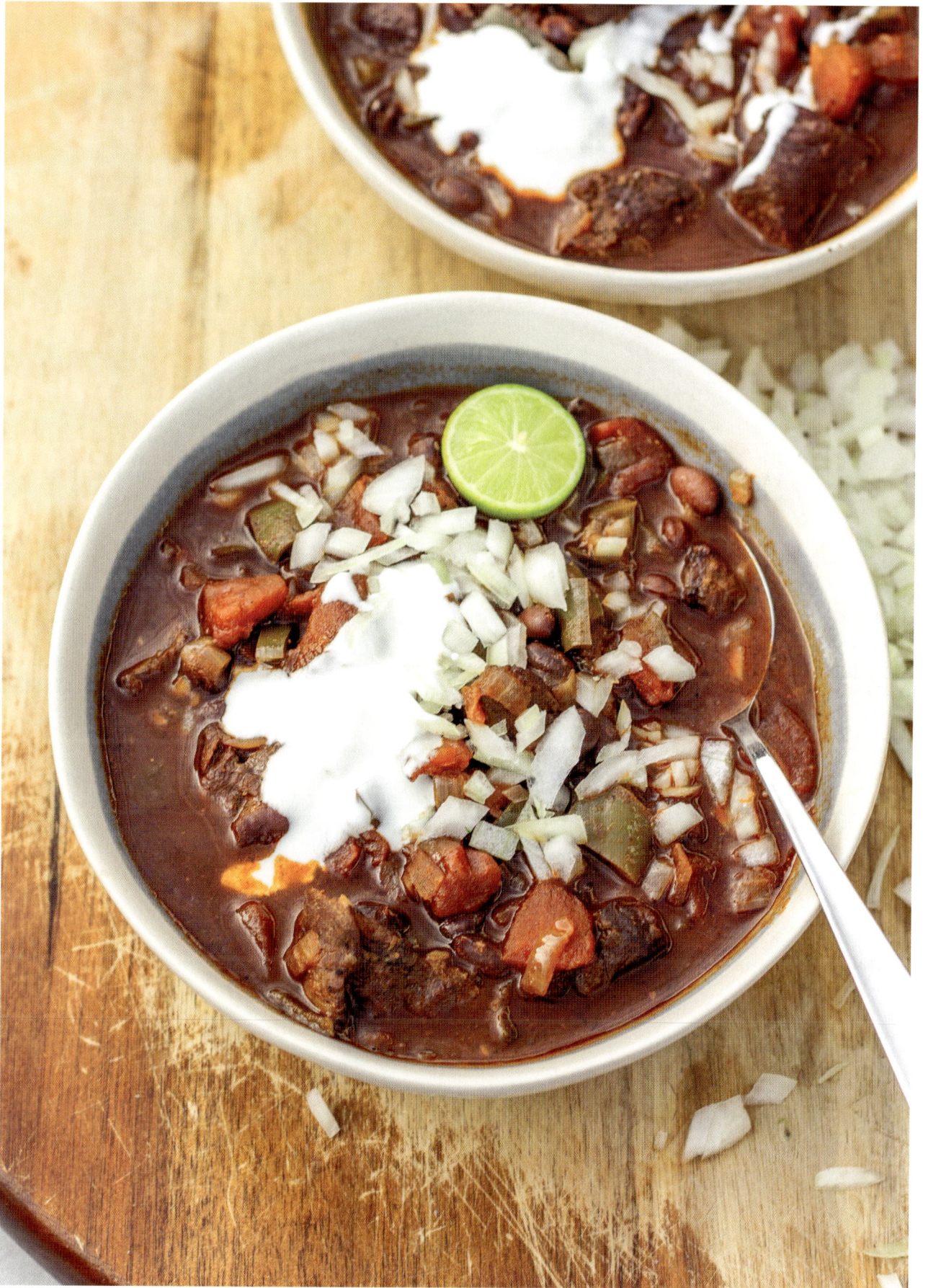

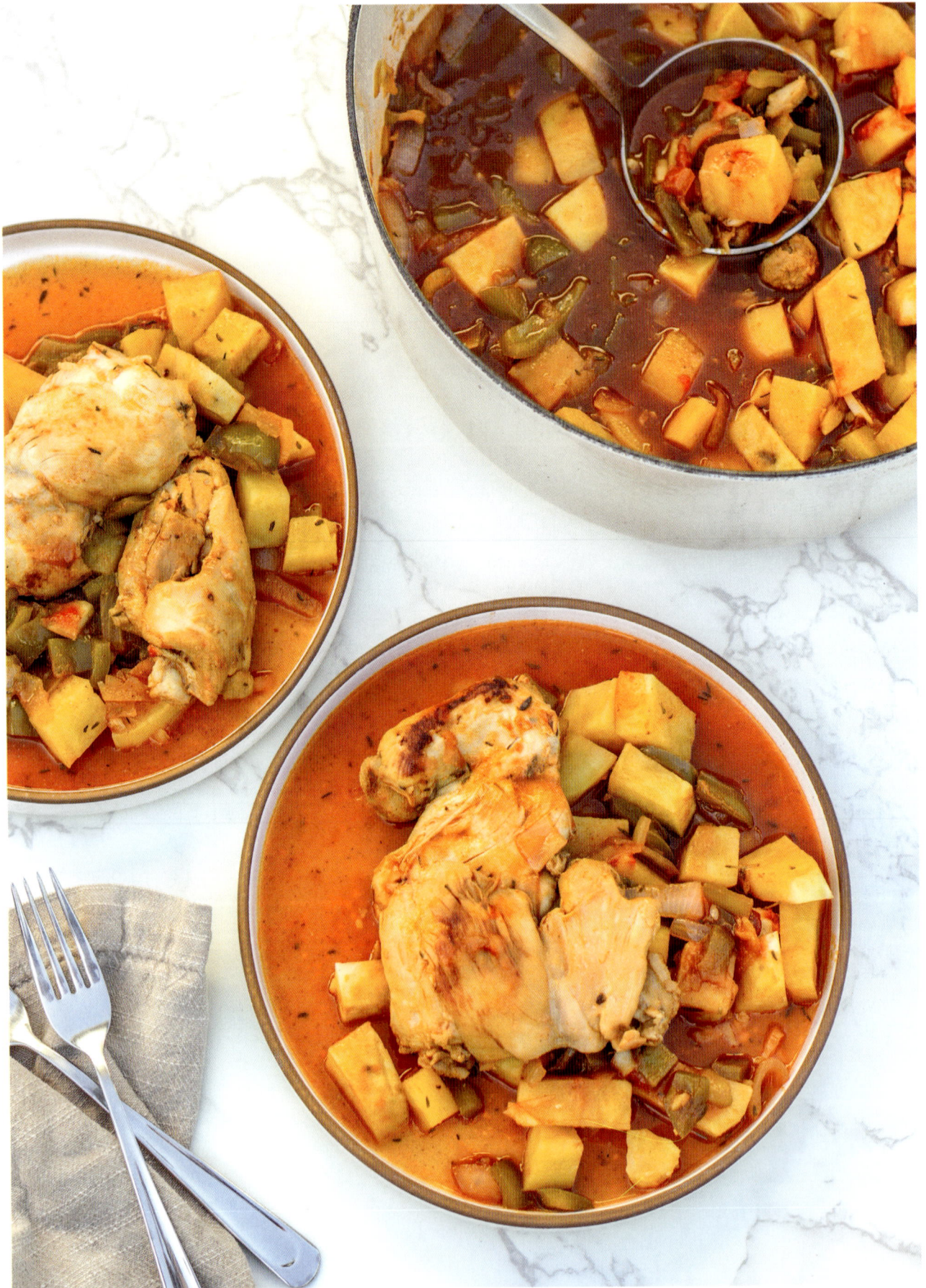

HAITIAN-STYLE CHICKEN STEW

SERVES 4

PREP TIME 5 minutes, plus at least 30 minutes to marinate chicken

COOK TIME 50 minutes

This stew is ridiculously flavorful with citrus and slightly spicy notes. On its own, this meal has 6 grams of fiber per serving, but I like to pair it with an additional crunchy veggie side, like my Garden House Salad (page 123). If you're looking to sneak some collagen into the meal, you can use bone broth instead of water in step 6.

Juice of 2 lemons (4 to 6 tablespoons)

Juice of 1 navel orange (about ¼ cup)

1 habanero pepper, thinly sliced (see note)

1 teaspoon garlic powder

1 teaspoon onion powder

1 teaspoon dried thyme leaves

1 teaspoon salt

1½ pounds boneless, skinless chicken thighs

1 tablespoon olive oil

½ medium yellow onion, diced

5 cloves garlic, minced

4 bell peppers (any color), diced

¼ cup tomato paste

2 medium sweet potatoes, peeled and cubed

1 cup water

1. Pour the orange and lemon juices into a mixing bowl. Add the habanero, garlic powder, onion powder, thyme, and salt. Stir to combine.

2. Place the chicken thighs in the marinade and press them down to ensure the marinade mostly covers each thigh. Cover the bowl and place in the fridge to marinate for at least 30 minutes or up to 24 hours. The longer it marinates, the more flavorful the chicken will be.

3. When ready to cook, remove the chicken from the marinade and pat dry. Do not discard the marinade; you will be using it in the stew.

4. Heat the olive oil in a Dutch oven or soup pot over medium-high heat. Add the chicken and cook for about 5 minutes on each side, until lightly browned. (It will not be fully cooked at this point.) Remove the chicken from the pot, place on a plate, and set aside.

5. Add the onion, garlic, and a heavy pinch of salt to the hot pot. Sauté for 3 minutes, or until the onion has softened. Add the bell peppers and sauté for 7 minutes, or until slightly softened. Sauté the tomato paste into the vegetable mixture until well incorporated.

6. Return the chicken to the pot and add the sweet potatoes, marinade, and water. Bring to a boil, then reduce to a simmer. Cover and cook for 30 minutes, or until the sweet potatoes are tender and the chicken is cooked through.

7. Ladle the stew into bowls and serve.

Note You can remove the habanero from the marinade before adding it to the stew in step 6 if you prefer a less spicy stew.

BEEF CHILI
WITH ALL THE TOPPINGS

SERVES 4

PREP TIME 5 minutes

COOK TIME 45 minutes

Chili is great, but chili with a *ton* of toppings is even better. At our house, we load up our chili with as many toppings as possible to add crunch and freshness to such a hearty meal. It helps that chili is universally a crowd-pleaser and easy to scale up or down if you have more mouths to feed. Plus, you get protein, fat, and fiber in one easy-to-prep dish. Each serving boasts 11 grams of fiber along with nearly 50 grams of protein. Needless to say, you're going to feel pretty satisfied after this meal.

CHILI

1 tablespoon olive oil

1 bell pepper (any color), diced

1 jalapeño pepper, diced (remove membranes and seeds if you prefer less heat)

1 medium yellow onion, diced

4 cloves garlic, minced

Salt

1½ pounds ground beef

1 tablespoon paprika

2 teaspoons garlic powder

2 teaspoons dried oregano leaves

1 teaspoon ground cumin

2 cups cooked kidney beans, canned or homemade (page 85)

1 (14-ounce) can crushed tomatoes

1 canned chipotle chili pepper in adobo sauce, diced

1 tablespoon adobo sauce (from the can)

1 cup water

TOPPINGS PER SERVING

2 tablespoons shredded cheddar cheese

2 tablespoons diced red or yellow onions

¼ avocado, sliced

1 tablespoon plain whole milk Greek yogurt, store-bought or homemade (page 81)

Juice of ½ lime (about 1 tablespoon)

1. Heat the olive oil in a Dutch oven or soup pot over medium heat. Add the bell pepper, jalapeño, onion, garlic, and a heavy pinch of salt. Sauté until the veggies are softened, about 5 minutes.

2. Add the ground beef, paprika, garlic powder, oregano, cumin, and another heavy pinch of salt. Break up the ground beef with a rubber spatula and cook until browned all the way through, 8 to 10 minutes.

3. Add the kidney beans, tomatoes, chipotle pepper, adobo sauce, and water. Give the mixture a stir and reduce the heat to a simmer. Cook for 30 minutes, stirring occasionally to prevent sticking.

4. Serve the chili in bowls and top with the cheese, raw onions, avocado slices, yogurt, and lime juice.

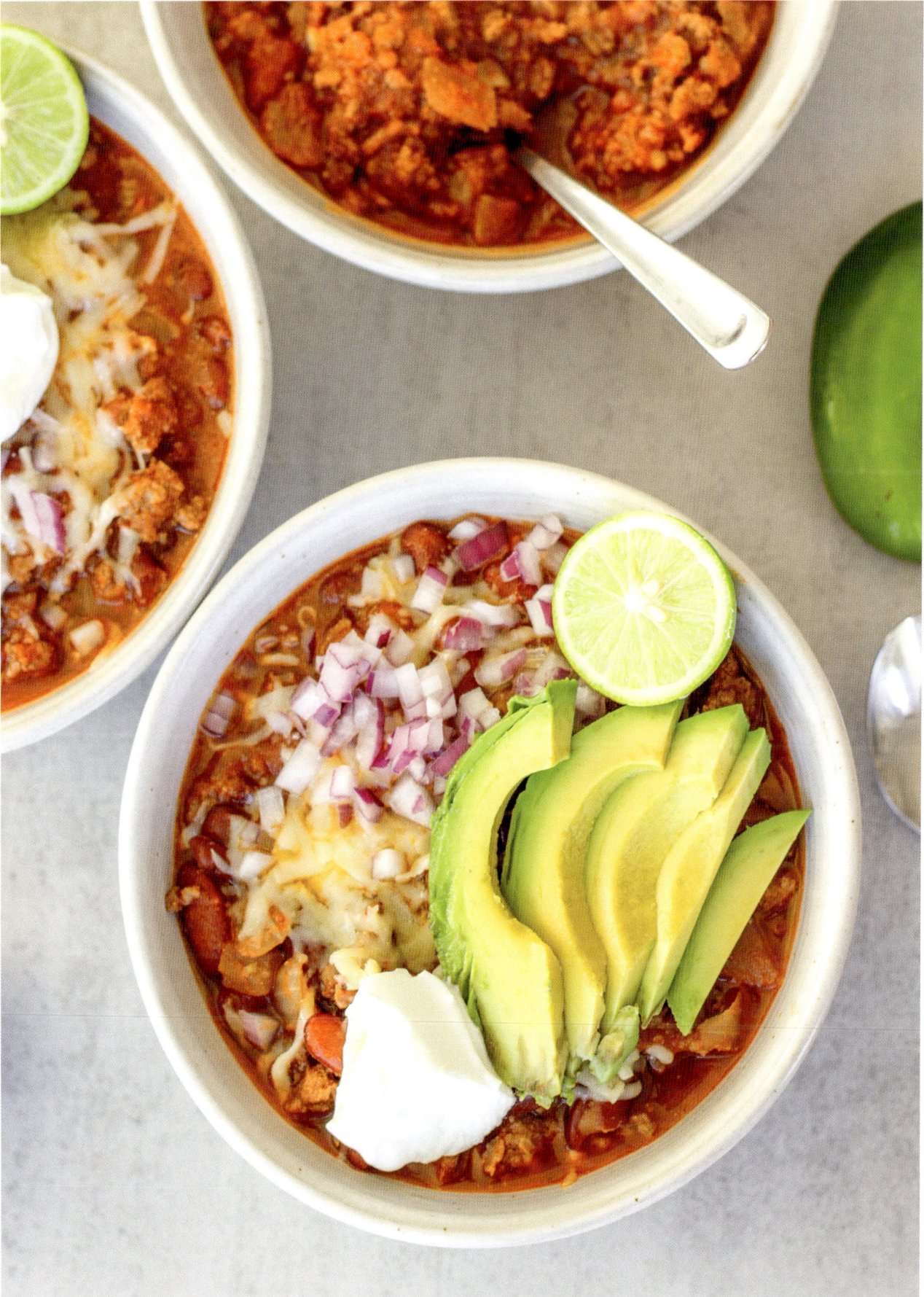

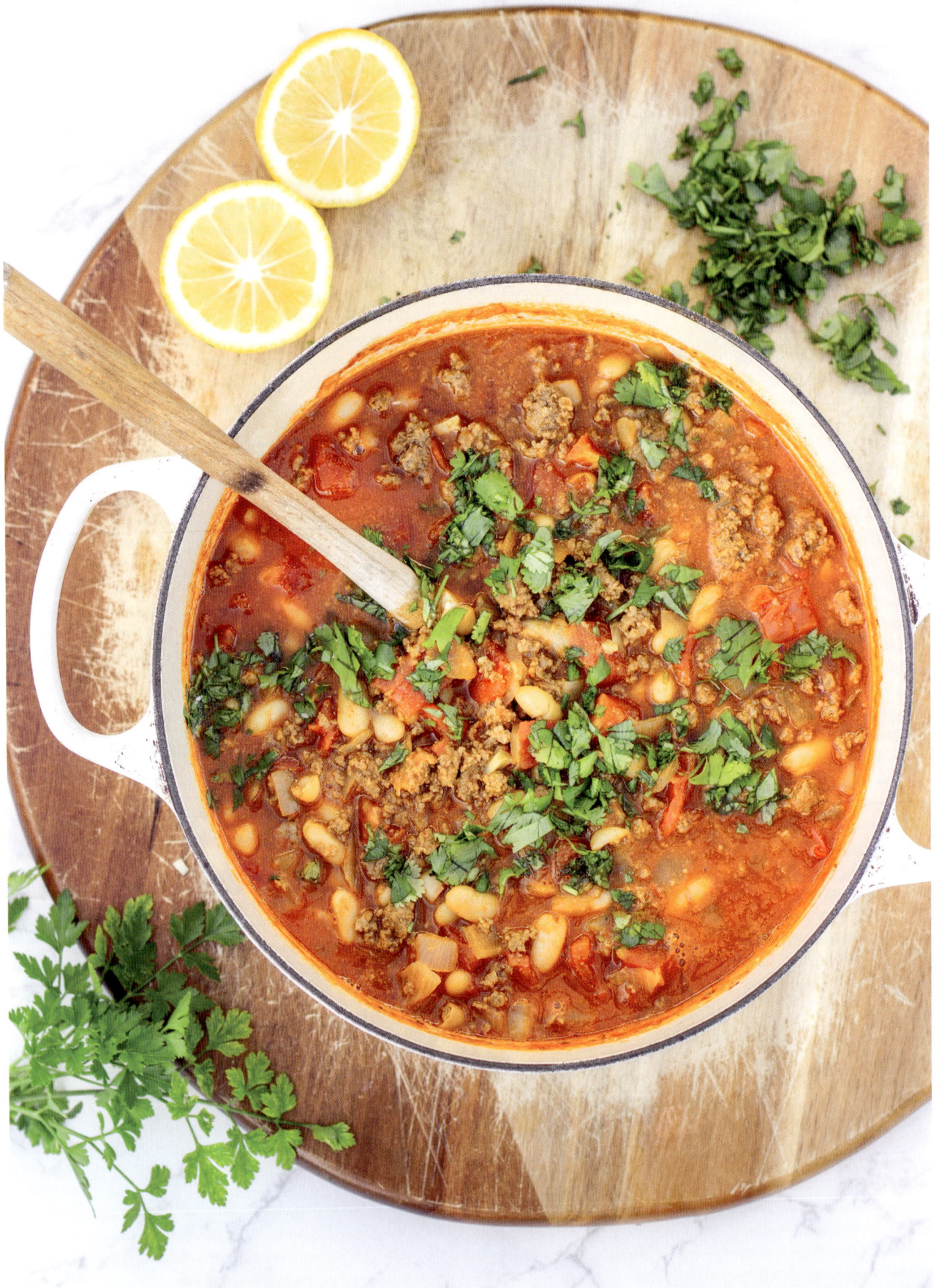

MOROCCAN-INSPIRED WHITE BEAN CHILI

SERVES 4

PREP TIME 10 minutes

COOK TIME 30 minutes

This is definitely not your average chili. Using ingredients like ginger, lemon, and cannellini beans makes this Moroccan-inspired version much lighter and brighter than traditional chili while still being ultra satisfying. I like having this meal during the spring months when the weather is starting to get a bit warmer, but there's still a chill in the air. It pairs really well with my Garden House Salad (page 123).

2 tablespoons olive oil

1 medium yellow onion, diced

4 cloves garlic, minced

1 pound ground beef

Salt

2 tablespoons tomato paste

2 teaspoons ground cumin

1 teaspoon paprika

¼ teaspoon ground ginger

¼ teaspoon turmeric powder

⅛ teaspoon cayenne pepper

1 (14-ounce) can diced tomatoes

½ cup chicken bone broth

1 (15-ounce) can cannellini beans, or 1¾ cups homemade cannellini beans (page 85)

¼ cup chopped fresh cilantro

¼ cup chopped fresh parsley

Juice of 1 lemon (2 to 3 tablespoons)

1. Heat the olive oil in a Dutch oven or soup pot over medium heat. Add the onion and garlic and sauté for 3 minutes, or until the onion is softened. Add the ground beef and a heavy pinch of salt and cook, breaking up the meat with a rubber spatula, until the meat is browned, about 8 minutes.

2. Add the tomato paste, cumin, paprika, ginger, turmeric, cayenne, and a heavy pinch of salt. Sauté until the meat is coated in the spices and tomato paste.

3. Add the diced tomatoes (with juices), broth, beans, and another pinch of salt. Stir to combine and reduce the heat to a simmer. Cook for 15 minutes, stirring occasionally to prevent the meat and beans from sticking to the pot.

4. Remove from the heat and stir in the cilantro, parsley, and lemon juice before serving.

HEARTY LENTIL AND SAUSAGE SOUP

SERVES 6

PREP TIME 5 minutes

COOK TIME 1 hour

In college, I ate veggie lentil soup all the time because it was so dang cheap to make. Lentils provide some protein and a lot of fiber, but in this grown-up version, I've packed my classic college lentil soup with a lot more nutrients (and flavor!). By adding sausage, bone broth, and Parmesan cheese, I was able to get the protein up to 40 grams per serving! Plus, the taste is rich and decadent—something my college self would have been very jealous of.

SOUP

1 tablespoon olive oil

1 pound mild Italian sausage, casings removed

1 medium yellow onion, diced

2 celery stalks, diced

2 medium carrots, diced

1 medium zucchini, diced

4 cloves garlic, minced

Salt

1 (14-ounce) can diced tomatoes

1½ cups brown lentils

1 bay leaf

1 teaspoon dried basil leaves

½ teaspoon red pepper flakes

6 cups chicken bone broth

TOPPINGS

¾ cup shredded Parmesan cheese

¾ cup minced fresh parsley

1. Heat the olive oil in a Dutch oven or soup pot over medium heat. Add the sausage and cook, breaking it up with a rubber spatula, until browned, 8 to 10 minutes.

2. Add the onion, celery, carrots, zucchini, garlic, and a heavy pinch of salt to the pot. Sauté until the veggies are softened, about 5 minutes.

3. Add the diced tomatoes (with juices), lentils, bay leaf, basil, and red pepper flakes, then pour in the broth. Bring to a boil, then reduce the heat to a simmer. Cover and cook for 45 minutes, or until the lentils are tender.

4. To serve, top each bowl of soup with 2 tablespoons of Parmesan and 2 tablespoons of parsley. Season with more salt to taste.

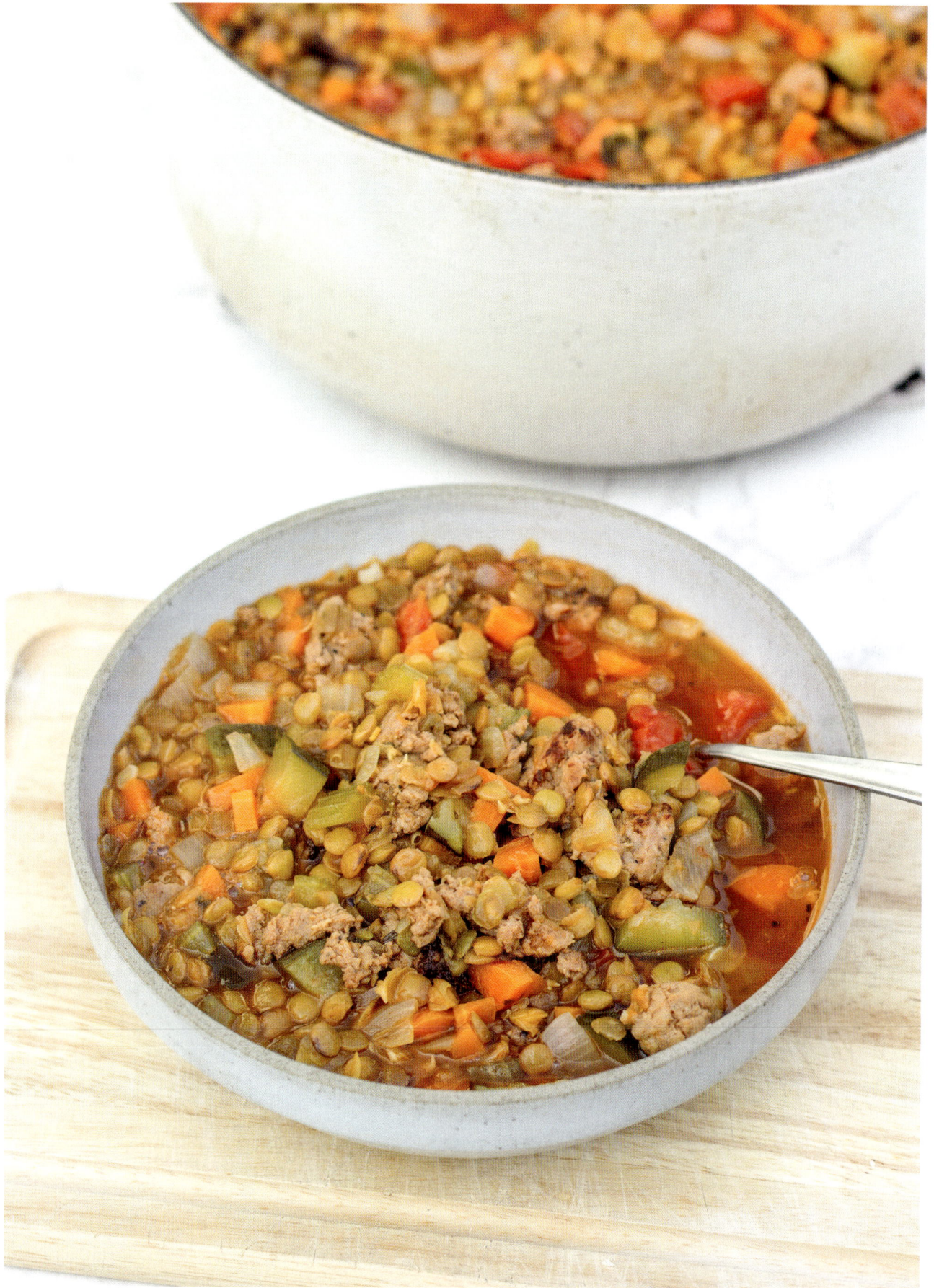

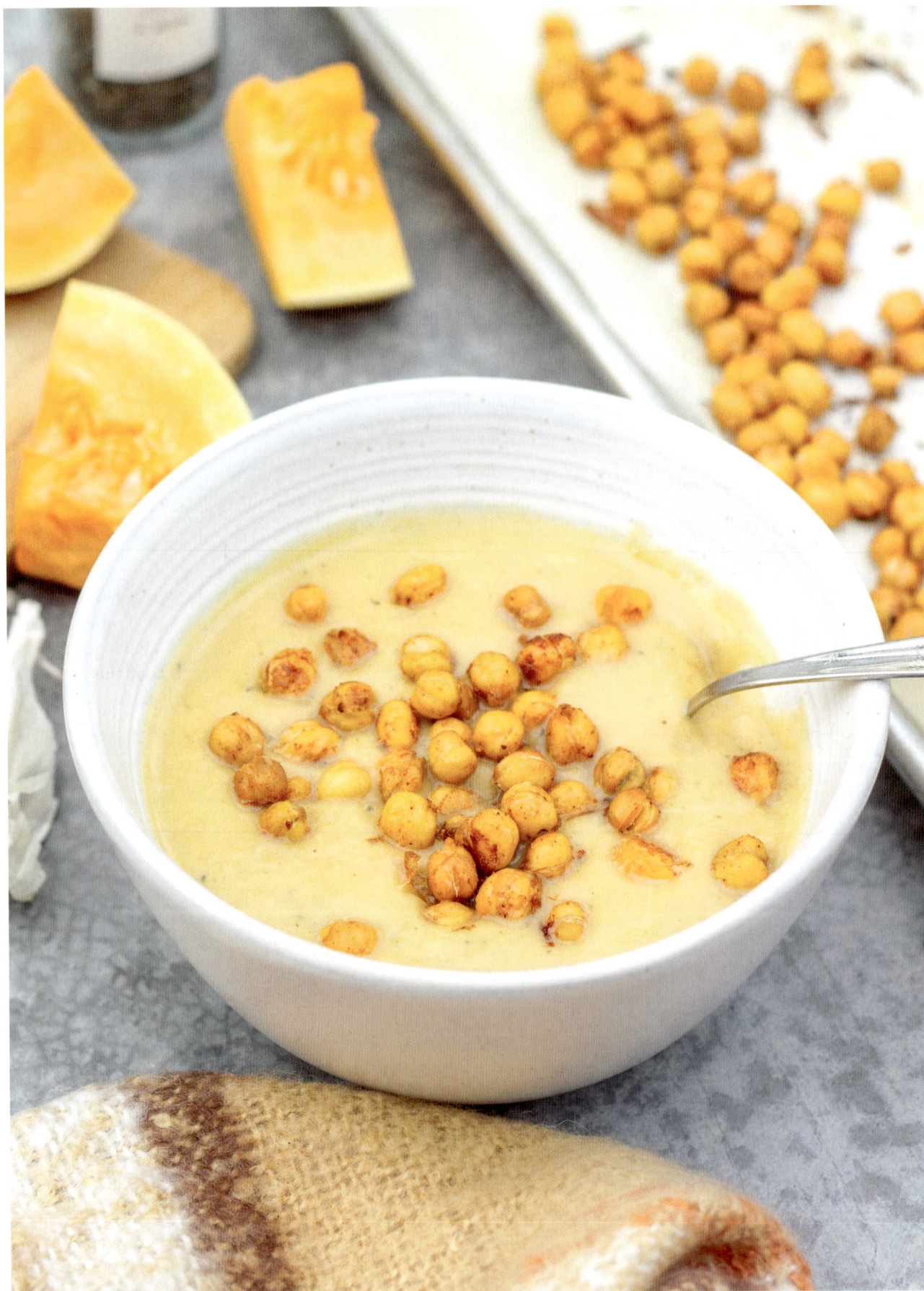

ROASTED BUTTERNUT SQUASH SOUP
WITH SPICED CHICKPEAS

SERVES 4

PREP TIME 10 minutes

COOK TIME 50 minutes

I love this soup. Roasting the butternut squash and red onion before cooking them in the broth brings out the natural sweetness of both ingredients and adds so much more flavor and complexity. This soup is hearty and rather filling on its own, but I recommend pairing it with a few ounces of your favorite grilled, baked, or sautéed protein to make sure you hit at least 30 grams of protein for the meal. My Balsamic Grilled Chicken (page 168) would be an excellent choice!

SOUP

1 medium butternut squash, peeled, seeded, and cut into 1-inch cubes

1 medium red onion, cut into 2-inch chunks

1 tablespoon plus 1 teaspoon olive oil, divided

1 teaspoon dried thyme leaves

Salt

4 cloves garlic, minced

4 cups chicken bone broth

¼ cup heavy cream or canned full-fat coconut milk

1 cup shredded sharp cheddar cheese

SPICED CHICKPEAS

1 cup cooked chickpeas, canned or homemade (page 85)

½ teaspoon paprika

¼ teaspoon cayenne pepper

1 tablespoon olive oil

Salt

1. Position one oven rack in the upper third and one in the lower third of the oven. Preheat the oven to 425°F and line two sheet pans with parchment paper.

2. Spread the butternut squash cubes and red onion pieces evenly on one of the prepared sheet pans. Drizzle with 1 tablespoon of the olive oil, then sprinkle with the thyme and a heavy pinch of salt. Using your hands, toss the ingredients to coat the vegetables. Roast on the bottom rack for 25 minutes.

3. Meanwhile, prepare the spiced chickpeas: Pour the chickpeas onto the second prepared pan. Sprinkle with the paprika, cayenne, olive oil, and a heavy pinch of salt, then toss to combine. Roast on the top rack for 20 to 25 minutes, until lightly browned and crunchy.

4. When the veggies are a few minutes away from being done, start the soup. Heat the remaining 1 teaspoon of olive oil in a Dutch oven or soup pot over medium heat. Add the garlic and sauté for 1 minute, or until fragrant. Add the roasted veggies, broth, and another heavy pinch of salt. Bring to a boil, then reduce to a simmer for 10 minutes.

5. Remove the pot from the heat. Using an immersion blender, blend the soup until smooth. (You can also carefully pour batches of the soup into a countertop blender and blend until smooth, then return the blended soup to the pot.)

6. Put the pot back on the burner and turn the heat to low. Stir in the heavy cream and cheese until the cheese is fully melted and well incorporated.

7. Top each serving of soup with some of the spiced chickpeas.

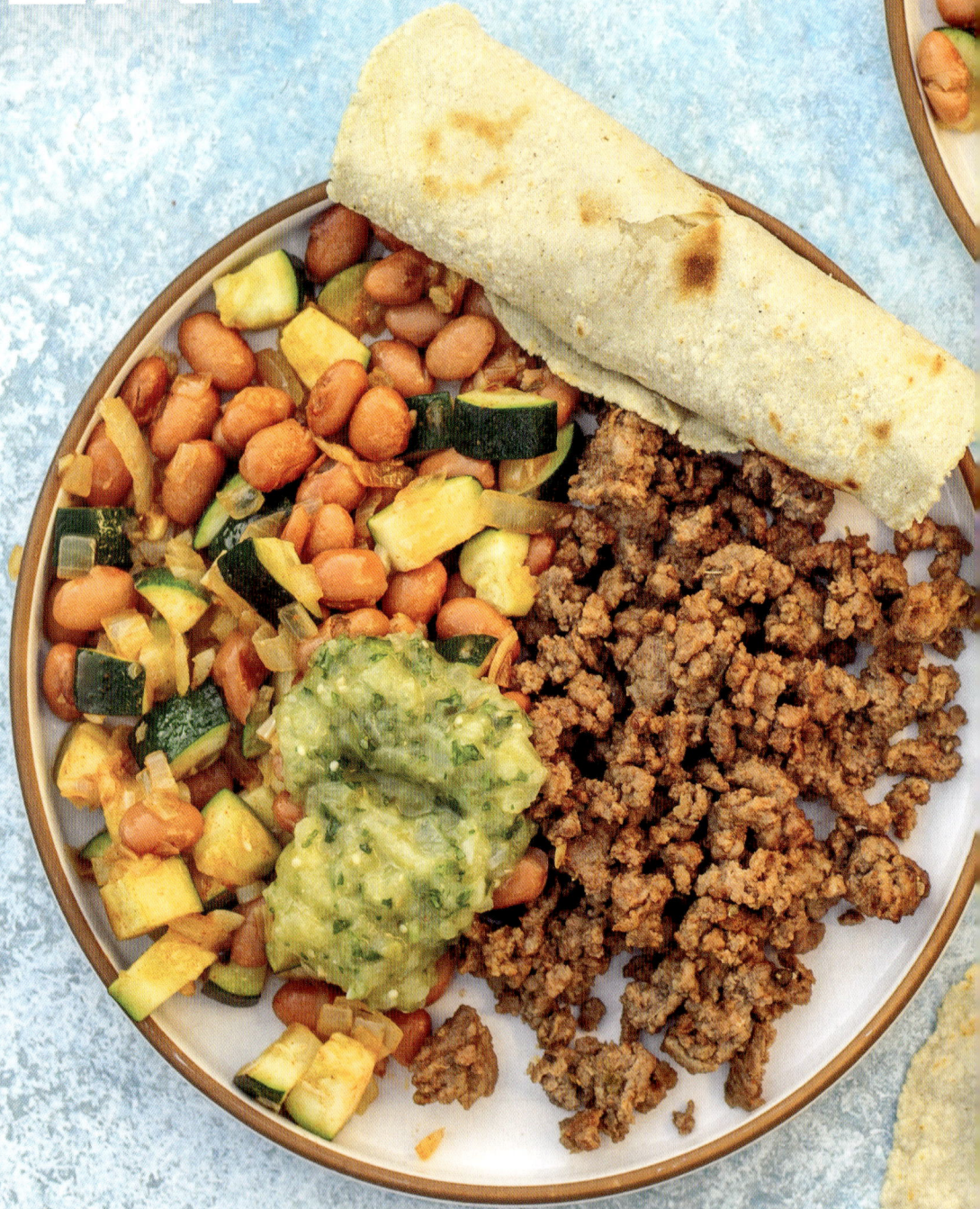

MEAT

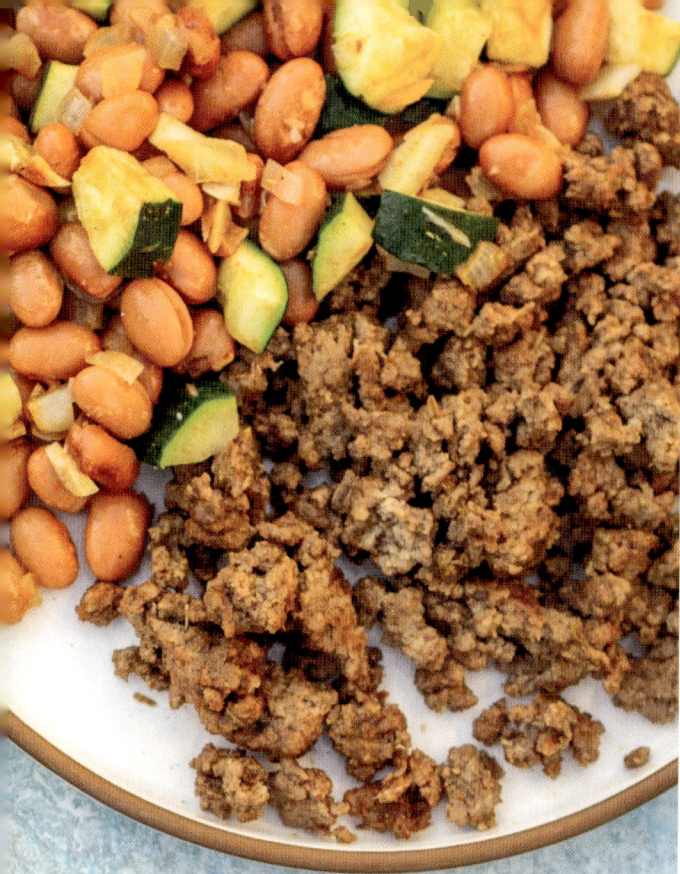

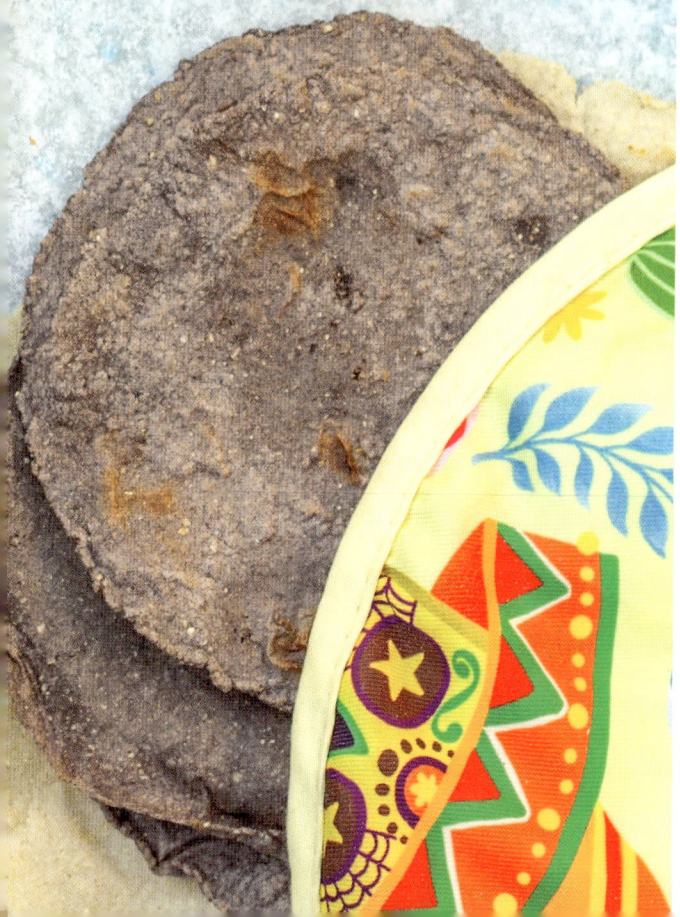

MINI BEEF ENCHILADA PIES

SERVES 4

PREP TIME 10 minutes

COOK TIME 35 minutes

My spin on the traditional enchilada is significantly higher in protein, lower in starchy carbs, and takes much less time to prep. By making enchiladas into "pie" form, you save a ton of time not having to meticulously roll each enchilada. If you already have enchilada sauce prepped in the freezer, this meal can be made in 45 minutes, making it perfect for a weeknight dinner. I like to make four individual pies, but you can also make one larger pie if you like (see note). This recipe is great paired with guacamole (page 237) for a boost of fiber.

1 teaspoon olive oil

½ medium yellow onion, diced

1 jalapeño pepper, finely diced (remove membranes and seeds if you prefer less heat)

Salt

1 pound ground beef

1 tablespoon dried oregano leaves

1 teaspoon paprika

1 teaspoon ground cumin

1 teaspoon garlic powder

1 teaspoon onion powder

2 cups red enchilada sauce, store-bought or homemade (page 74)

8 (6-inch) corn tortillas, store-bought or homemade (page 77)

½ cup Mexican-style shredded cheese

1. Preheat the oven to 400°F. Have on hand four individual-sized ceramic or glass baking dishes, about 5 by 7 inches.

2. In a medium-sized pan over medium heat, put the olive oil, onion, jalapeño, and a heavy pinch of salt. Sauté for 3 to 5 minutes, until the onion has softened. Add the ground beef, oregano, paprika, cumin, garlic powder, onion powder, and another heavy pinch of salt. Break up the meat using a rubber spatula and cook until the beef is fully browned, 8 to 10 minutes.

3. Spread ¼ cup of the enchilada sauce in each baking dish. Top with the cooked beef mixture, dividing it evenly among the dishes. Top the beef layer with two tortillas each, overlapping them slightly. Finally, top the tortillas in each dish with another ¼ cup of sauce and 2 tablespoons of cheese.

4. Bake for 15 minutes, or until the cheese is melted and slightly bubbled. Allow to cool for 5 to 10 minutes before serving.

Note To make one large enchilada pie, coat the bottom of a 9-inch square glass or ceramic baking dish with half of the enchilada sauce. Next, add the beef mixture, followed by the tortillas and the remaining sauce. Sprinkle on the cheese. Bake for 20 minutes, or until the cheese is melted and slightly bubbled. Allow to cool for 5 to 10 minutes before serving.

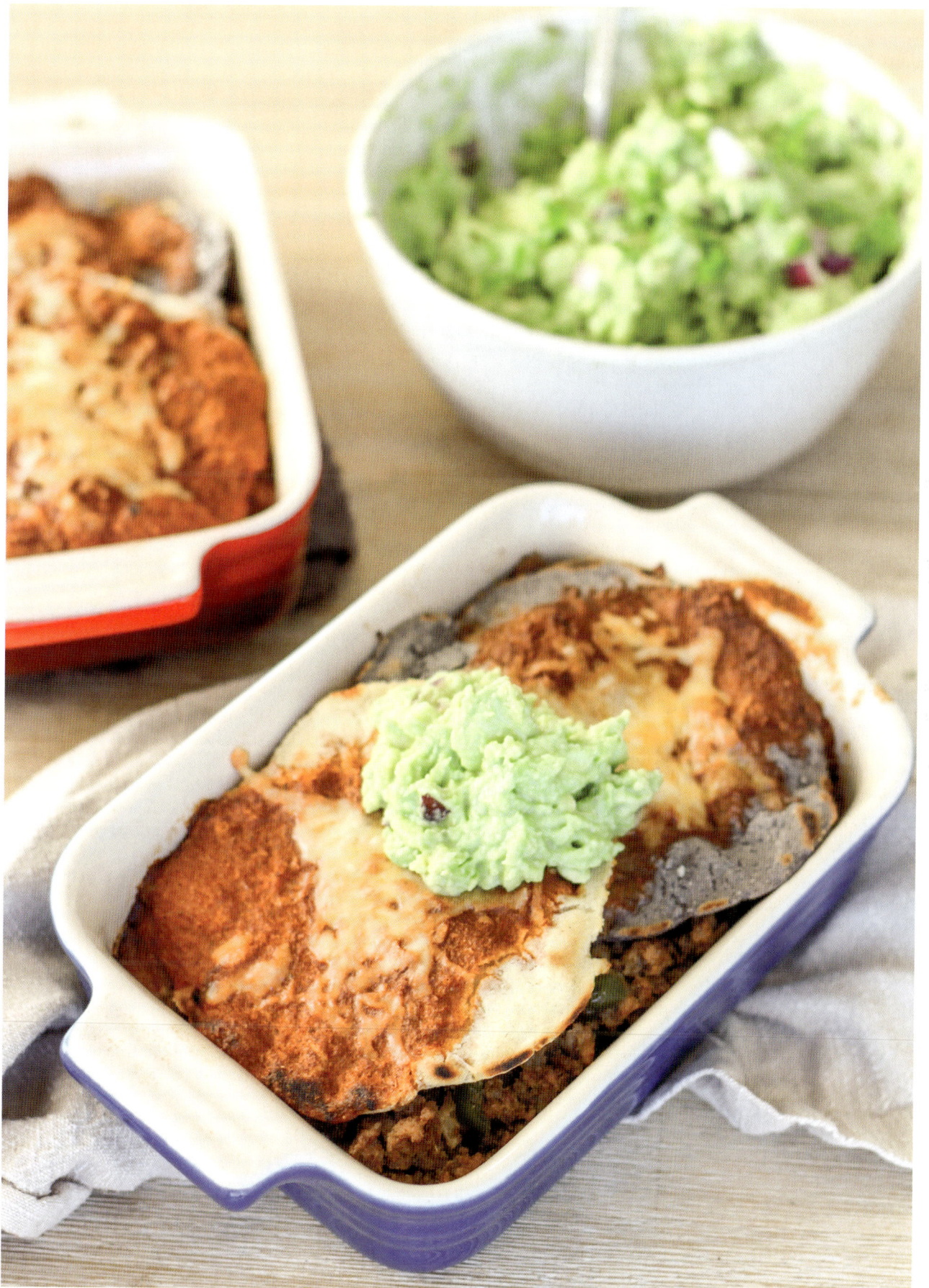

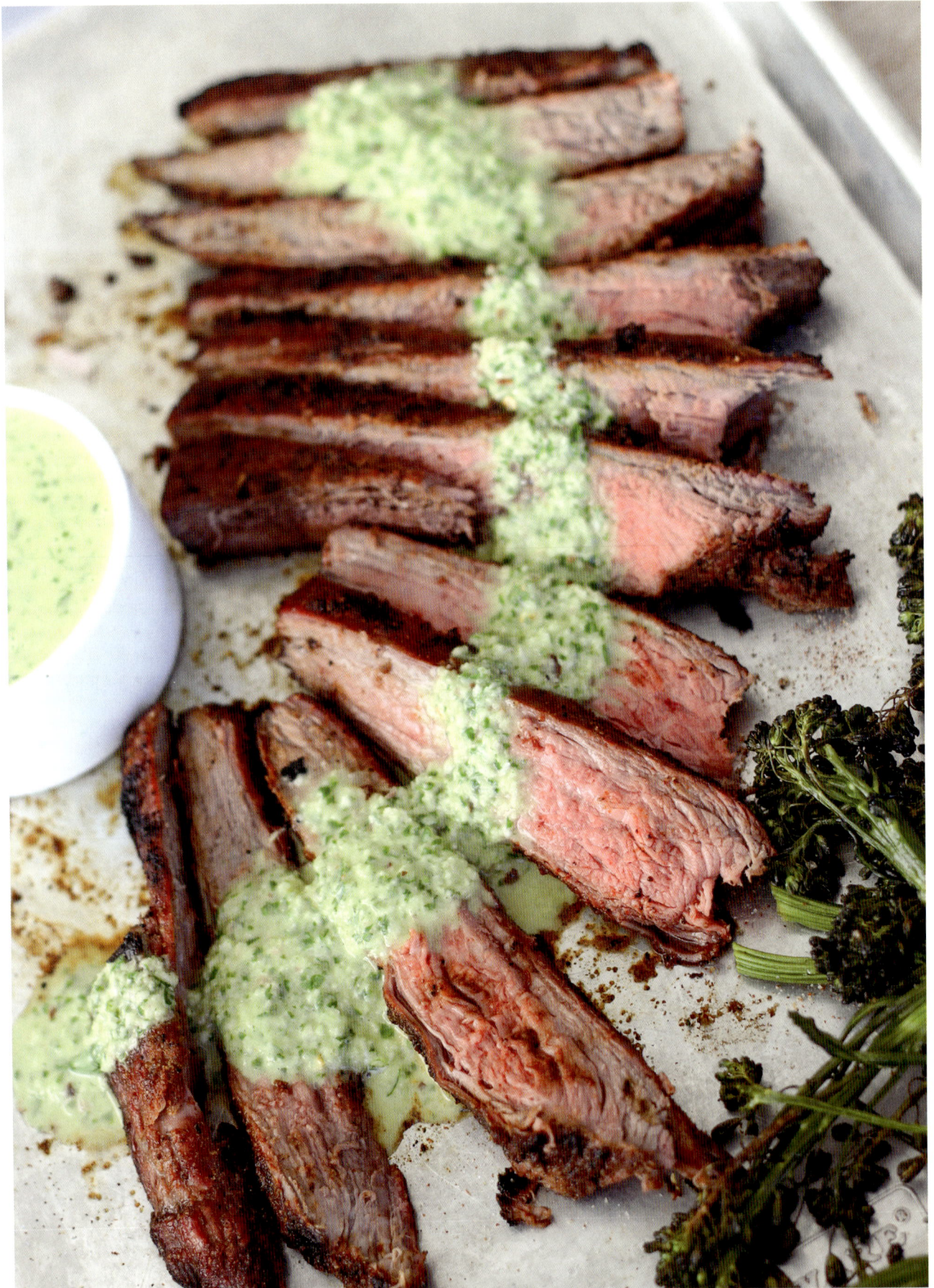

GRILLED FLANK STEAK
WITH CHIMICHURRI

SERVES 4

PREP TIME 10 minutes

COOK TIME 10 minutes

Chimichurri is an herby salsa that adds a springy freshness to a grilled steak. We don't cook steak often, but when we do, my husband always requests it with chimichurri. If you have leftover chimichurri, you can save it to mix into coleslaw or use it as the dressing for a salad. Serve this steak with the vegetable side of your choice; Crispy Broccolini (page 218) is a great option.

STEAK

1 teaspoon paprika

1 teaspoon garlic powder

1 teaspoon onion powder

½ teaspoon salt

1 pound flank steak

CHIMICHURRI

¼ cup olive oil

¼ cup red wine vinegar

Juice of 1 lemon (2 to 3 tablespoons)

½ cup chopped fresh cilantro

½ cup chopped fresh parsley

¼ cup chopped fresh oregano

¼ cup diced red onions or shallots

3 cloves garlic, chopped

¼ teaspoon salt

¼ teaspoon red pepper flakes

1. Preheat a grill to medium-high heat (425°F to 450°F).

2. Combine the paprika, garlic powder, onion powder, and salt in a small bowl. Sprinkle half of the spice mixture on one side of the flank steak and rub it in. Flip the steak over, sprinkle the other half of the spice mixture on the other side of the steak, and rub it in.

3. Once the grill is hot, grill the steak for 5 minutes on each side, or until the internal temperature is 145°F (the meat will be medium done). If you prefer your steak medium-rare, pull it off the grill when the temperature reaches 135°F. (Flank steak is best cooked to no more than medium; otherwise, it becomes tough.) Allow the steak to rest for 10 minutes before slicing.

4. While the steak is resting, put all of the chimichurri ingredients in a blender. Blend on medium-high speed until emulsified.

5. Thinly slice the steak against the grain. Split among four plates and top with the chimichurri.

SWISS SMASH BURGERS

SERVES 2 or 4

PREP TIME 10 minutes

COOK TIME 15 minutes

My husband could have burgers literally every single day for the rest of his life and never get bored. I, on the other hand, don't love burgers as much...with this recipe being an exception. Smash burgers are crispier than a traditional thicker burger. They also cook up much faster, with only a few minutes of cook time on each side. This recipe makes either four single-patty burgers or two double-patty burgers. A single patty with one slice of cheese provides about 30 grams of complete protein. However, if you require more protein, you can make it a double for about 60 grams of protein. This recipe is great served with my Oven-Roasted Sweet Potato Fries (page 221).

BURGERS

1 tablespoon olive oil

1 medium yellow onion, thinly sliced

6 large cremini mushrooms, thinly sliced

Salt

1 head iceberg lettuce

1 pound 85% lean ground beef

Ground black pepper

4 deli slices Swiss cheese (¾ to 1 ounce each)

BURGER SAUCE

½ cup plain whole milk Greek yogurt, store-bought or homemade (page 81)

¼ cup zero-sugar ketchup

1 teaspoon garlic powder

Salt

1. Preheat a griddle to high heat for 10 minutes. While the griddle heats up, cook the onion and mushrooms.

2. Heat the olive oil in a large skillet over medium heat. Add the onion, mushrooms, and a heavy pinch of salt. Sauté for 10 minutes, or until the onion and mushrooms are very soft.

3. Make the burger sauce: Put the yogurt, ketchup, garlic powder, and a heavy pinch of salt in a small bowl and whisk to combine.

4. Cut the iceberg lettuce into "buns." (Refer to the visual step-by-step example, opposite.)

5. Make the burgers: Divide the ground beef into four equal portions and shape each into a ball. Check the temperature of the griddle: You know it's hot enough when you sprinkle a drop of water onto it and it immediately sizzles away.

6. Place two beef balls on the hot griddle, allowing at least 5 inches between them, and press down firmly with a large flat surface, such as the back of a skillet or a large spatula (without holes). The burgers should be no more than ½ inch thick. Sprinkle the tops with a pinch of salt and pepper. Cook the burgers for 2 minutes, then flip. Top each patty with a slice of Swiss cheese. Cook for another 2 minutes, then remove from the griddle. Repeat with the remaining beef balls and cheese slices.

7. Assemble the burgers: Lay a lettuce "bun" on a plate and top it with a burger patty. If making a double-patty burger, top this patty with a second one. Spread 3 to 4 tablespoons of burger sauce on the burger and top with one-quarter of the onion and mushroom mixture (or one-half if making a double). Finally, top with another lettuce "bun." Repeat with the remaining ingredients to assemble the other burgers.

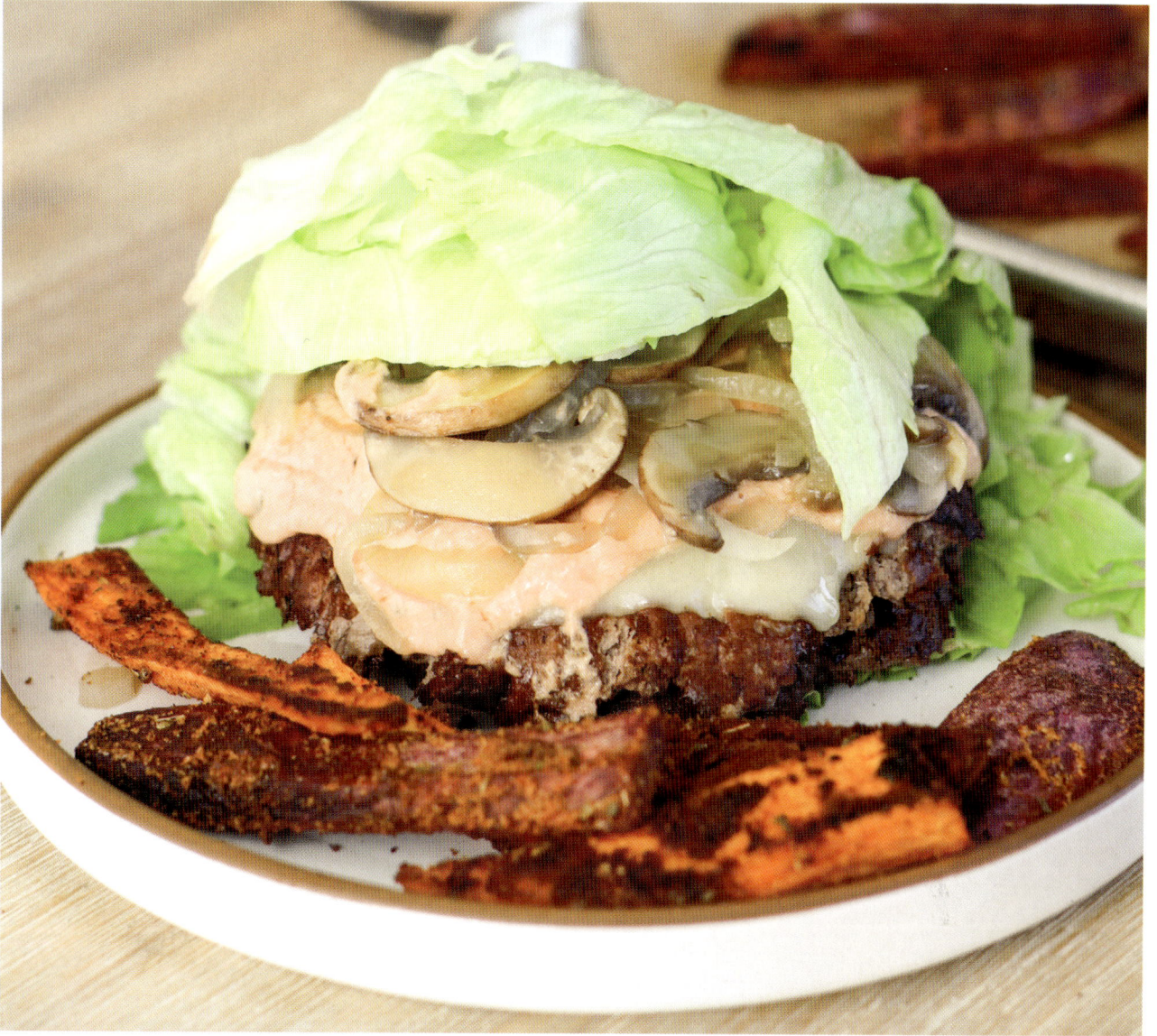

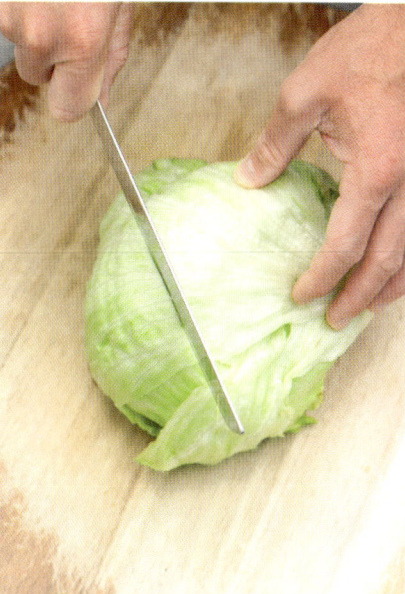

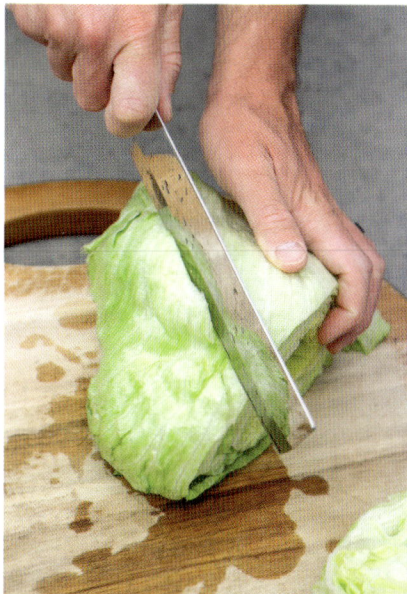

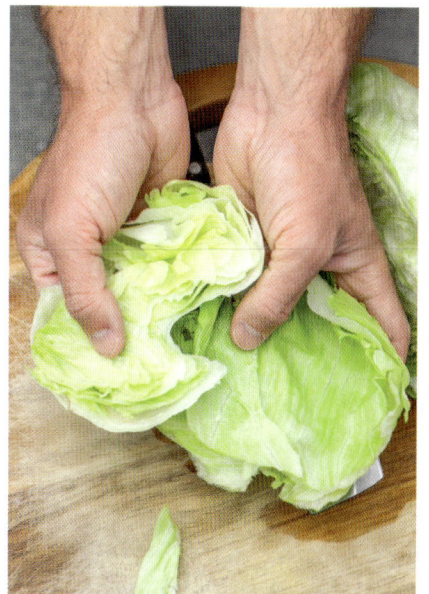

JUMBO MEATBALLS
WITH ROASTED VEGGIES

SERVES 4

PREP TIME 15 minutes

COOK TIME 45 minutes

Clients always ask me, "What should I order at an Italian restaurant?" I admit it can be tricky because of the prevalence of pasta and pizza. But one of the easiest tools for high-protein add-ons is the appetizers section of the menu, where you typically can find meatballs in some form. Large, hearty meatballs are perfect for sharing but are even better as the main feature of a meal. When done properly, they are high in protein and packed with flavor, and they're easy to make at home. Instead of high–glycemic load pasta, I like to pair these restaurant-style jumbo meatballs with micronutrient-packed roasted veggies and a simmered homemade marinara sauce.

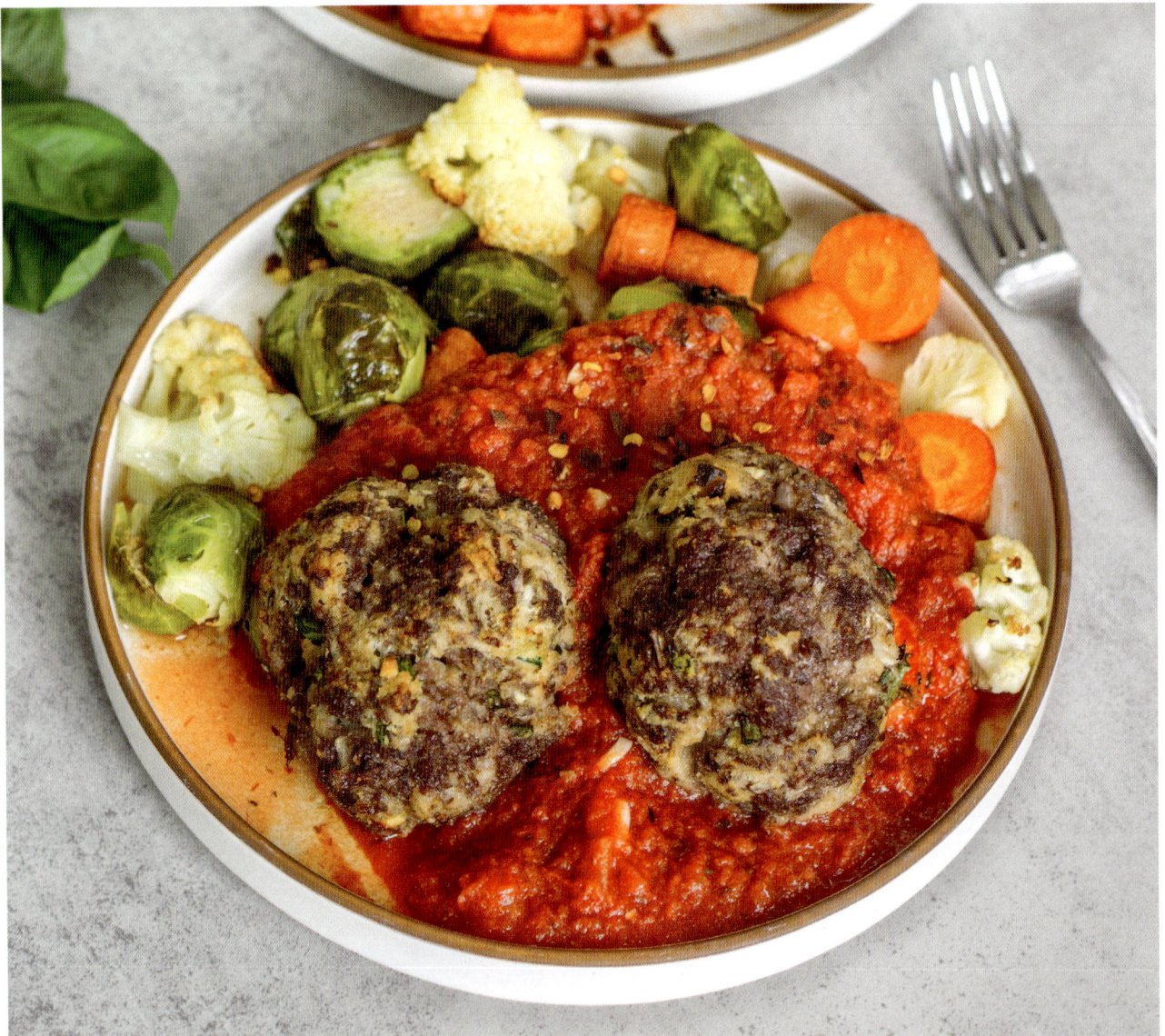

MEATBALLS

½ cup almond flour

⅔ cup whole milk

1¼ pounds ground beef

¼ medium yellow onion, grated

2 cloves garlic, minced

2 tablespoons chopped fresh parsley

1 teaspoon dried basil leaves

1 teaspoon salt

¼ teaspoon red pepper flakes

ROASTED VEGGIES

2 cups chopped cauliflower (bite-sized pieces)

2 cups Brussels sprouts, halved

4 medium carrots, sliced into 1-inch rounds

1 tablespoon olive oil

Salt

MARINARA SAUCE

1 teaspoon olive oil

5 cloves garlic, minced

¼ teaspoon red pepper flakes

1 (28-ounce) can crushed tomatoes

1 teaspoon dried basil leaves

Salt

FOR GARNISH (OPTIONAL)

Shredded Parmesan cheese

Fresh basil

1. Position one oven rack in the upper third and one in the lower third of the oven. Preheat to 400°F. Line two sheet pans with parchment paper.

2. Make the meatballs: Mix the almond flour and milk in a large mixing bowl. Wait 5 minutes, then add the remaining meatball ingredients. Mix thoroughly with your hands. Form eight evenly sized meatballs and place on one of the prepared sheet pans.

3. Roast the veggies: On the second sheet pan, spread out the cauliflower, Brussels sprouts, and carrots. Drizzle with the olive oil and sprinkle with a heavy pinch of salt. Put both pans in the oven, with the veggies on the upper rack and the meatballs on the lower, and bake for 35 to 40 minutes, until the veggies are crispy on the edges and the meatballs register at 165°F. You may need to take the veggies out a few minutes before the meatballs are done.

4. Prepare the sauce: Heat the olive oil in a large saucepan over medium heat. Add the garlic and red pepper flakes and sauté for 1 to 2 minutes, until the garlic is browned and fragrant. Carefully pour the tomatoes into the pan. The oil will tend to splatter a bit, so stand back to avoid any splashes. Add the basil and a heavy pinch of salt and give it a stir. Turn the heat down to medium-low and simmer for 20 minutes while the meatballs and veggies are roasting.

5. When the meatballs are done, transfer them to the pan with the sauce and simmer for an additional 5 minutes.

6. Split the roasted veggies among four bowls or plates and top each with two meatballs and some of the sauce. If desired, garnish with Parmesan and/or fresh basil.

ITALIAN-STYLE POT ROAST

SERVES 6

PREP TIME 5 minutes

COOK TIME 3 to 5 hours

Being mostly vegetarian growing up, I never experienced a cozy pot roast meal. It wasn't until my late twenties when I finally had my first bite of a slow-cooked pot roast, and I was instantly hooked. The long cook time helps transform the relatively inexpensive cut of meat into a tender, juicy, restaurant-worthy meal. I love traditional pot roast, but this Italian-style alternative has so much flavor and makes a sauce that's perfect to pair with mashed cauliflower or roasted veggies. Try serving it with my Crispy Broccolini (page 218) for a perfect, warming dinner pairing.

4 slices bacon, diced

1 (2¼-pound) chuck roast

Salt and pepper

½ medium yellow onion, diced

4 medium carrots, diced

2 celery stalks, diced

5 cloves garlic, minced

½ to 1 teaspoon red pepper flakes, based on spice preference

2 cups beef bone broth

1 (14-ounce) can crushed tomatoes

1 sprig fresh rosemary, or 1 teaspoon dried rosemary leaves

1 sprig fresh thyme, or 1 teaspoon dried thyme leaves

1 teaspoon dried basil leaves

1 teaspoon dried oregano leaves

1 teaspoon garlic powder

1 bay leaf

1. In a Dutch oven over medium-high heat, cook the bacon until browned and crispy, 8 to 10 minutes. Remove with a slotted spoon and place on a large plate lined with a paper towel. Leave the bacon fat in the pot.

2. Season all sides of the beef with a heavy sprinkle of salt and pepper. Sear the beef in the pot until browned on all sides, 8 to 10 minutes per side. Once browned, remove the roast and place on the plate with the bacon.

3. Add the onion, carrots, celery, garlic, red pepper flakes, and a heavy pinch of salt to the pot. Sauté for about 5 minutes, until the veggies are softened.

4. Add the broth, tomatoes, rosemary, thyme, basil, oregano, garlic powder, bay leaf, and another heavy pinch of salt. Give the mixture a stir before returning the beef and bacon to the pot.

5. Bring to a boil, then reduce to a simmer. Cover and cook for at least 2 hours or up to 4 hours. When it is ready, the meat will be very tender and easily pull apart with a fork.

6. Remove the bay leaf before serving the meat and veggies.

Note You can prep all of the ingredients and transfer them to a slow cooker to cook on low for 8 to 10 hours instead of simmering on the stovetop in step 5. This is a great option if you have to prep the meal in the morning and leave for work while it cooks.

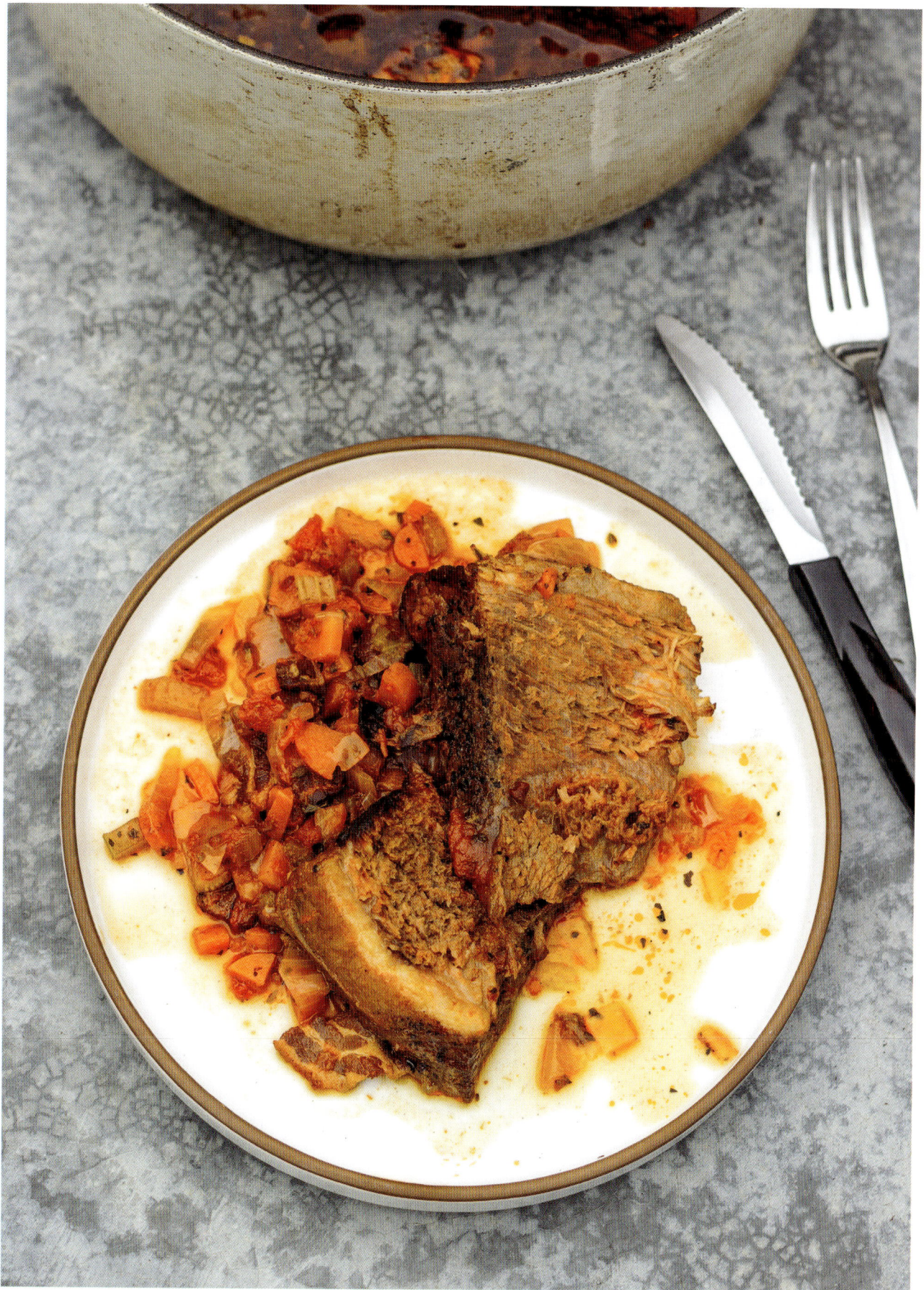

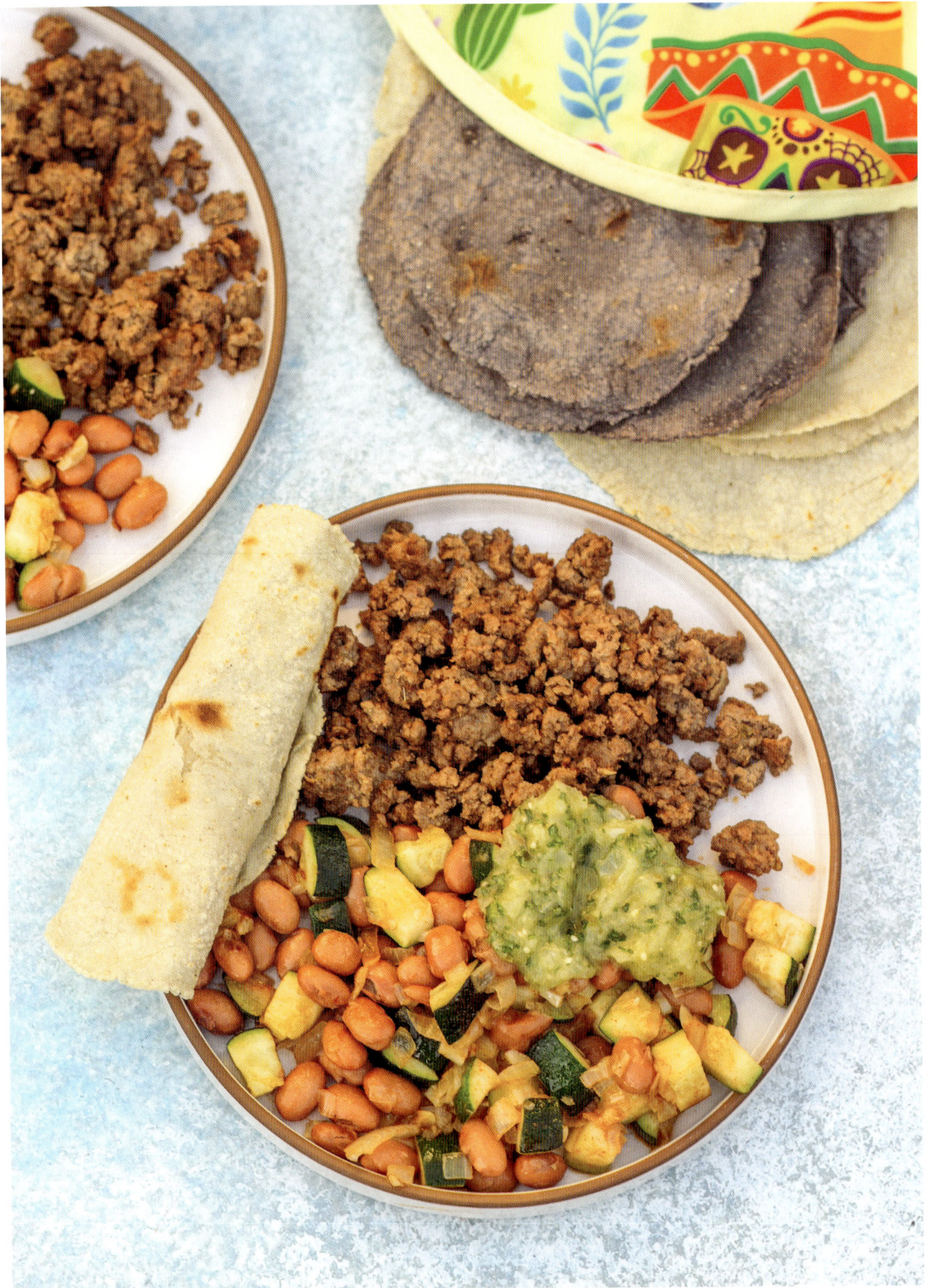

WEEKNIGHT GROUND BEEF TACOS
WITH SALSA VERDE

SERVES 4

PREP TIME 5 minutes

COOK TIME 15 minutes

This is a super fast yet impressive weeknight dinner. From start to finish, the whole meal takes only about 20 minutes to make, but it's loaded with flavor. Because these tacos are so hearty, I serve them in a freeform style: Just dump all of the ingredients on a plate and scoop the mixture onto a tortilla as you take each bite. You'll likely have too much filling for two tortillas, but you can eat the rest of the meal like a taco bowl. If you're very carb sensitive, you can turn the entire meal into a taco bowl to reduce the glycemic load. Just eliminate the tortillas and serve the rest of the ingredients over Spiced Cauliflower Rice (page 230).

SALSA VERDE

5 tomatillos, husks removed (about 1 pound)

1 jalapeño pepper, cut in half down the center (remove membranes and seeds if you prefer less heat)

½ medium yellow onion, cut into 3 thick circles

5 cloves garlic

2 teaspoons olive oil, divided

Salt

Juice of 1 lime (about 2 tablespoons)

1 cup fresh cilantro leaves

¼ teaspoon ground cumin

TACOS

1½ pounds 90% lean ground beef

1 teaspoon garlic powder

1 teaspoon dried oregano leaves

1 teaspoon paprika

1 batch Pinto Beans and Veggies (page 226)

8 (6-inch) corn tortillas, store-bought or preferably homemade (page 77)

1. Preheat the oven to 425°F and line a sheet pan with parchment paper.

2. Roast the veggies for the salsa: Spread the tomatillos, jalapeño, onion, and garlic on the prepared pan. Drizzle 1 teaspoon of the olive oil over the onion and garlic. Sprinkle a heavy pinch of salt over all of the ingredients. Bake for 15 minutes.

3. While the veggies are in the oven, start the meat. Heat the remaining 1 teaspoon of olive oil in a large skillet over medium heat. Add the ground beef, garlic powder, oregano, paprika, and a heavy pinch of salt. Use a rubber spatula to break up the meat into very small pieces while it cooks. Cook until completely browned, 7 to 10 minutes. Remove the pan from the heat while you prepare the rest of the ingredients.

4. Carefully pour the roasted veggies into a food processor or blender. Add the lime juice, cilantro, cumin, and a pinch of salt. Process on low speed until you have a mostly smooth but still slightly chunky salsa.

5. Split the taco meat and prepared Pinto Beans and Veggies evenly among four serving plates. Place two tortillas on each plate. Pour the salsa into a serving bowl so each person can top their tacos with as much salsa as they prefer.

LAMB KEFTA
WITH GRILLED ZUCCHINI

SERVES 4

PREP TIME 5 minutes, plus 30 minutes to chill (not including time to make dip)

COOK TIME 10 minutes

Kefta is a seasoned ground meat dish originating from the Middle East. For this recipe, I used ground lamb, but you can swap it out for ground beef if you prefer. Lamb is a fattier meat, so you don't need to pair it with as many sides to feel satisfied. I've found that a simple grilled zucchini and roasted bell pepper dip makes the perfect pairing for lamb.

1¾ pounds ground lamb

2 tablespoons finely chopped yellow onions

4 cloves garlic, minced

2 teaspoons paprika

2 teaspoons ground cumin

1¼ teaspoons salt

1 teaspoon ground cinnamon

½ teaspoon ground ginger

¼ teaspoon cayenne pepper

4 medium zucchini, cut lengthwise into ½-inch-thick planks

1 batch Roasted Red Pepper Dip (page 229), for serving

1. Put all of the ingredients except the zucchini in a mixing bowl. Use your hands to thoroughly mix until well combined. Cover and refrigerate for at least 30 minutes or up to 24 hours.

2. Preheat a grill to medium-high heat (425°F to 450°F).

3. Form the meat mixture into 16 elongated meatballs (a little less than 2 ounces each). They should look like slightly rounded-out footballs. Place the lamb kefta on the grill along with the zucchini. Cook for 5 minutes before flipping. Cook for another 5 minutes, or until the internal temperature of the kefta is 165°F and the zucchini has grill marks on both sides.

4. Serve immediately with the dip.

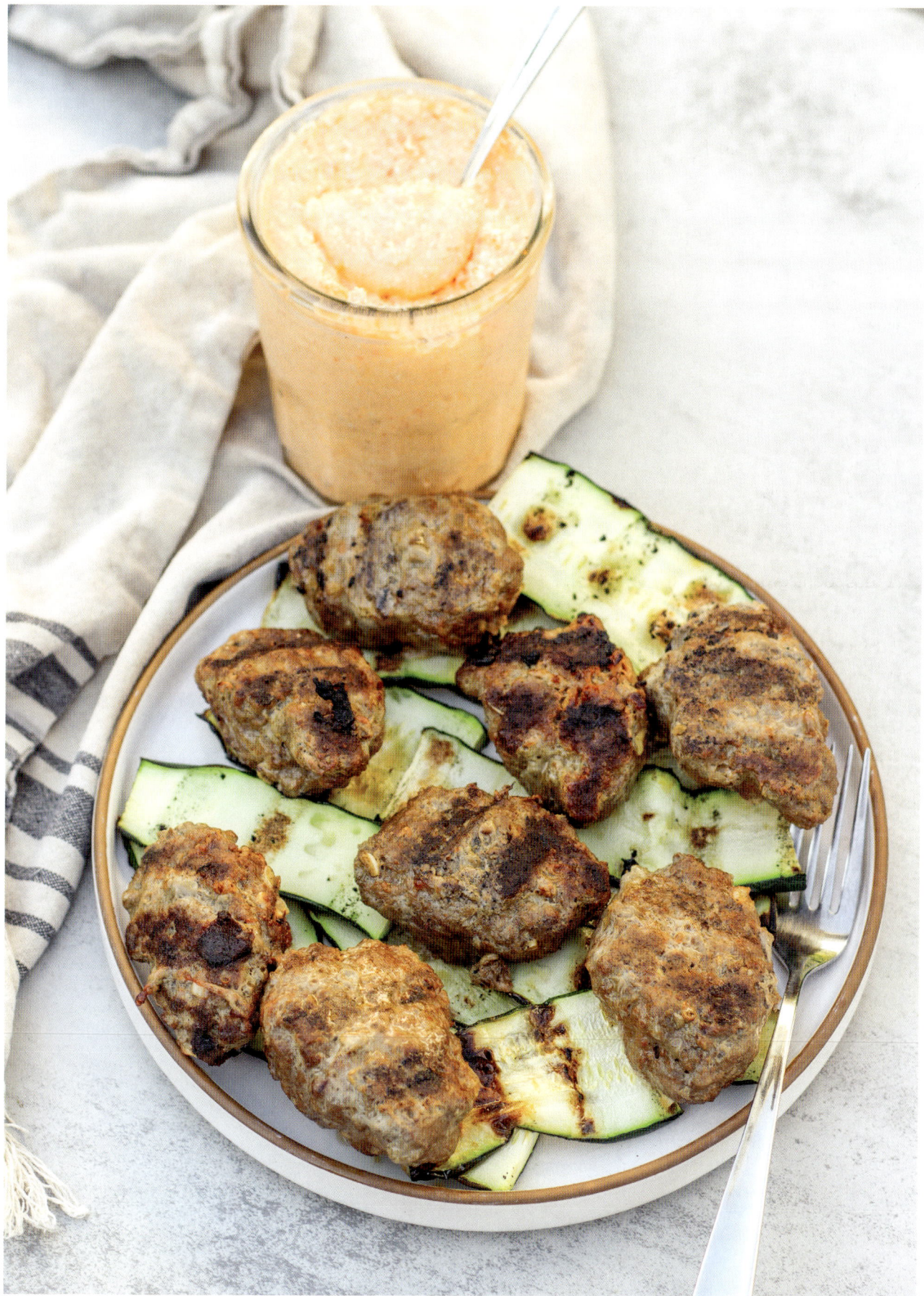

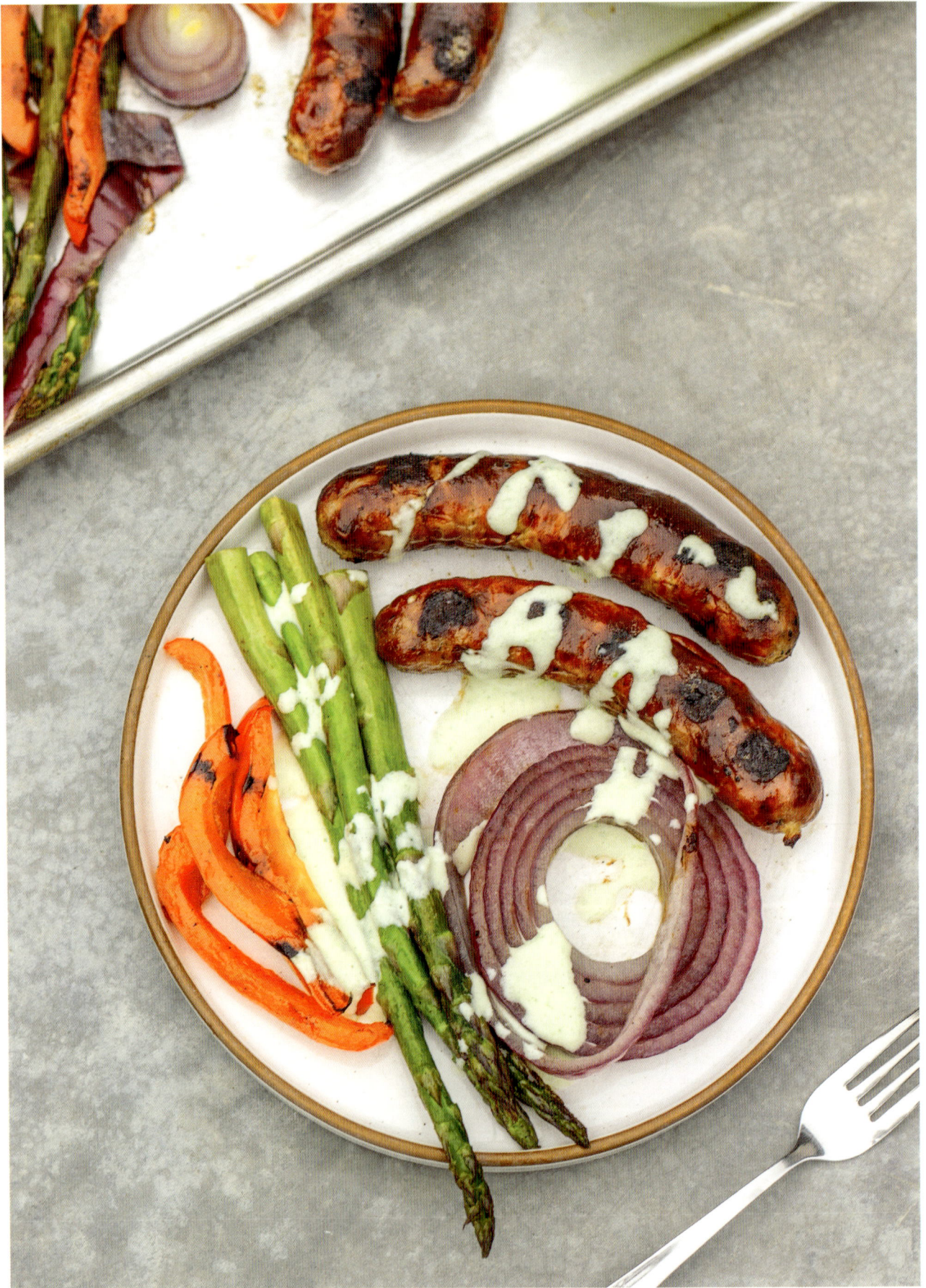

GRILLED SAUSAGE AND VEG
WITH GREEN DRESSING DRIZZLE

SERVES 4

PREP TIME 5 minutes

COOK TIME 15 minutes

Sausage tends to be a fattier protein, which means it is best paired with simple veggie sides. The green dressing was the result of me cleaning out the fridge and using up the plethora of parsley from our garden. Although probably not the usual combination you would think of, this dressing is a perfectly light and flavorful complement to the grilled sausage. Because all of the cooking is done on a grill, this is a great meal to make in the middle of the summer when you can't fathom the idea of switching on the oven.

SAUSAGE AND VEG

2 red bell peppers, thinly sliced

1 medium red onion, cut into 1-inch-thick circles

1 pound asparagus, bottom 2 inches trimmed

1 tablespoon olive oil

Salt

8 precooked uncured beef Polish sausages

GREEN DRESSING

½ cup plain whole milk Greek yogurt, store-bought or homemade (page 81)

Juice of ½ lemon (1 to 1½ tablespoons)

1 tablespoon olive oil

¼ cup chopped green onions

¼ cup shredded Parmesan cheese

½ teaspoon garlic powder

½ teaspoon onion powder

Heavy pinch of salt

Special equipment: grill mat or basket (optional; see note) and immersion blender

1. Preheat a grill to medium-high heat (425°F to 450°F).

2. Spread the bell peppers, red onion, and asparagus on a sheet pan and drizzle with the olive oil and a heavy pinch of salt. Lay the asparagus, onion, and bell pepper on the grill mat, if using, or directly on the grill. Next, place the sausages on the grill. Cover and cook for 5 minutes, then flip the veggies and sausages and set a new timer for 5 minutes. After 10 minutes total, remove the veggies and sausages from the grill and put on a plate.

3. Make the dressing: In a 2-cup glass measuring cup or a small bowl, blend all of the dressing ingredients with an immersion blender until the ingredients are well combined and the dressing has turned a light green.

4. Serve the veggies and sausages with the dressing.

Note I like to use a grill mat when cooking sliced veggies so they don't fall through the grate. If you don't have a grill mat or basket, simply grill the veggies whole and slice before serving.

LAMB BURGERS
WITH TZATZIKI

SERVES 4

PREP TIME 15 minutes

COOK TIME 10 minutes

When I learned that lamb is one of the most nutrient-dense foods you can eat, I started testing out a variety of meals with it. Because we eat so many burgers at home, I knew I had to turn lamb into a burger also. This recipe is packed with flavors not normally found in your typical double-double. Lamb is a fattier meat, so I love pairing these burgers with a refreshing Cauliflower Avocado Tabbouleh (page 234) to lighten up the meal while providing some fiber. If you want to add even more flavor, I highly recommend serving them with Roasted Red Pepper Dip (page 229) too. This is my husband's favorite combo!

BURGERS

1½ pounds ground lamb

¼ cup crumbled feta cheese

¼ cup minced fresh parsley

2 cloves garlic, minced

1 teaspoon dried oregano leaves

1 teaspoon ground cumin

¼ teaspoon red pepper flakes

Grated zest of ½ lemon

TZATZIKI

1 cup plain whole milk Greek yogurt, store-bought or homemade (page 81)

1 clove garlic, minced

Juice of ½ lemon (1 to 1½ tablespoons)

1 tablespoon minced fresh mint

Pinch of salt

1. Preheat a grill to medium-high heat (425°F to 450°F).

2. Place all of the burger ingredients in a bowl and mix thoroughly with your hands until combined. Form into four patties about 1 inch thick. Grill for 5 minutes on each side. The burgers are done when the internal temperature reaches 145°F. Remove from the grill and set aside.

3. While the burgers are resting, make the tzatziki: Mix together all of the ingredients in a small bowl or measuring cup. Add more salt to taste.

4. Serve the burgers with a drizzle of tzatziki sauce.

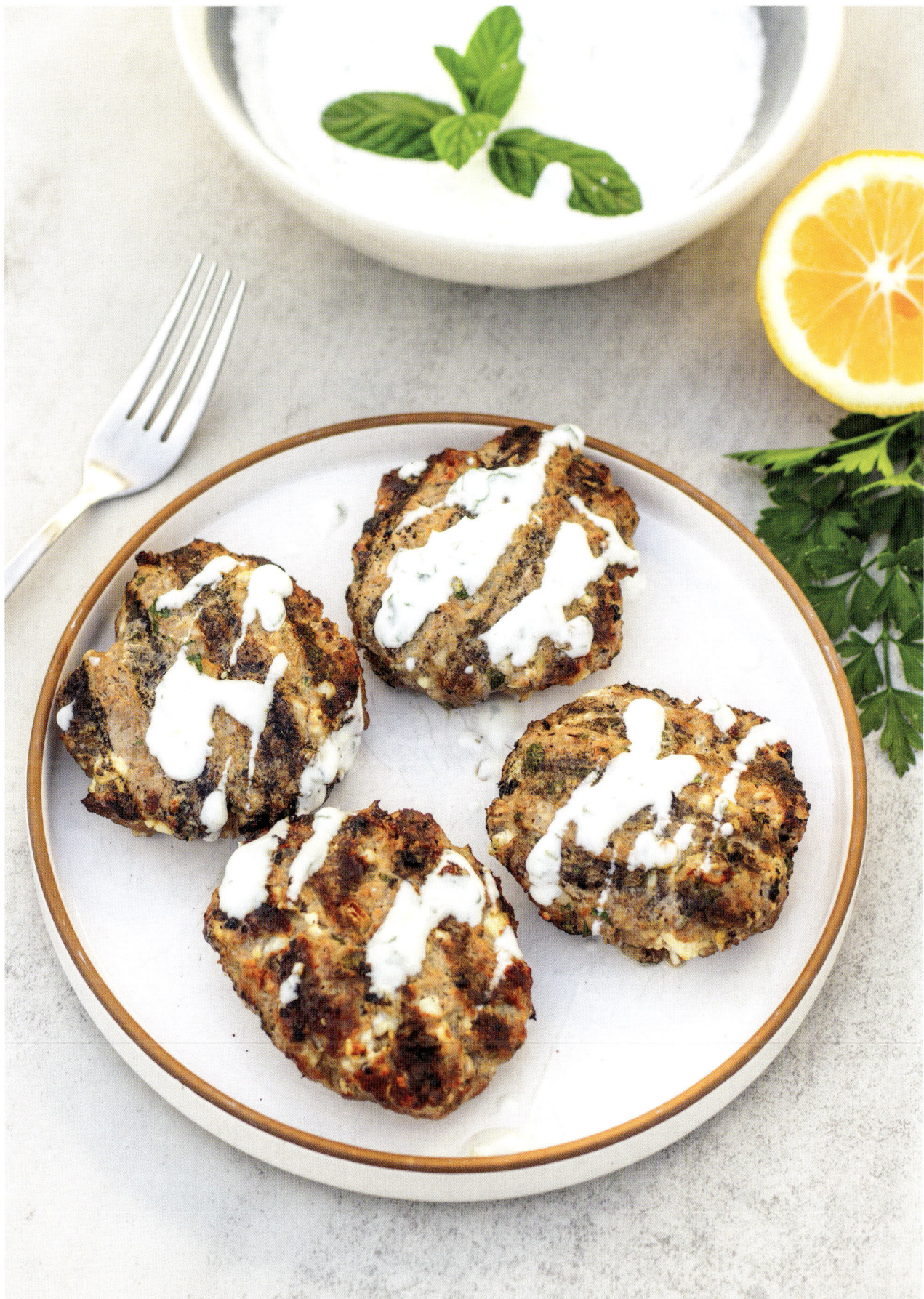

Note You can eat this Bolognese on its own with a spoon or serve it with pasta. The best pasta options for satiety and blood sugar control (and that actually taste like pasta) are those made from chickpeas or lentils. Look for a brand with minimal ingredients and cook according to the package instructions. For an even lower-carb option, some of my favorites are zucchini noodles, thinly sliced cabbage, hearts of palm pasta, or roasted broccoli and cauliflower. For any of these, aim for 1 to 2 cups per serving.

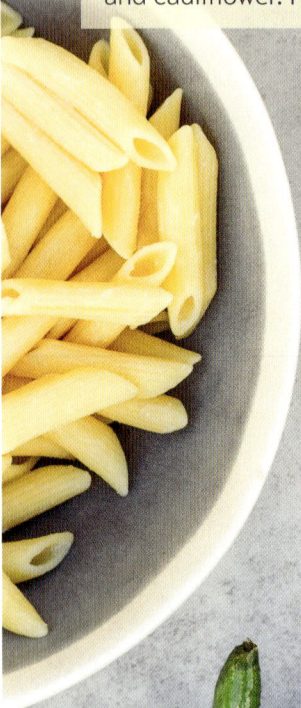

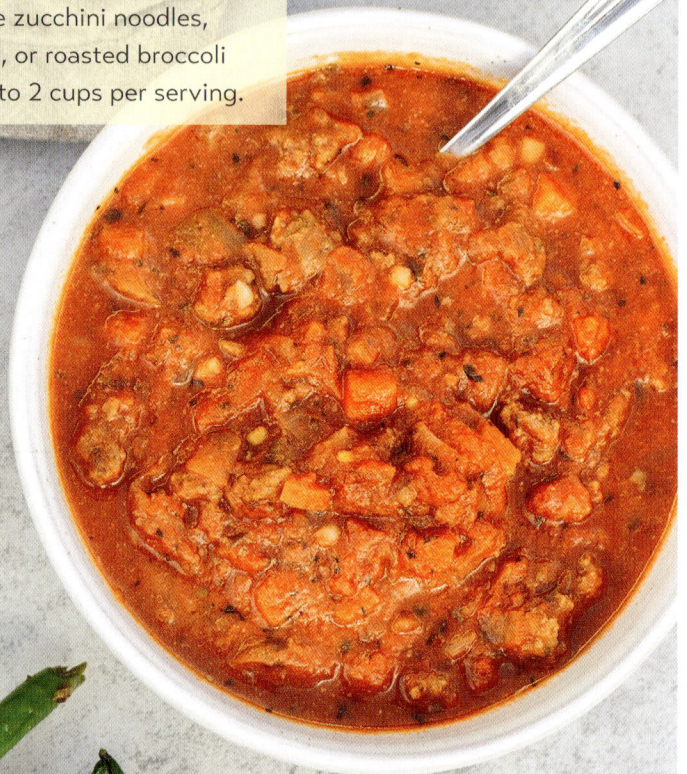

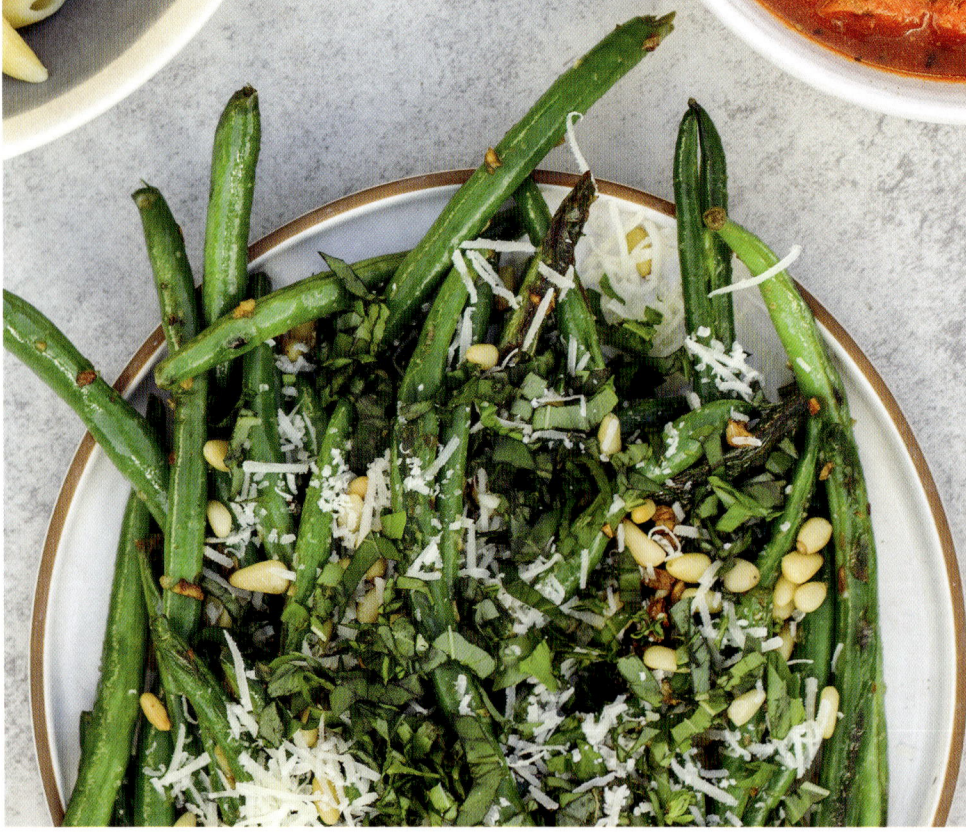

SLOW-COOKED BOLOGNESE
WITH GARLICKY BASIL GREEN BEANS

SERVES 4

PREP TIME 5 minutes

COOK TIME 2 to 4 hours

This Bolognese is a staple at our house. The low-and-slow cooking method helps break down the beef into super tender, flavorful bites. Even though it takes a long time to simmer, the prep time is very short. I like to make this meal when I have a few extra minutes at lunchtime to get dinner started. It's also a great recipe to double or triple to eat as leftovers throughout the week. Typically, Bolognese is served with spaghetti, but I like to pair it with quick sautéed beans in a pesto-style sauce for a delicious low-glycemic alternative. To serve this with pasta instead, start the pasta at the same time as the green beans.

BOLOGNESE

1 tablespoon olive oil

2 medium carrots, finely chopped

1 medium yellow onion, chopped

4 cloves garlic, minced

1 pound ground beef

Salt

1 (28-ounce) can crushed tomatoes

1 cup whole milk

¼ cup tomato paste

2 teaspoons dried basil leaves

2 teaspoons dried oregano leaves

1 bay leaf

1 teaspoon dried thyme leaves

1 teaspoon garlic powder

½ teaspoon red pepper flakes

GREEN BEANS

1 tablespoon olive oil

1 pound green beans, trimmed and halved

Salt

4 cloves garlic, minced

½ cup thinly sliced fresh basil leaves

¼ cup shredded Parmesan cheese

¼ cup pine nuts

1. Start the Bolognese: Heat the olive oil in a Dutch oven over medium-high heat. Add the carrots, onion, and garlic and sauté for 2 minutes, or until fragrant. Add the ground beef and a heavy pinch of salt and cook, breaking up the beef with a rubber spatula as it cooks, until it is browned and cooked all the way through, about 8 minutes.

2. Add the remaining Bolognese ingredients. Bring the mixture to a boil, then reduce the heat to low, cover, and simmer for at least 2 hours or up to 4 hours. The longer the sauce simmers, the more tender the meat will become; however, it's still quite tender after 2 hours if you're short on time.

3. About 15 minutes before serving, start the green beans: Heat the olive oil in a large skillet over medium-high heat. Add the beans and a heavy pinch of salt. Cook without stirring for 2 minutes, until you see a slight browning of the green beans, then move the beans around and let them sit for another 2 minutes to sear the other side. Add the garlic and stir continuously for 30 seconds to 1 minute, until the garlic is softened and slightly browned. Remove the pan from the heat and stir in the basil, Parmesan, and pine nuts.

4. Serve the Bolognese with the veggies.

MINI MEATLOAF SHEET PAN DINNER

SERVES 4

PREP TIME 15 minutes

COOK TIME 30 minutes

Sheet pan dinners are perfect for weeknights because they're fast and very easy to clean up. Everything is contained to one cooking vessel! Splitting the meat mixture into mini loaves also cuts down on the cook time while providing the classic cozy flavors you know and love. This meal makes an appearance on our menu every week when Brussels sprouts are in season. For unsweetened BBQ sauce and ketchup, I love the brand Primal Kitchen.

½ cup diced yellow onions

1½ tablespoons zero-sugar ketchup

1 large egg

1 tablespoon Worcestershire sauce

3 tablespoons whole milk

½ cup almond flour

1½ pounds ground beef

1 teaspoon dried basil leaves

1 teaspoon dried oregano leaves

1 teaspoon paprika

Salt

4 large carrots, peeled and roughly chopped

1 pound Brussels sprouts, halved

1 tablespoon olive oil

½ cup unsweetened BBQ sauce, plus extra for dipping

1. Preheat the oven to 375°F and line a sheet pan with parchment paper.

2. In a mixing bowl, whisk together the onions, ketchup, egg, Worcestershire, milk, and almond flour. Add the ground beef, basil, oregano, paprika, and a heavy pinch of salt. Mix thoroughly with your hands, then allow to rest while you prepare the veggies.

3. Place the carrots and Brussels sprouts on the sheet pan and drizzle with the olive oil. Sprinkle with a heavy pinch of salt and toss to combine. Make sure the veggies are not overlapping and leave spaces for the mini meatloaves.

4. Form the meat mixture into four loaf shapes and place on the sheet pan with the veggies. Brush the BBQ sauce on the outsides of the meatloaves. Bake the veggies and meatloaves for 30 minutes, or until the internal temperature of the meatloaves reaches 165°F.

5. Serve the veggies and meatloaves with additional BBQ sauce for dipping.

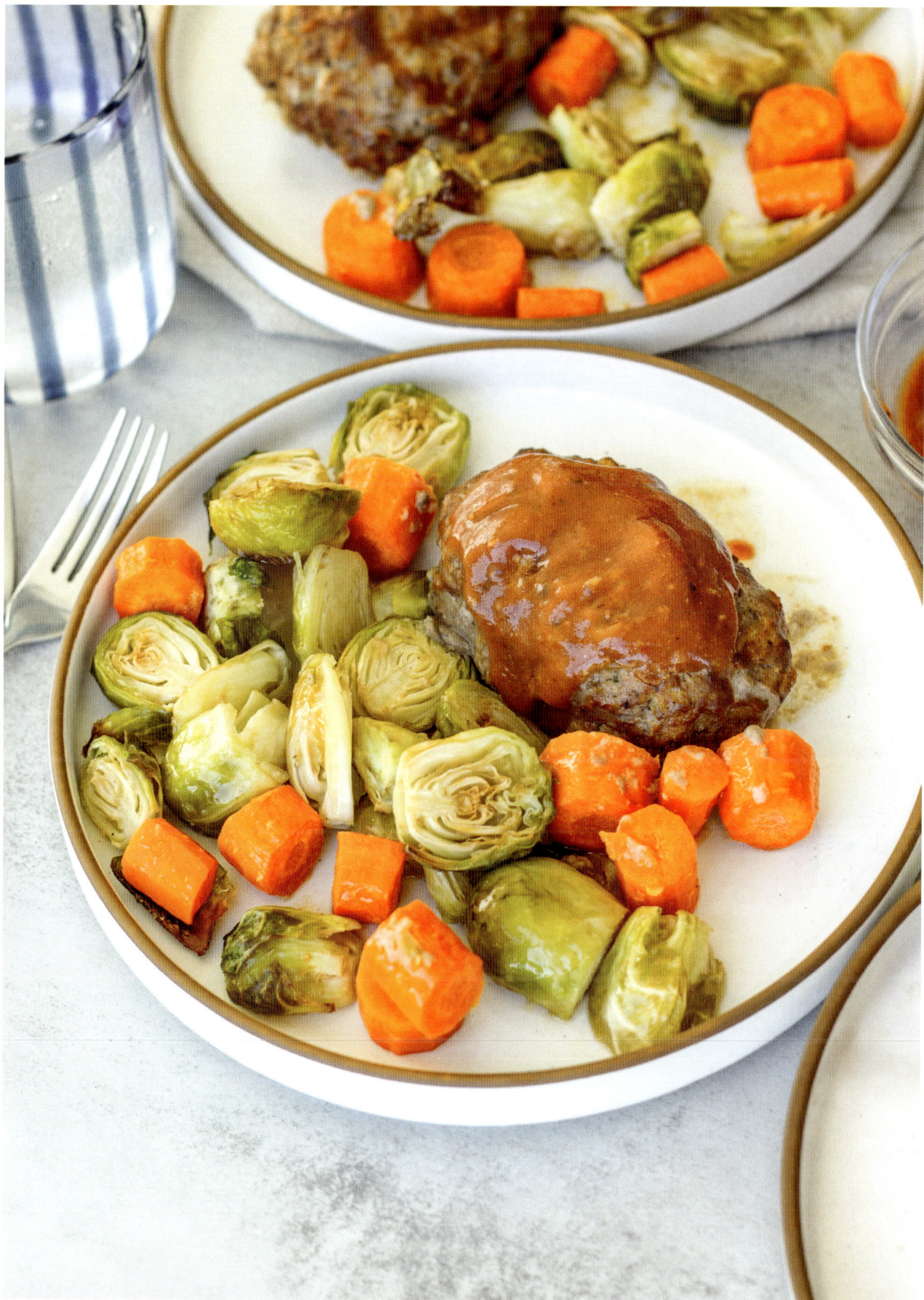

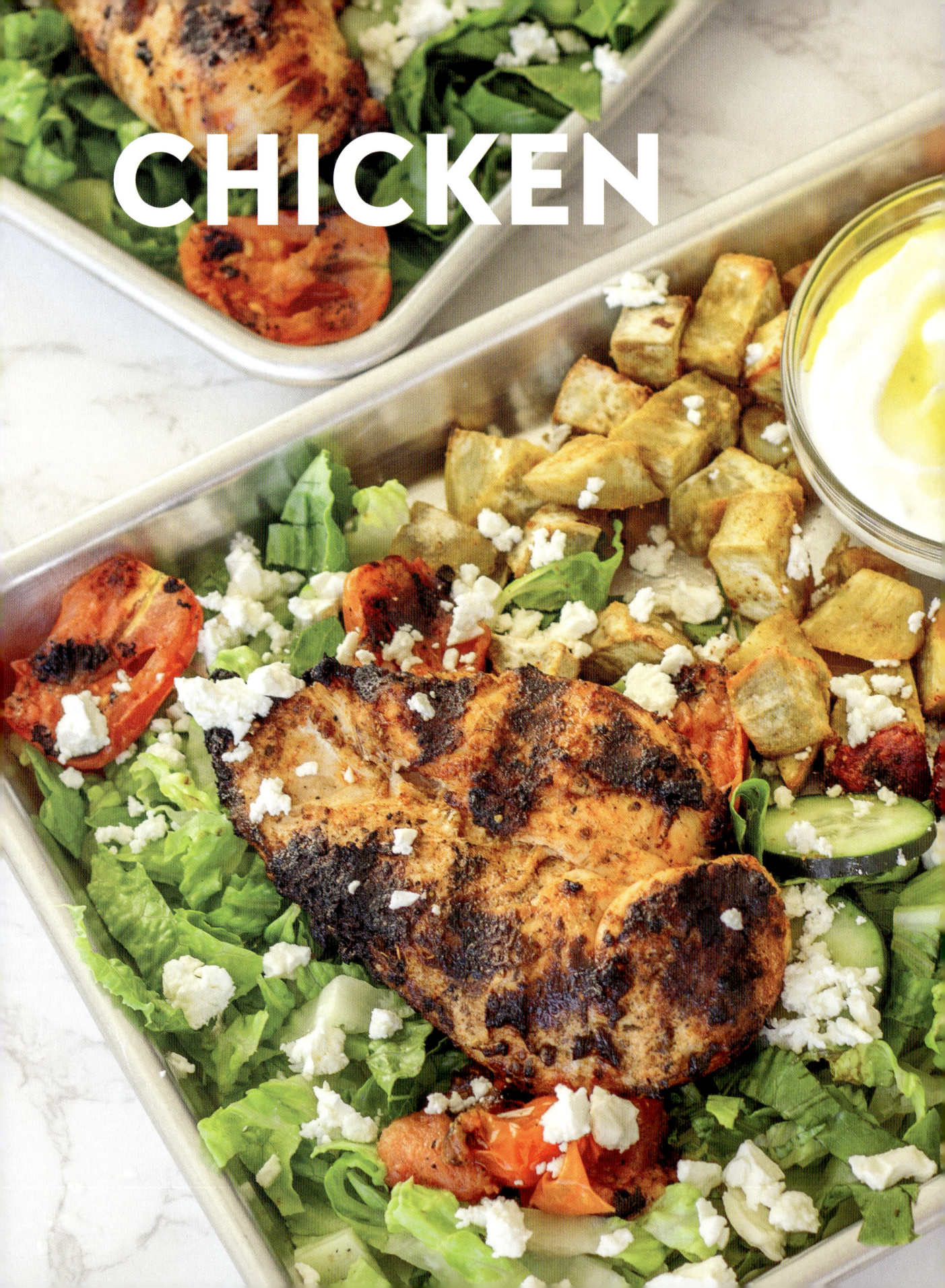

CHICKEN

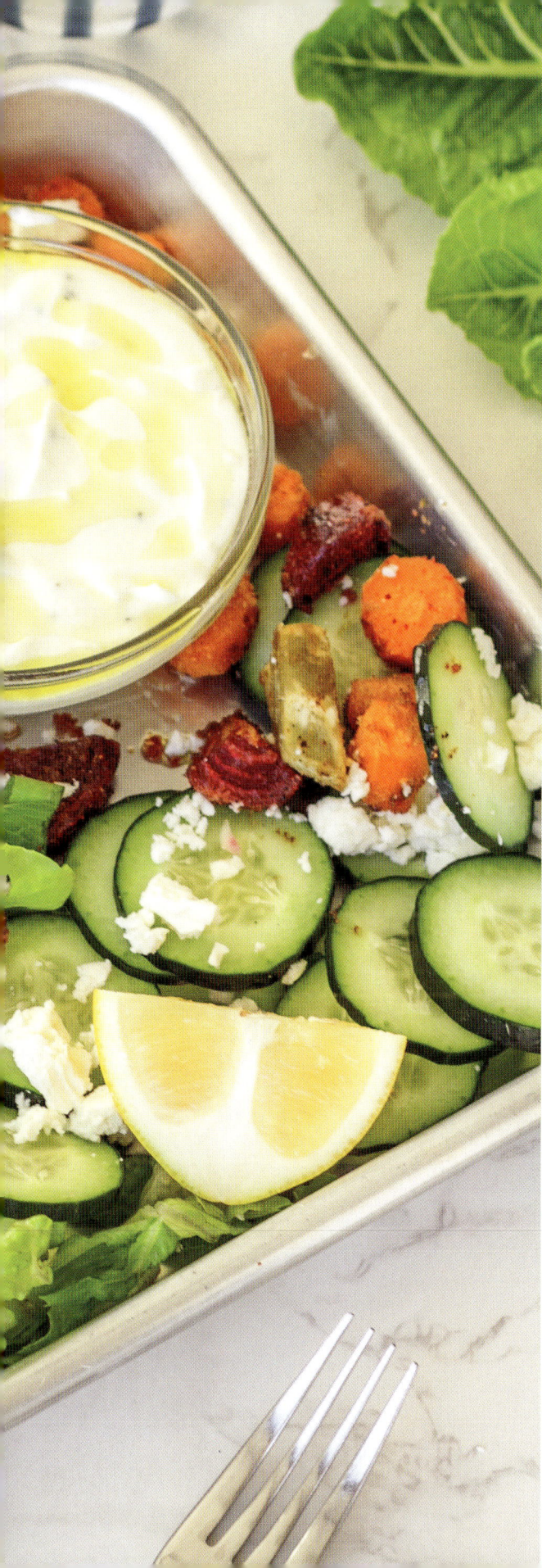

MINI CHICKEN ENCHILADA PIES

SERVES 4

PREP TIME 10 minutes

COOK TIME 30 minutes

Like my Mini Beef Enchilada Pies recipe on page 140, this dish is higher in protein and lower in starchy carbs than traditional enchiladas. You can shred leftover rotisserie chicken or my Easy Poached Chicken to use in this recipe. I like to make four individual pies, but you can make one larger pie if you like (see the note below). This dish pairs well with a dollop of homemade guacamole (see my recipe on page 237).

2 teaspoons olive oil

2 medium zucchini, diced

1 bell pepper (any color), diced

½ medium yellow onion, diced

3 cloves garlic, minced

Salt

½ batch Easy Poached Chicken (page 80), or 3 cups rotisserie chicken, shredded

1 jalapeño pepper, finely diced (remove membranes and seeds if you prefer less heat)

1 tablespoon dried oregano leaves

1 teaspoon ground cumin

1 teaspoon garlic powder

1 teaspoon onion powder

1 teaspoon paprika

2¼ cups red enchilada sauce, store-bought or homemade (page 74), divided

¾ cup Mexican-style shredded cheese, divided

8 (6-inch) corn tortillas, store-bought or homemade (page 77)

1. Preheat the oven to 400°F. Have on hand four individual-sized ceramic or glass baking dishes, about 5 by 7 inches each.

2. Heat the olive oil in a medium-sized skillet over medium heat. Add the zucchini, bell pepper, onion, garlic, and a heavy pinch of salt. Sauté for 5 minutes, or until the veggies have softened.

3. Add the chicken, jalapeño, oregano, cumin, garlic powder, onion powder, paprika, and ¼ cup of the enchilada sauce. Stir to combine and cook for 5 to 7 minutes, until all of the ingredients are warmed through. Sprinkle with ¼ cup of the cheese and stir until evenly distributed.

4. Spread ¼ cup of the enchilada sauce in each baking dish. Spoon one-quarter of the cooked chicken and veggie mixture into each dish. Top the chicken layer with two tortillas each, overlapping them slightly. Finally, top the tortillas in each dish with another ¼ cup of enchilada sauce and 2 tablespoons of cheese.

5. Bake for 15 minutes, or until the cheese is melted and slightly bubbled. Allow to cool for 5 to 10 minutes before serving.

Note To make one large enchilada pie, coat the bottom of a 9-inch square glass or ceramic baking dish with 1 cup of the enchilada sauce. Next, add the chicken mixture, followed by the tortillas and the remaining cup of sauce. Sprinkle on the cheese and bake for 20 minutes, or until the cheese is melted and slightly bubbled. Allow to cool for 5 to 10 minutes before serving.

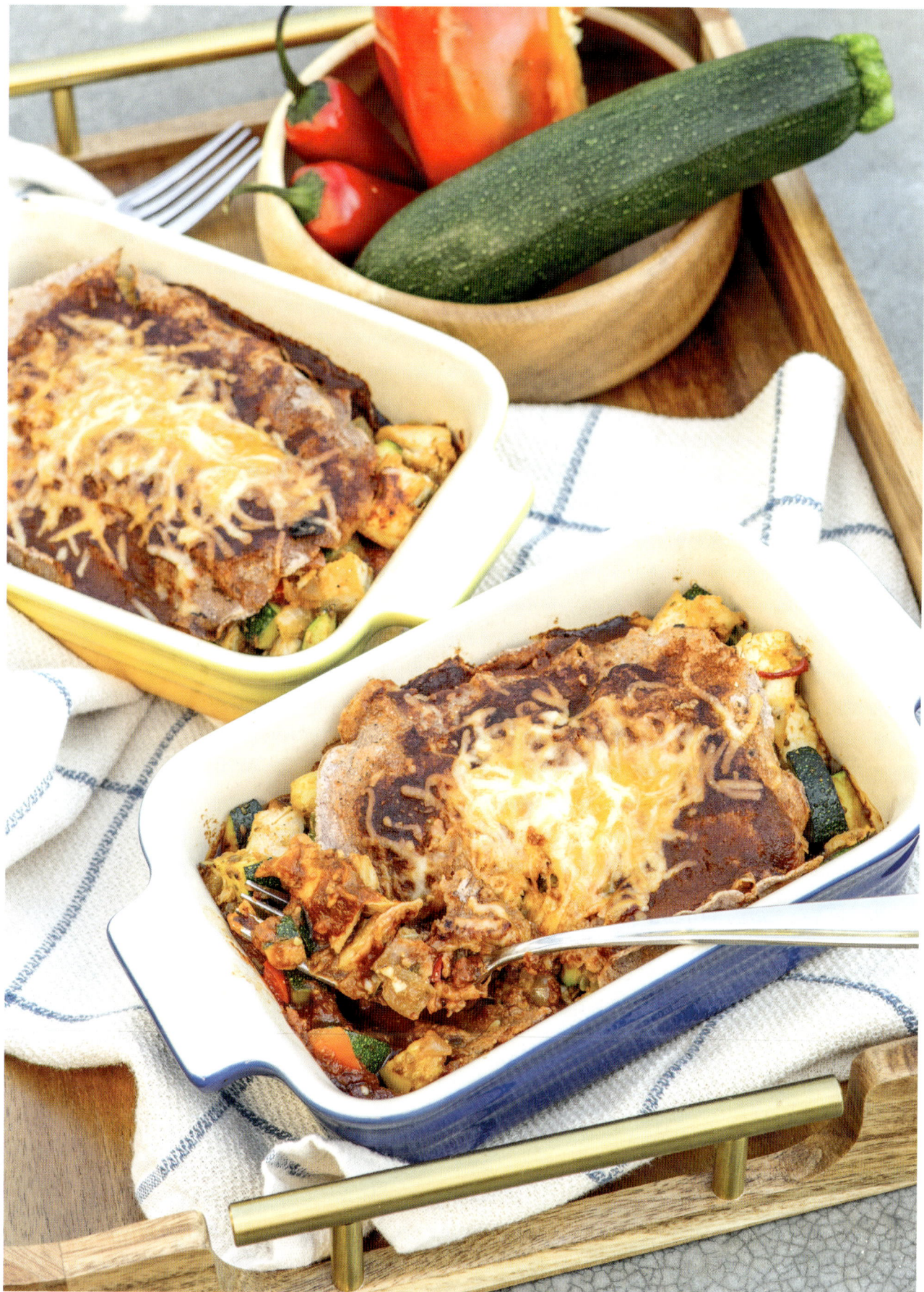

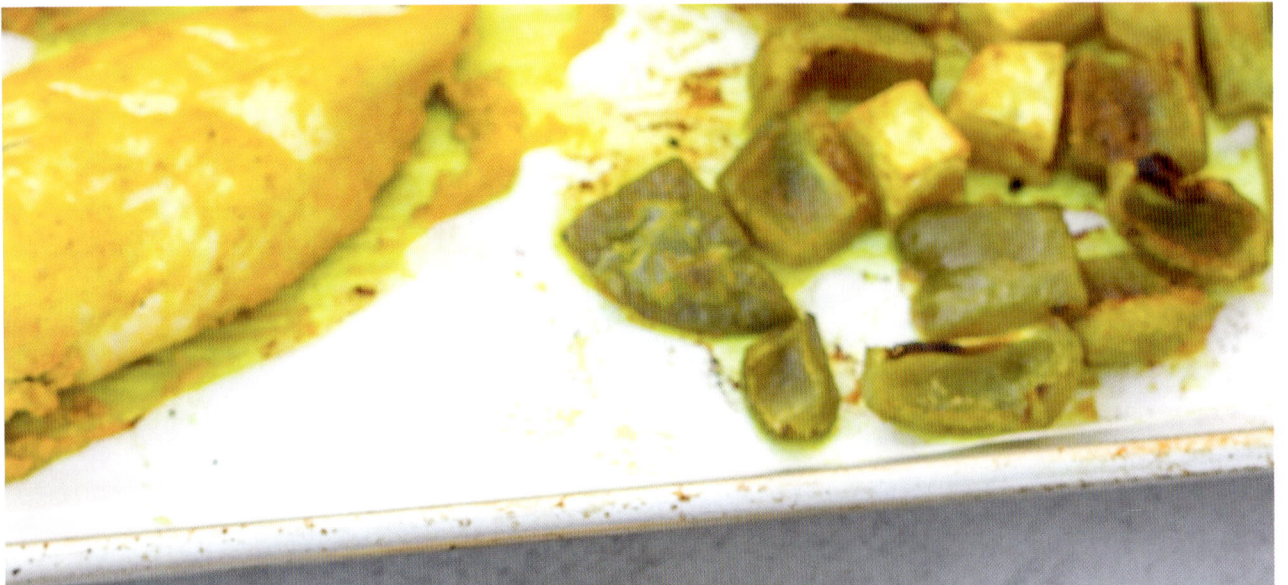

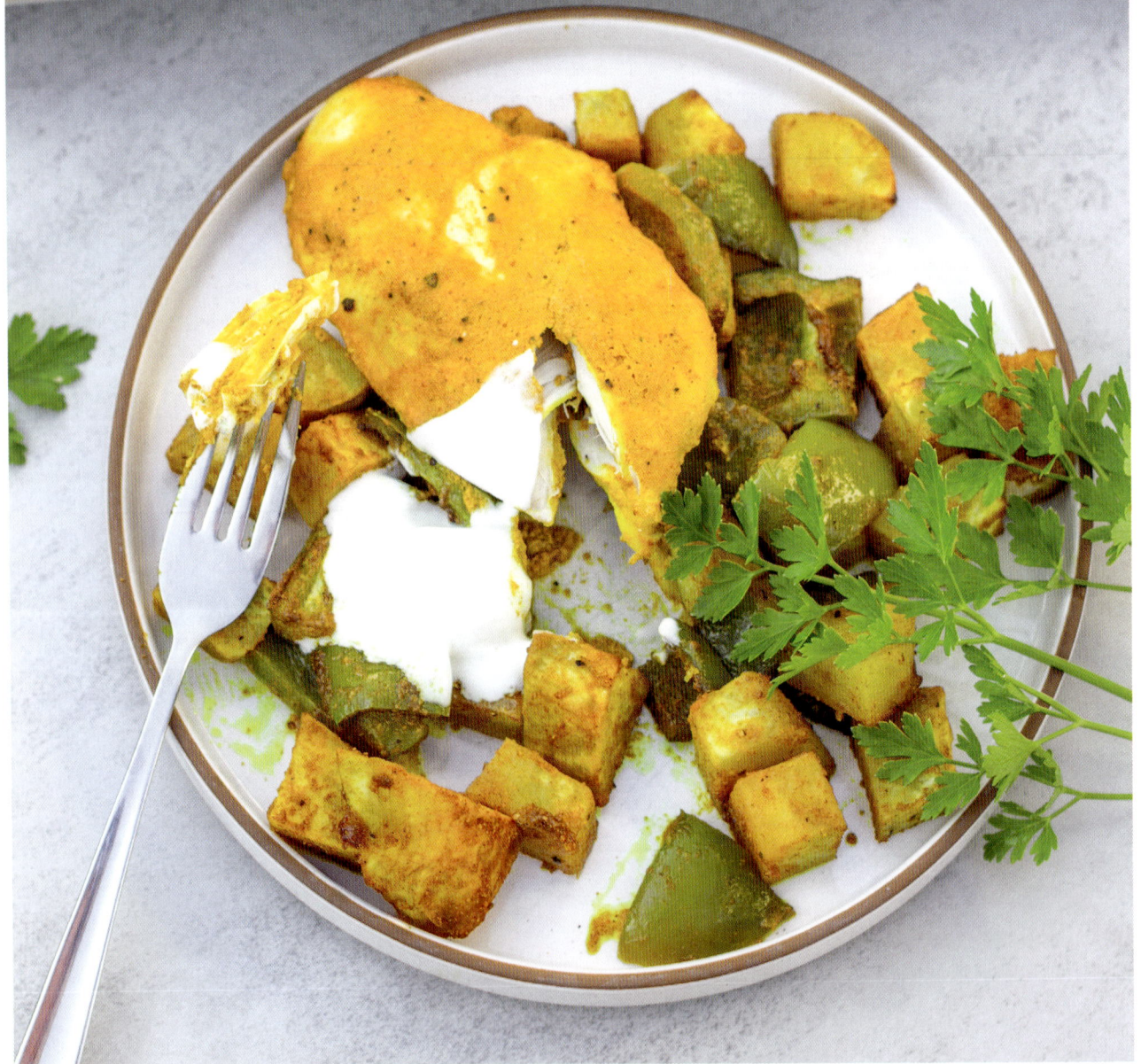

MOROCCAN-STYLE CHICKEN AND VEGGIES

SERVES 4

PREP TIME 5 minutes, plus 30 minutes to marinate chicken

COOK TIME 20 minutes

Marinating skinless chicken in yogurt helps keep it tender and delicious. It can be marinated the night before you plan to cook it, which helps limit day-of prep time.

SPICE MIX

2 teaspoons ground coriander

2 teaspoons ground cumin

2 teaspoons garlic powder

2 teaspoons salt

1 teaspoon ground cinnamon

1 teaspoon turmeric powder

½ teaspoon cayenne pepper

½ teaspoon ground black pepper

CHICKEN AND VEGGIES

1 pound boneless, skinless chicken breasts or thighs

1 cup plain whole milk Greek yogurt, store-bought or homemade (page 81), divided

Juice of 1 lemon (2 to 3 tablespoons)

2 medium sweet potatoes, peeled and cut into 1-inch chunks

2 bell peppers (any color), cut into 1- to 2-inch chunks

2 tablespoons olive oil

Fresh parsley, for garnish

1. In a small bowl, combine all of the ingredients for the spice mix.

2. In a large zip-top plastic bag, combine the chicken, yogurt, lemon juice, and half of the spice mix. With the bag sealed shut, massage the ingredients into the chicken so that everything is evenly distributed. Place in the fridge to marinate for at least 30 minutes or up to 24 hours.

3. Preheat the oven to 425°F. Line a sheet pan with parchment paper.

4. Put the sweet potatoes, bell peppers, olive oil, and the remaining half of the spice mix on one half of the prepared sheet pan. Toss to combine. On the other half of the pan, arrange the chicken, carefully shaking off the excess marinade. (Discard the marinade.)

5. Bake for 20 minutes, or until the internal temperature of the chicken reaches 165°F.

6. Top the chicken with the remaining ½ cup of yogurt and garnish with parsley.

BALSAMIC GRILLED CHICKEN

SERVES 4

PREP TIME 5 minutes, plus 30 minutes to marinate chicken

COOK TIME 16 minutes

I'm not the biggest fan of chicken breast because I find it very hard to cook right. It always seems to come out too dry or undercooked. That's why I love a good marinade. It infuses the chicken with flavor while preventing it from drying out during the cooking process. This Balsamic Grilled Chicken uses pantry items that you probably already have on hand for a protein-packed main dish. Make sure to pair it with one of my veggie sides, like the Garden House Salad (page 123) or Cauliflower Avocado Tabbouleh (page 234), to make it a complete meal.

⅓ cup olive oil

¼ cup balsamic vinegar

1 tablespoon dried basil leaves

2 teaspoons garlic powder

1 teaspoon salt

4 boneless, skinless chicken breasts (about 2 pounds)

1. In a large zip-top plastic bag, combine the olive oil, balsamic, basil, garlic powder, and salt by lightly swirling or shaking the bag. Add the chicken breasts and seal the bag, being careful to squeeze out as much air as possible. Place in the refrigerator to marinate for at least 30 minutes or up to 24 hours.

2. Preheat a grill to medium heat (350°F to 375°F). Once preheated, place the chicken breasts on the grill, making sure to shake off any excess marinade first. (Discard the marinade.) Cook for 8 minutes, then flip and grill for another 8 minutes, or until the internal temperature of the chicken is 165°F.

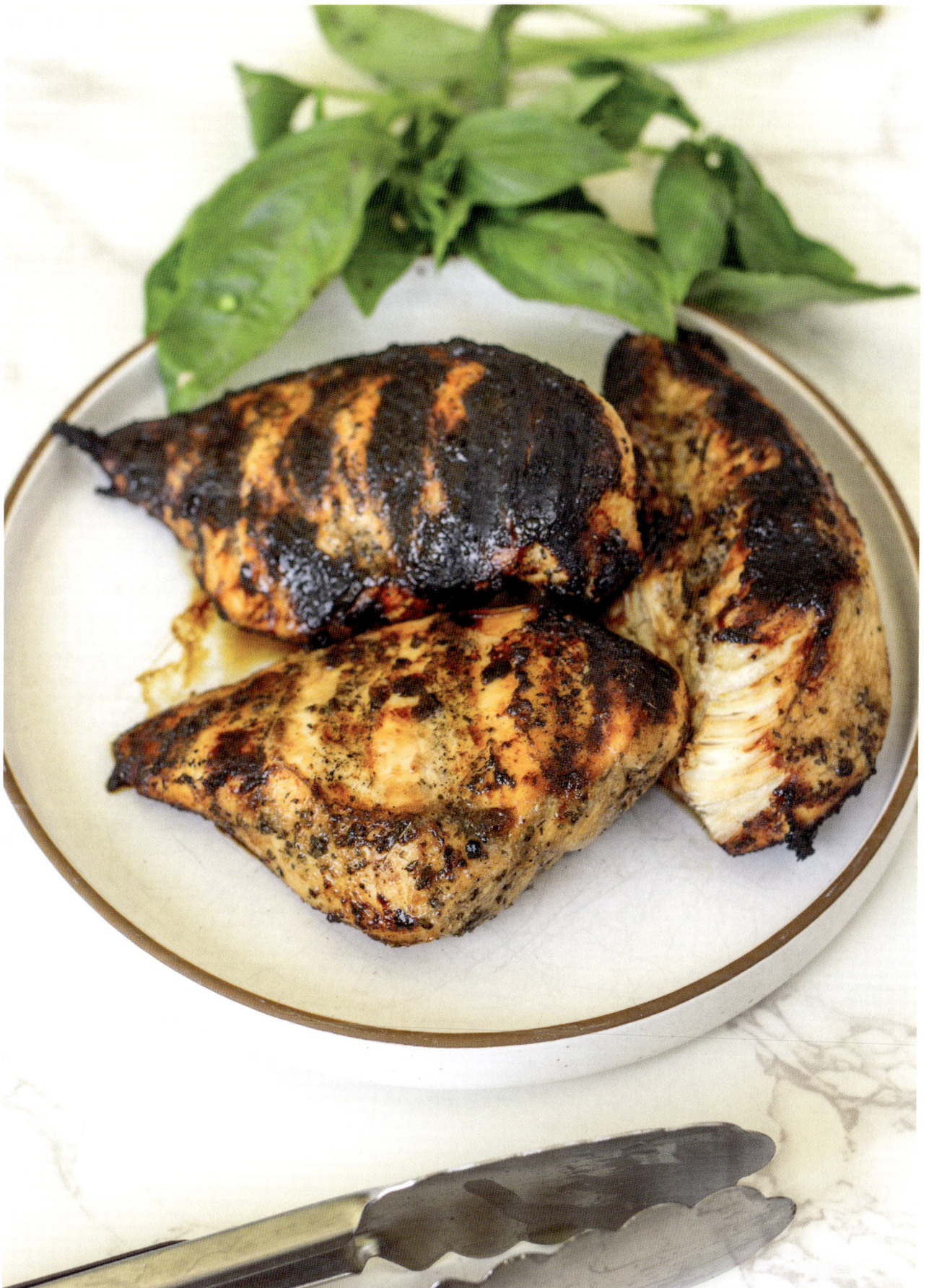

SPICED CHICKEN AND CHICKPEAS
WITH QUICK PICKLED CARROTS

SERVES 4

PREP TIME 10 minutes, plus 30 minutes to marinate chicken

COOK TIME 30 minutes

I created this meal when clearing my fridge of leftovers. I had chicken, pickled carrots, fresh mozzarella, and crispy baked chickpeas on hand. At first, it seemed like a typical fridge cleanout dinner that was eaten out of necessity. But after taking a bite, I realized this combination was worthy of its own recipe that I could make again and again. It's slightly sour, crunchy, and so flavorful. Best part, it makes an amazing lunch the next day.

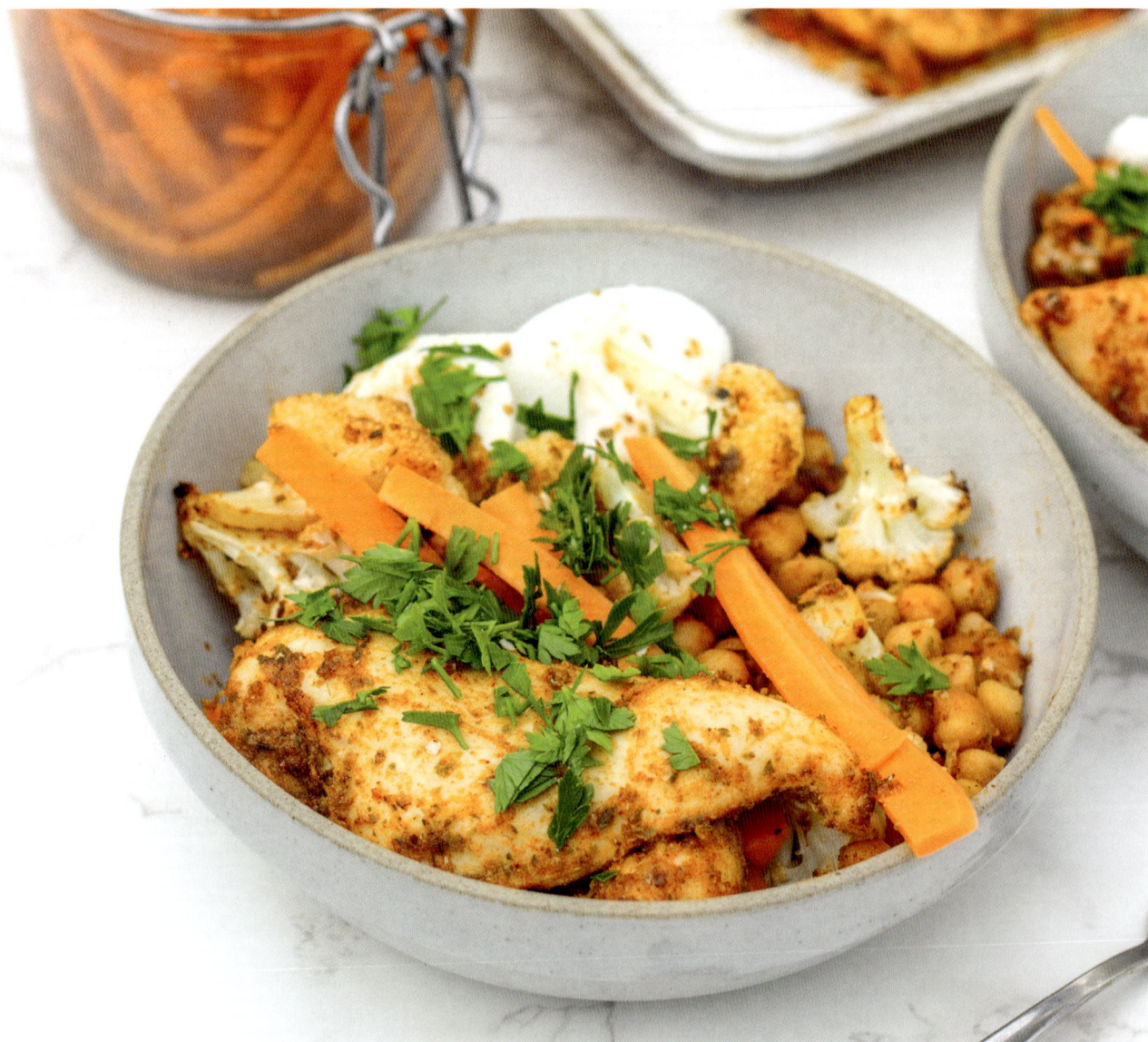

SPICED CHICKEN AND CHICKPEAS

2 teaspoons garlic powder

2 teaspoons onion powder

2 teaspoons dried oregano leaves

2 teaspoons smoked paprika

1 teaspoon salt

¼ teaspoon cayenne pepper

4 small boneless, skinless chicken breasts (about 1¼ pounds)

2 tablespoons olive oil, divided

Juice of 1 lemon (2 to 3 tablespoons)

1 cup cooked chickpeas, canned or homemade (page 85)

1 small head cauliflower, chopped into florets

QUICK PICKLED CARROTS

1 cup apple cider vinegar

½ cup water

2 cloves garlic, sliced

1 teaspoon dried oregano leaves

½ teaspoon salt

4 medium carrots, cut into matchsticks

OTHER TOPPINGS

8 ounces fresh mozzarella cheese, thinly sliced

1 cup chopped fresh parsley

1. Put the garlic powder, onion powder, oregano, paprika, salt, and cayenne in a small bowl and stir to combine. Pour half of the mixture into a large zip-top plastic bag.

2. Add the chicken, 1 tablespoon of the olive oil, and the lemon juice. Seal the bag and massage the marinade into the chicken. Refrigerate for at least 30 minutes or up to 24 hours.

3. While the chicken marinates, make the quick pickled carrots: Bring the vinegar and water to a boil in a sauce pot. Add the garlic, oregano, and salt. Give it a stir, reduce the heat to a simmer, and cook for 1 minute. Remove the pot from the heat and allow to cool for 10 minutes. Put the carrots in a 1-quart mason jar and pour the cooled vinegar mixture into the jar. Let sit at room temperature, uncovered, for 30 minutes.

4. Preheat the oven to 425°F and line a sheet pan with parchment paper.

5. Put the chickpeas, cauliflower, remaining half of the spice mixture, and remaining tablespoon of olive oil on the prepared sheet pan. Toss with your hands to combine and spread out the ingredients. Arrange the marinated chicken on the pan, nestling it among the chickpeas and cauliflower. Bake for 25 minutes, or until the chickpeas and cauliflower are lightly browned and crispy and the internal temperature of the chicken reaches 165°F.

6. Split the chicken and veggie mixture among four bowls. Top each bowl with one-quarter of the pickled carrots, 2 ounces of mozzarella, and ¼ cup of parsley.

COZY COCONUT CHICKEN AND VEGGIES

SERVES 4

PREP TIME 5 minutes

COOK TIME 32 minutes

I accidentally created this recipe when I was planning to make a curry and then realized that I didn't have all of the necessary ingredients. Instead of curry powder, I tried seasonings like cumin, garlic powder, and paprika to make a Mexican-inspired "stew." Thankfully, this recipe uses many pantry and freezer staples for a quick and easy weeknight meal. I recommend starting the cauliflower rice while the chicken is cooking so that all of the components are ready to serve at the same time. If you're physically active or working toward a fitness goal, you can add a diced sweet potato when you add the zucchini in step 3.

2 teaspoons ground cumin

2 teaspoons garlic powder

2 teaspoons dried oregano leaves

2 teaspoons paprika

¼ teaspoon cayenne pepper

Salt

1½ pounds boneless, skinless chicken thighs

1 tablespoon olive oil

1 jalapeño pepper, diced (remove membranes and seeds if you prefer less heat)

½ medium yellow onion, diced

2 medium zucchini, cut into 1-inch cubes

2 medium carrots, cut into 1-inch cubes

1 (14-ounce) can full-fat coconut milk

1 (14-ounce) can crushed tomatoes

8 ounces frozen peas

4 cups fresh cauliflower rice, store-bought or homemade (see note, page 234), for serving

1. In a small bowl, stir together the cumin, garlic powder, oregano, paprika, cayenne, and 1 teaspoon of salt. Lay the chicken thighs on a plate or in a bowl and sprinkle half of the spice mixture over them, ensuring that all sides are covered.

2. Heat the olive oil in a Dutch oven or medium-sized pot over medium heat. Add the chicken thighs and cook for 7 minutes, then flip the thighs. Continue cooking for another 7 minutes, or until the chicken is cooked all the way through and the internal temperature is 165°F. Remove the chicken and place on a plate.

3. Dump the jalapeño and onion into the pot. Sprinkle with a heavy pinch of salt. Sauté for 3 minutes, or until the onion is softened. Add the zucchini and carrots and sauté for another 5 minutes, until slightly softened. Pour in the coconut milk, tomatoes, peas, and remaining half of the spice mixture and give it a stir. Return the chicken thighs to the pot. Raise the heat to bring the mixture to a boil, then reduce to a simmer. Cover and cook for 10 minutes, or until the zucchini and carrots are fork-tender.

4. To serve, put 1 cup of prepared cauliflower rice in each of four bowls. Ladle the chicken and veggies into the bowls, ensuring that each bowl gets the same amount of chicken.

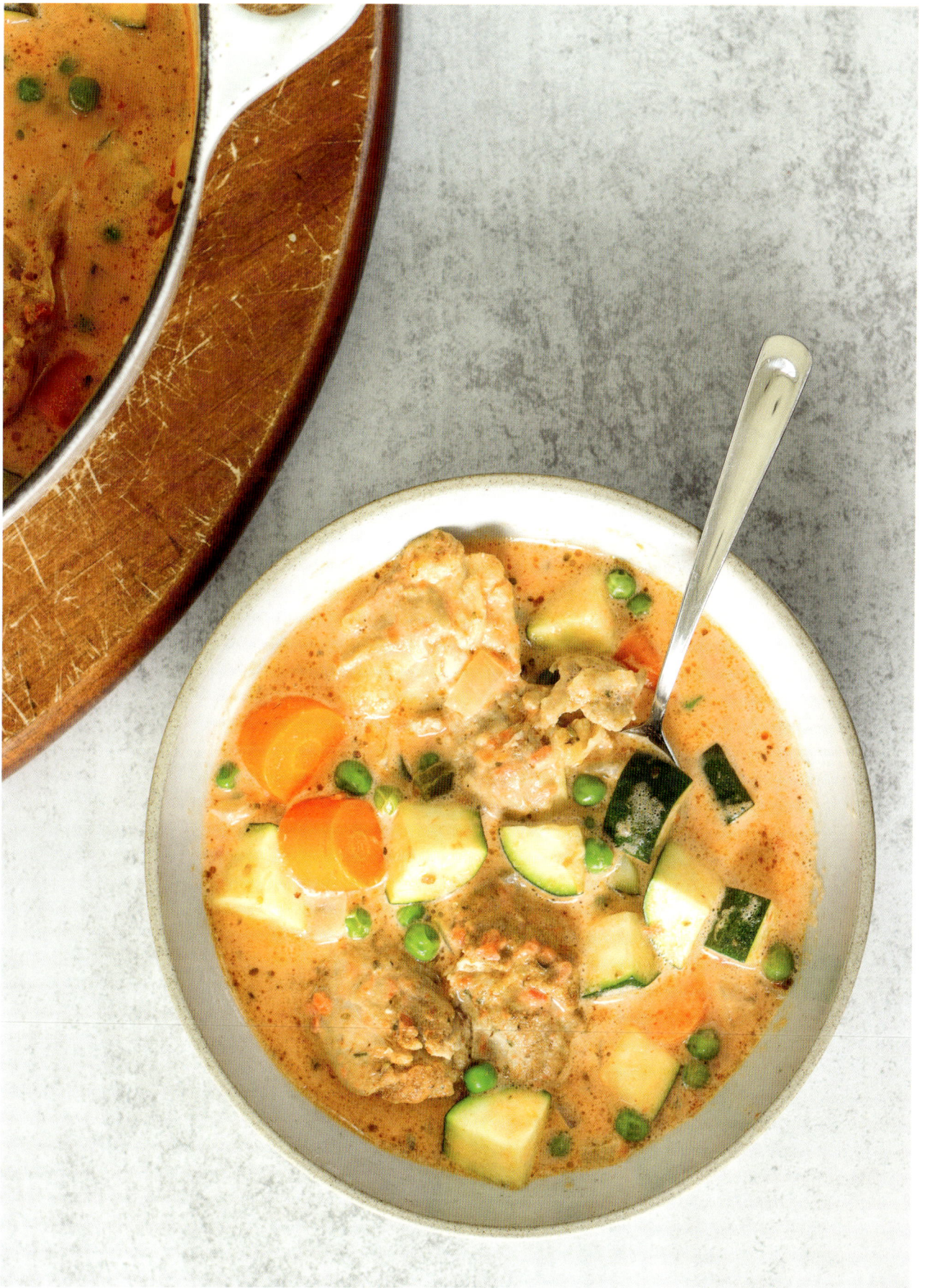

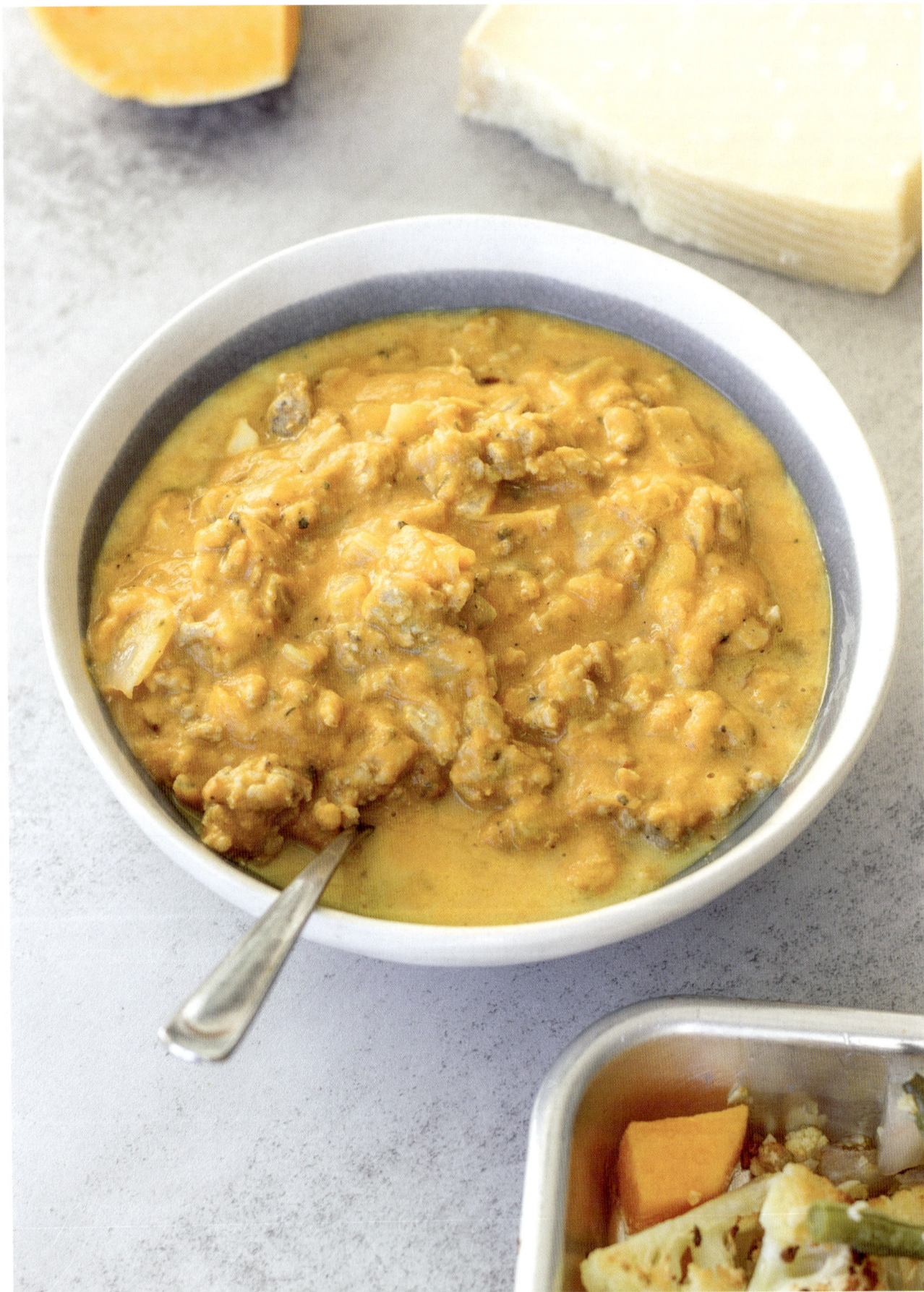

PUMPKIN, CHICKEN, AND ROASTED VEGGIE BOWL

SERVES 4

PREP TIME 10 minutes

COOK TIME 30 minutes

I know I'm not unique in feeling like fall is in the air when the calendar hits August. Even though the days are still hot, there's a definite change to the atmosphere letting us know that sweater weather and latte season are nearly here. This recipe screams fall—or should I say Autumn? ;) Not only is this dish loaded with micronutrient-dense veggies and satiety-promoting protein, but it has the perfect balance of flavor and creamy goodness too. I also love that this recipe is a super fast and easy weeknight meal that can be prepped in less than an hour.

1 medium head cauliflower, chopped into florets

2 cups cubed butternut squash

2 cups trimmed and halved green beans

1 small red onion, cut into thick strips

6 cloves garlic, minced

1 teaspoon olive oil, plus extra for drizzling

Salt

1 small yellow onion, diced

1½ pounds ground chicken

½ teaspoon ground nutmeg

½ teaspoon dried oregano leaves

¼ teaspoon ground cinnamon

⅛ teaspoon red pepper flakes

1 cup chicken bone broth

1 cup canned pumpkin puree

¼ cup heavy cream

1 cup shredded Parmesan cheese

1. Preheat the oven to 425°F and line a sheet pan with parchment paper.

2. Put the cauliflower, squash, green beans, red onion, and one-third of the minced garlic on the prepared pan. Top with a drizzle of olive oil and a heavy pinch of salt and toss to combine. Roast for 25 to 30 minutes, until the veggies are slightly browned and crispy.

3. In a medium-sized skillet, heat the 1 teaspoon of olive oil over medium heat. Add the yellow onion, remaining two-thirds of the garlic, and a pinch of salt. Sauté for 3 minutes, or until the veggies are softened and fragrant.

4. Add the chicken, nutmeg, oregano, cinnamon, red pepper flakes, and another heavy pinch of salt. Cook the chicken, breaking it up with a rubber spatula as it cooks, until browned, about 10 minutes.

5. Add the broth, pumpkin, and heavy cream and stir to combine. Bring the mixture to a boil, then reduce to a simmer and cook for 10 minutes. After 10 minutes, turn off the heat and stir in the Parmesan and one more heavy pinch of salt.

6. Serve the pumpkin chicken in bowls with the roasted veggies.

SUMMER GRILLED CHICKEN BOWL

SERVES 4

PREP TIME 10 minutes, plus 30 minutes to marinate chicken

COOK TIME 25 minutes

This recipe uses up some of the best ingredients that late summer has to offer: fresh carrots, beets, tomatoes, and sweet potatoes. I balanced the roasted and grilled components with crunchy and refreshing lettuce and cucumber. The recipe is quite simple but creates a beautiful display, making it perfect for get-togethers and dinner parties. Leftovers also store well, so feel free to double the recipe for your next day's lunch.

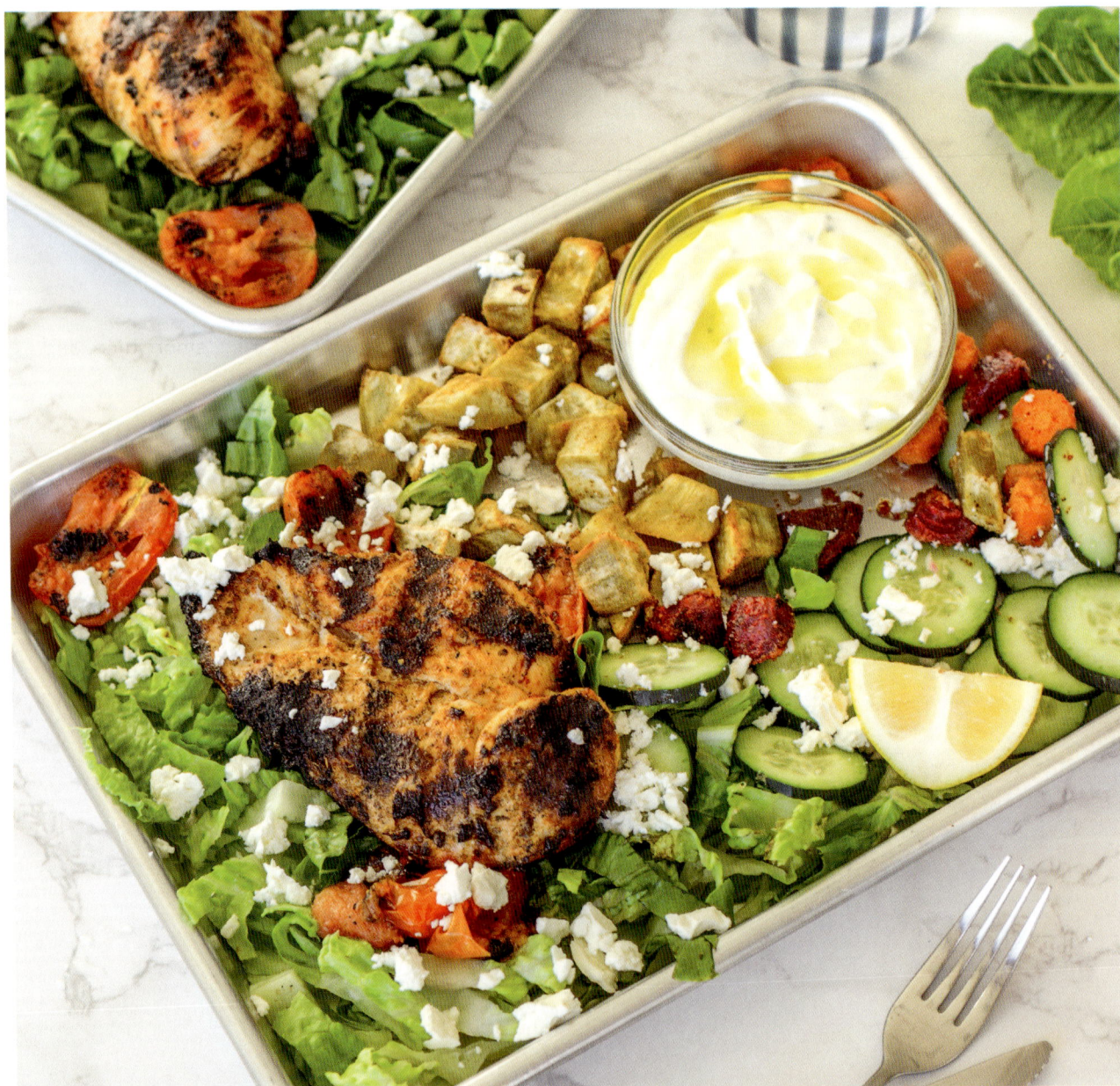

GRILLED CHICKEN

1 tablespoon olive oil

Grated zest and juice of
1 lemon (2 to 3 tablespoons)

1 teaspoon garlic powder

1 teaspoon dried oregano
leaves

1 teaspoon paprika

½ teaspoon salt

1¼ pounds boneless,
skinless chicken breasts
(about 4 small)

ROASTED VEGGIES

3 medium sweet potatoes,
peeled and cut into cubes

4 medium carrots, cut into
1-inch chunks

2 medium beets, peeled and
cut into 1-inch chunks

1 tablespoon olive oil

1 teaspoon ground cumin

1 teaspoon garlic powder

⅛ teaspoon cayenne pepper

Salt

GARLIC YOGURT SAUCE

1 cup plain whole milk Greek
yogurt, store-bought or
homemade (page 81)

2 tablespoons olive oil

2 cloves garlic, minced

Juice of ½ lemon (1 to
1½ tablespoons)

Salt and pepper

OTHER INGREDIENTS

1 large tomato, sliced, or 8 to
10 cherry or grape tomatoes

Olive oil

Salt

1 medium cucumber, thinly
sliced

4 cups finely chopped
romaine lettuce

½ cup crumbled feta cheese

1. Marinate the chicken: Place the olive oil, lemon zest and juice, garlic powder, oregano, paprika, salt, and chicken in a large zip-top plastic bag. Seal the bag and mix well, ensuring that each chicken breast is evenly coated. Place in the fridge to marinate for 30 minutes or up to 24 hours.

2. Preheat the oven to 425°F and line a sheet pan with parchment paper.

3. Roast the veggies: Place the sweet potatoes, carrots, and beets on the prepared pan. Drizzle the olive oil and sprinkle the cumin, garlic powder, cayenne, and a heavy pinch of salt over the veggies. Toss to evenly coat and roast for 25 minutes.

4. Grill the chicken: Preheat a grill to medium-high heat (425°F to 450°F). Once hot, place the chicken on the grill, making sure to gently shake off the excess marinade first. Cover the grill and set a timer for 8 minutes. Discard the marinade.

5. While the chicken cooks, coat the tomato slices with a little olive oil and a pinch of salt. Place on the grill for 4 minutes. Once done, remove the tomatoes and place on a plate.

6. After 8 minutes, flip the chicken and grill for another 8 minutes, or until the internal temperature reaches 165°F. Once done, remove the chicken from the grill and let it rest for 10 minutes while you prepare the rest of the ingredients.

7. Make the sauce: Put the yogurt, olive oil, garlic, lemon juice, and a heavy pinch each of salt and pepper in a measuring cup. Stir with a fork to combine.

8. Evenly divide the cucumber slices, lettuce, and feta among four bowls or plates. Top with the roasted veggies, grilled chicken, and grilled tomatoes. Serve with the garlic yogurt sauce.

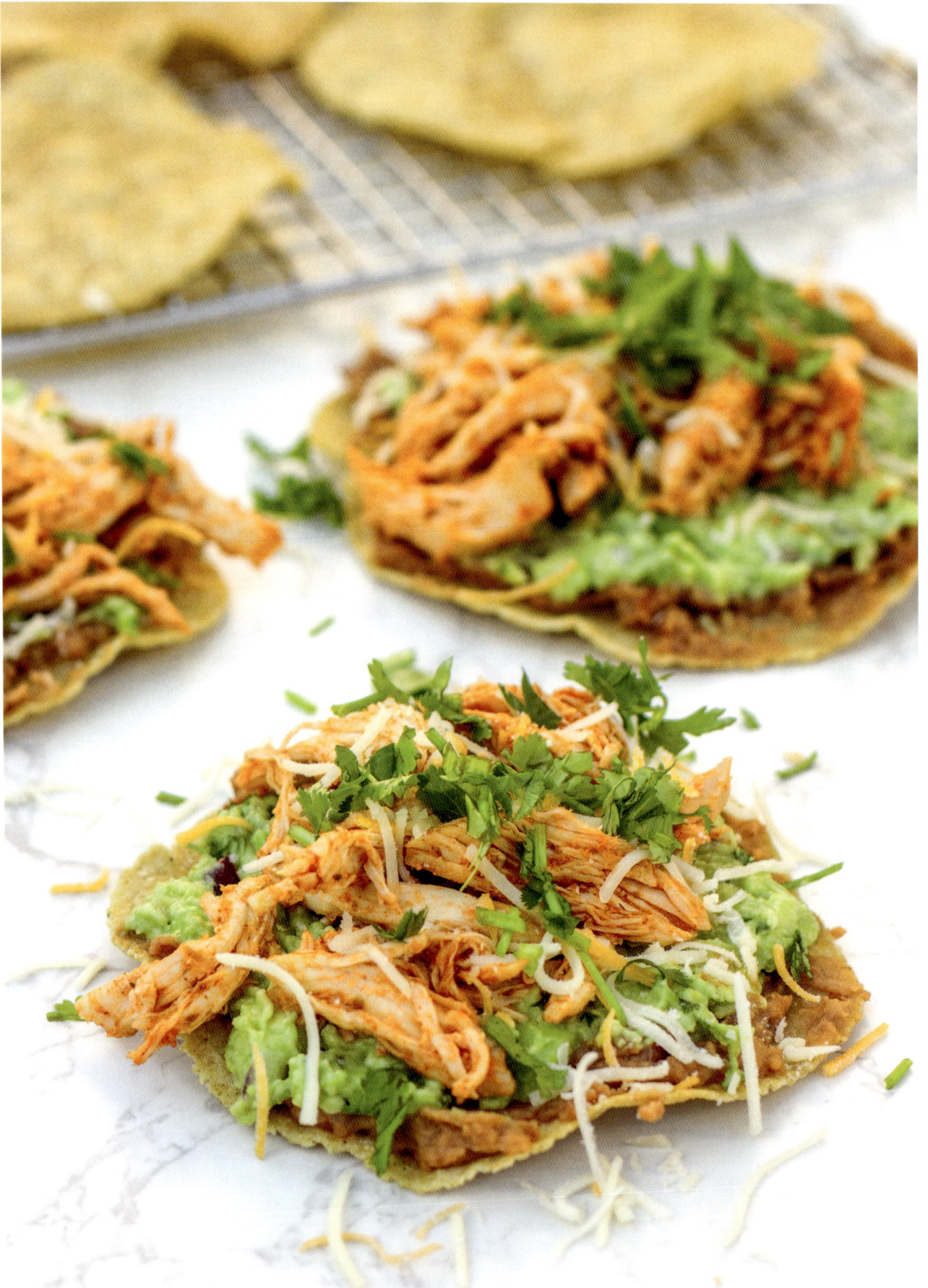

CHICKEN TOSTADAS

SERVES 4

PREP TIME 10 minutes
(not including time to
make guacamole)

COOK TIME 20 minutes

Crunchy tostadas are always a crowd-pleaser. They look impressive, but they're actually super simple to throw together. I like to make my own tostadas by baking homemade corn tortillas in the oven with a little bit of avocado oil and salt. The end result is light and crunchy without all of the inflammatory seed oils you normally would find in store-bought tostada shells.

8 (6-inch) corn tortillas, store-bought or homemade (page 77)

Avocado oil, for brushing

Salt

1 cup chicken bone broth

1 tablespoon tomato paste

1 tablespoon honey

Juice of ½ lime (about 1 tablespoon)

½ teaspoon ground cumin

½ teaspoon dried oregano leaves

½ teaspoon smoked paprika

¼ teaspoon garlic powder

¼ teaspoon onion powder

¼ teaspoon cayenne pepper

½ batch Easy Poached Chicken (page 80), or 3 cups rotisserie chicken, shredded

1 (16-ounce) can refried beans

2 cups Guacamole (page 237)

½ cup Mexican-style shredded cheese

Chopped fresh cilantro, for garnish

1. Preheat the oven to 400°F.

2. Lightly brush both sides of each tortilla with avocado oil. Sprinkle with a pinch of salt. Place on a sheet pan and bake for 4 minutes, or until the tortillas start to get lightly browned. Flip the tortillas and bake for another 4 minutes, or until the other sides start to get lightly browned. Remove from the oven and allow to cool on a plate or wire rack while you prepare the rest of the ingredients.

3. Put the broth, tomato paste, honey, lime juice, cumin, oregano, paprika, garlic powder, onion powder, cayenne, and a heavy pinch of salt in a medium-sized saucepan over medium-high heat. Stir to combine, then reduce to a simmer for 5 minutes, or until the sauce starts to thicken. Add the chicken and toss to coat each piece. Simmer for another 5 minutes to warm the chicken through.

4. Assemble the tostadas: Lay two tortillas side by side on a plate. Spread 2 to 3 tablespoons of refried beans on each base. Layer on ¼ cup of guacamole and 2 ounces of chicken, then top with 1 tablespoon of cheese. Garnish with cilantro. Repeat the process with the remaining ingredients to make eight tostadas.

CHICKEN MARINARA DIPPERS

SERVES 4

PREP TIME 20 minutes

COOK TIME 20 minutes

This simple weeknight meal combines my love for a good marinara sauce with classic chicken tenders. It's a great family-friendly meal option that even my toddler loves! I recommend pairing this dish with the Garden House Salad on page 123.

½ cup almond flour

½ cup shredded Parmesan cheese

1 teaspoon garlic powder

1 teaspoon onion powder

Salt

1 large egg

1¼ pounds boneless, skinless chicken breasts, cut into tenders or strips

2 tablespoons olive oil

½ medium yellow onion, diced

4 cloves garlic, minced

1 (28-ounce) can crushed tomatoes

1 teaspoon dried basil leaves

¼ teaspoon dried oregano leaves

1. Preheat the oven to 425°F and line a sheet pan with parchment paper.

2. Put the almond flour, Parmesan, garlic powder, onion powder, and ½ teaspoon of salt on a large plate. Mix with your fingers to combine. In a bowl, whisk the egg. Line it up so that the egg bowl is first, then the almond flour plate, and then your prepared sheet pan.

3. Bread the chicken: Dip a chicken tender in the egg bowl and shake off any excess egg. Then place it on the almond flour plate and dredge it in the mixture, pressing it into the chicken. Shake off the excess flour and place on the sheet pan. Repeat the process with the remaining chicken strips.

4. Bake the chicken for 18 minutes, or until the internal temperature reaches 165°F and the breading is golden.

5. While the chicken cooks, make the marinara sauce: In a large saucepan over medium heat, combine the olive oil and onion. Sauté for 3 minutes, or until the onion is softened. Add the garlic and a heavy pinch of salt. Sauté for 1 minute before adding the tomatoes, basil, oregano, and another heavy pinch of salt. Stir to combine and reduce the heat to a simmer. Let the sauce simmer, stirring occasionally, while the chicken finishes baking.

6. Serve the chicken strips with a bowl of marinara sauce for dipping.

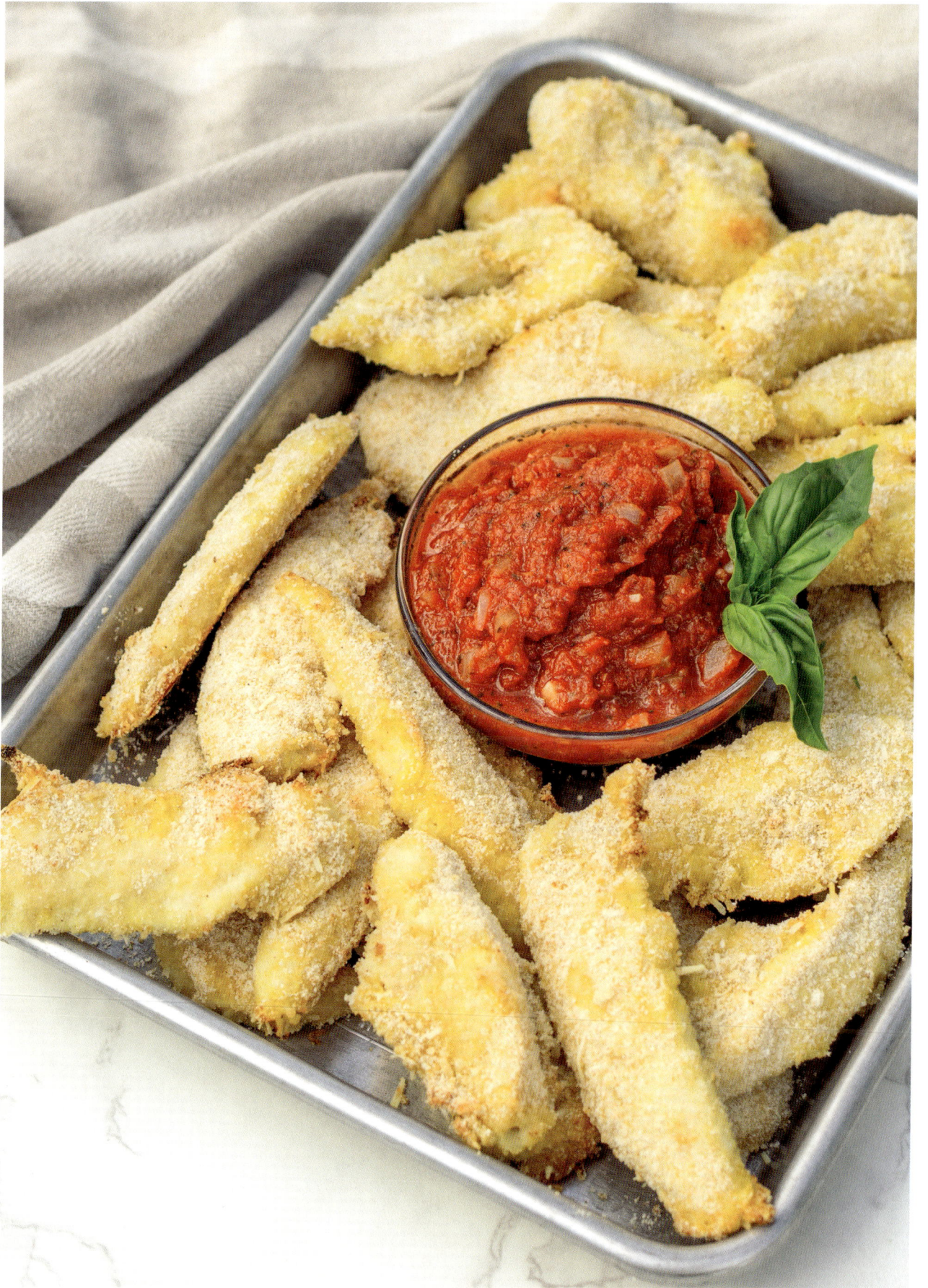

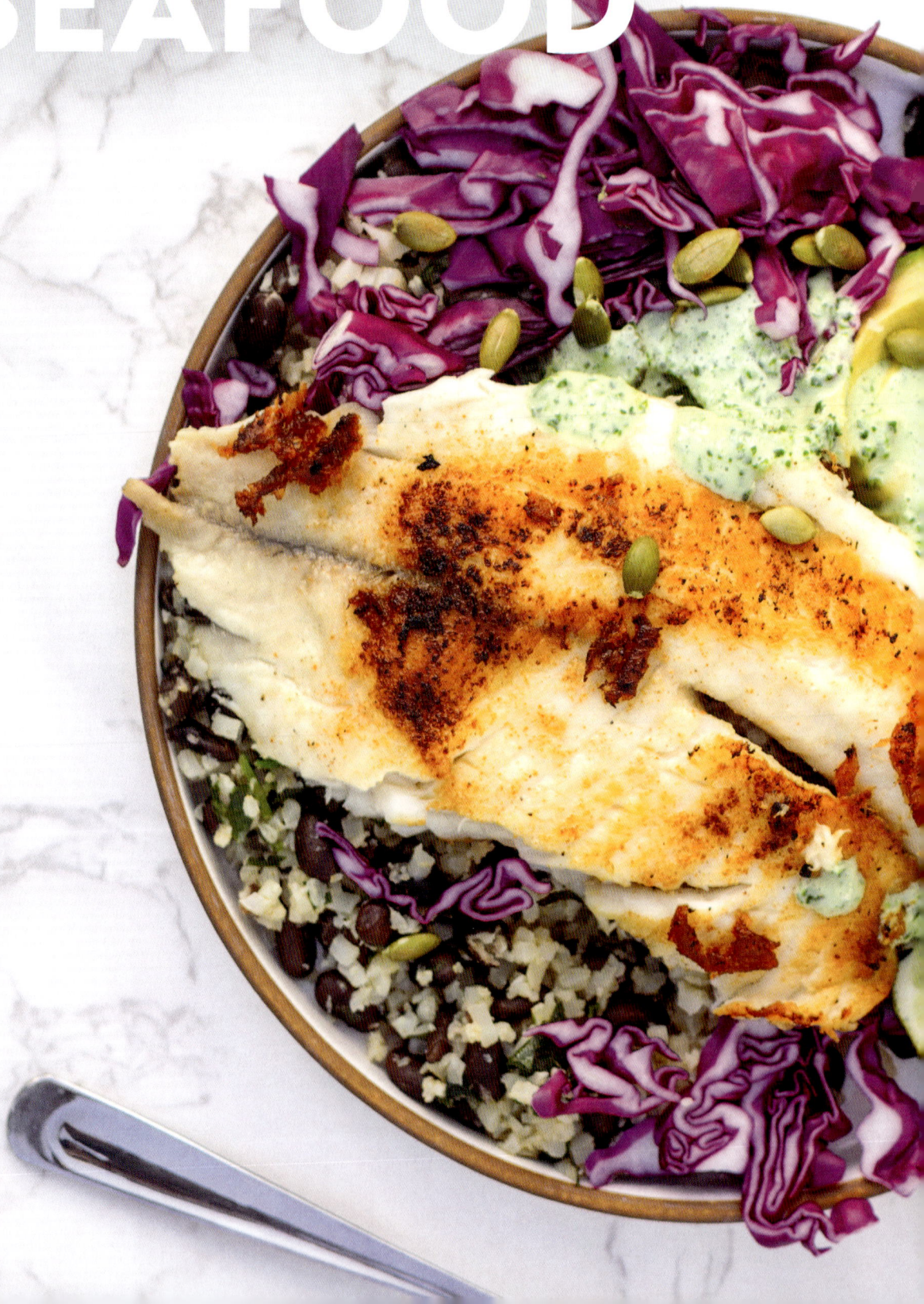

SEAFOOD

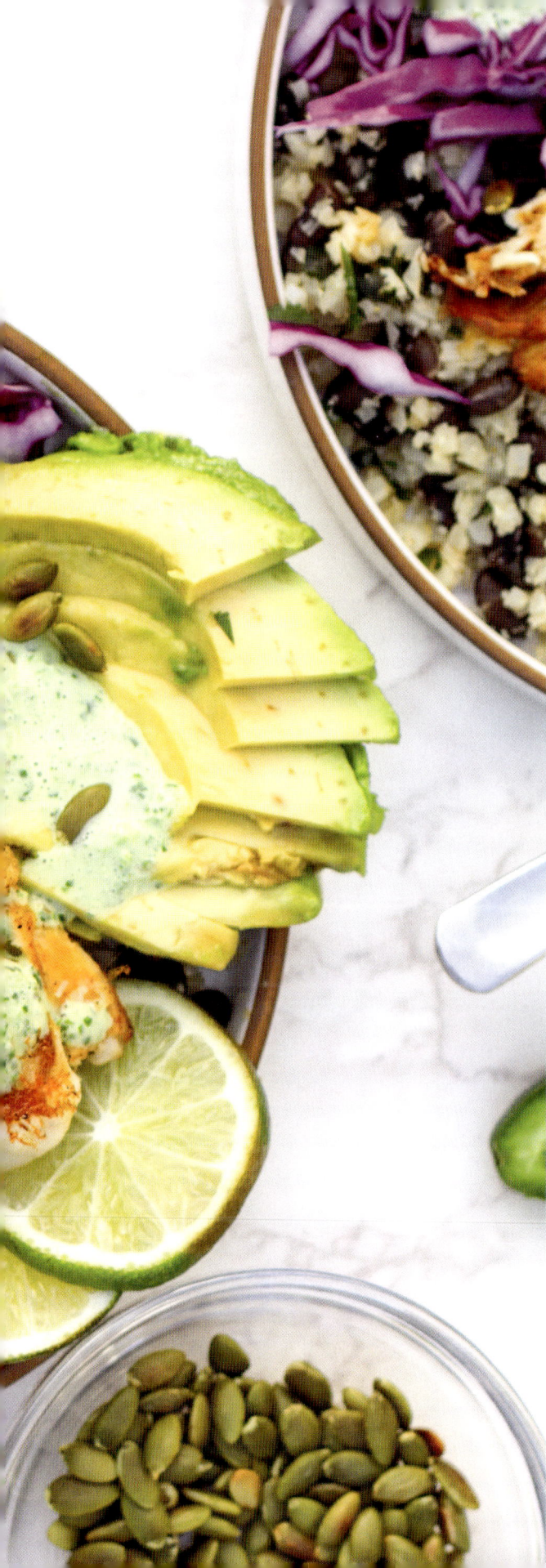

GREEK SALMON WITH ASPARAGUS AND CRISPY SWEET POTATOES

SERVES 4

PREP TIME 5 minutes

COOK TIME 25 minutes

This is an easy, nutrient-dense weeknight meal that you need to add to your rotation. Because everything is cooked on two sheet pans, the cleanup is minimal, leaving more time for you to enjoy your meal. Plus, salmon is rich in protein and also a great source of anti-inflammatory omega-3 fatty acids. These are essential fats, meaning we must get them from our diet.

¼ cup olive oil

Juice of ½ lemon (1 to 1½ tablespoons)

4 cloves garlic, minced

1 teaspoon dried dill weed

1 teaspoon dried oregano leaves

½ teaspoon salt

2 medium sweet potatoes, peeled and cut into ¼-inch-thick rounds

4 (6-ounce) skin-on salmon fillets

1 pound asparagus, bottom 2 inches trimmed

1. Position one oven rack in the upper third and one in the lower third of the oven. Preheat the oven to 400°F and line two sheet pans with parchment paper.

2. In a small bowl, mix together the olive oil, lemon juice, garlic, dill, oregano, and salt.

3. On the first prepared pan, evenly lay out the sweet potato rounds so they aren't overlapping. Brush one-quarter of the olive oil mixture over the sweet potatoes. Bake on the upper rack for 25 minutes, flipping the rounds halfway through, until they are lightly browned along the edges.

4. While the sweet potatoes bake, prepare the salmon and asparagus: On the second prepared pan, arrange the salmon and asparagus, making sure that the asparagus spears are evenly spaced and not overlapping. Brush the remaining olive oil mixture over the salmon and asparagus. When the sweet potatoes have 12 minutes left to cook, put the salmon and asparagus in the oven on the lower rack and bake for the remaining 12 minutes, or until the internal temperature of the salmon reaches 145°F.

5. Remove both pans from the oven and serve immediately.

Note If you have time, I suggest soaking the sliced sweet potatoes in cold water for 30 minutes, then draining and patting them dry before baking. This helps the potatoes get a bit crispier. If you don't have time, though, you can throw them straight into the oven, and they'll still taste great.

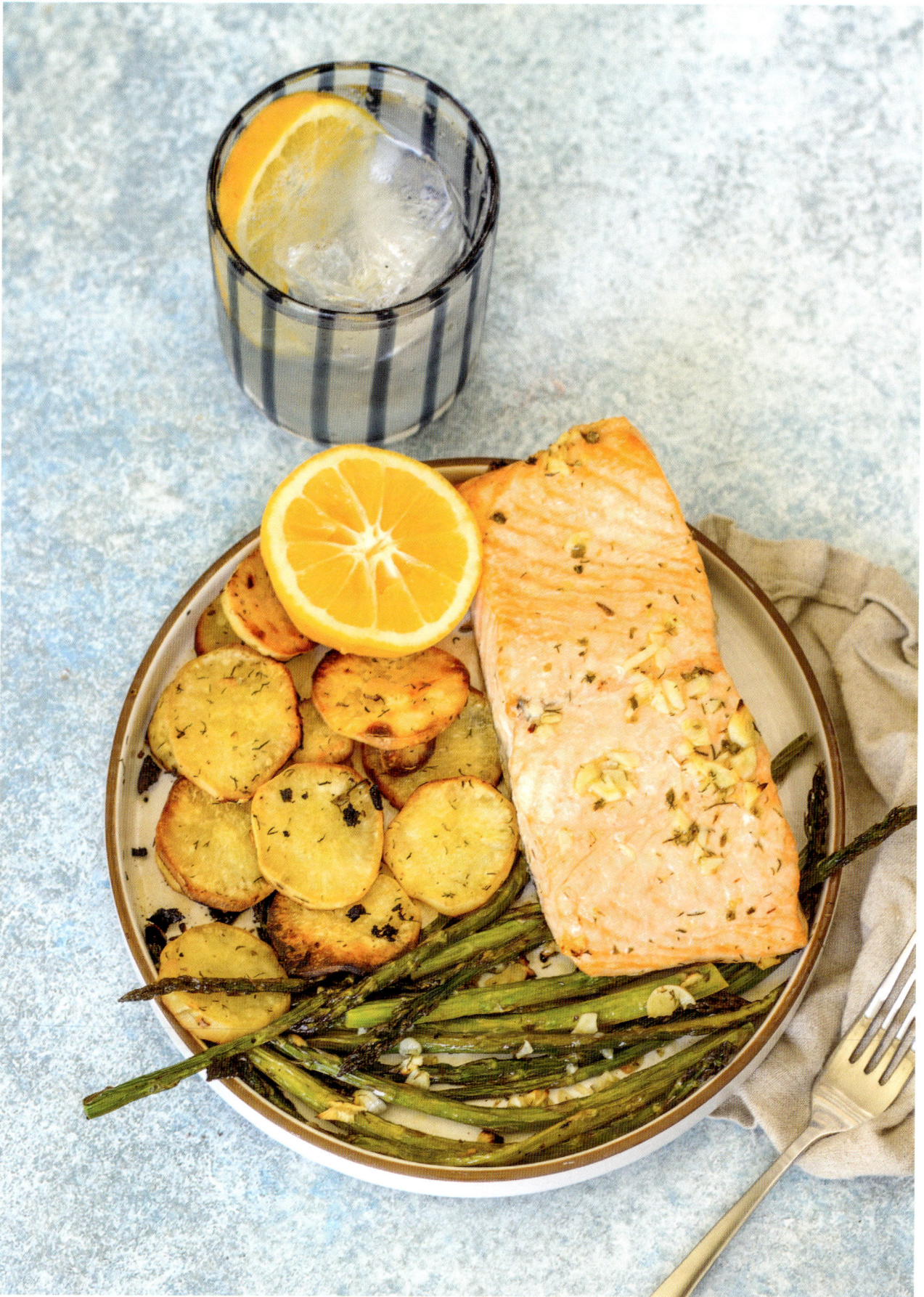

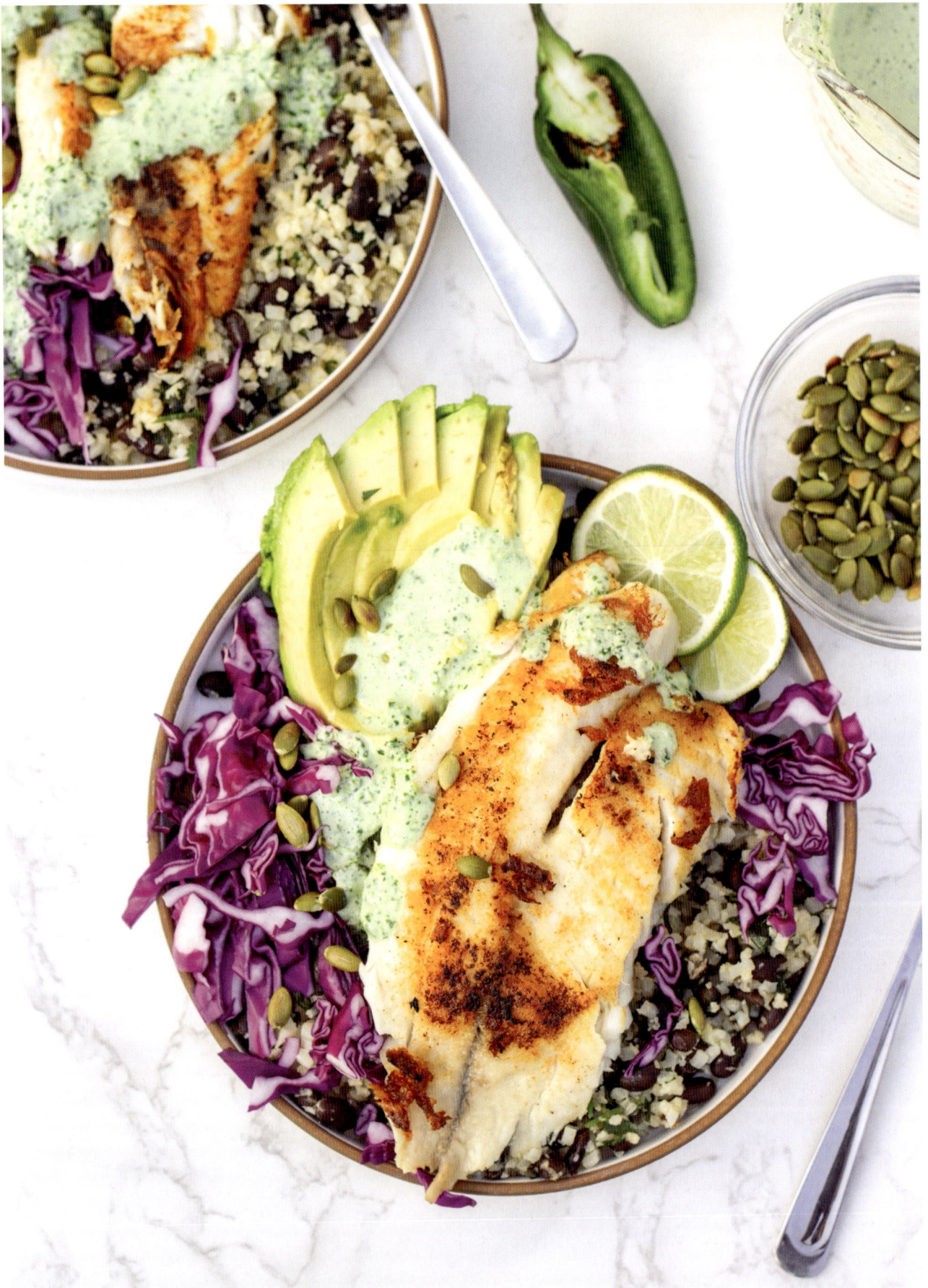

FISH TACO BOWLS

SERVES 4

PREP TIME 10 minutes

COOK TIME 15 minutes

This recipe might look complicated, but if you time it right, you can make it in less than 30 minutes. Start with the rice and beans, and while that component cooks, prep the fish. You can whip up the sauce in a matter of seconds if you have an immersion blender—a tool that I highly recommend investing in because it's super simple to use and keeps cleanup to a minimum. The sauce is well worth the few extra minutes of prep. My husband, Trevor, says that it reminds him of his favorite Peruvian restaurant from his hometown of Hermosa Beach. This is very high praise from him indeed.

CILANTRO LIME CAULIFLOWER RICE AND BEANS

1 teaspoon olive oil

4 cloves garlic, minced

4 cups cauliflower rice

1 cup cooked black beans, canned or homemade (page 85)

1 teaspoon ground cumin

Salt

½ cup chopped fresh cilantro

Grated zest and juice of 1 lime (about 2 tablespoons)

SPICED FISH

2 teaspoons paprika

1 teaspoon ground cumin

1 teaspoon garlic powder

1 teaspoon onion powder

1 teaspoon salt

1½ pounds white fish, such as cod, tilapia, halibut, or mahi mahi, cut into 4 (6-ounce) fillets

1 tablespoon olive oil

JALAPEÑO CILANTRO SAUCE

1 cup chopped fresh cilantro

½ cup plain whole milk Greek yogurt, store-bought or homemade (page 81)

Juice of 1 lime (about 2 tablespoons)

½ jalapeño pepper, chopped (remove membranes and seeds if you prefer less heat)

½ teaspoon garlic powder

¼ teaspoon ground cumin

¼ teaspoon salt

TOPPINGS

4 cups thinly sliced purple cabbage

2 avocados, peeled and sliced

4 tablespoons pumpkin seeds, toasted (see page 108)

Lime slices

1. Make the "rice" and beans: Heat the olive oil in a large skillet or wok over medium heat. Add the garlic and sauté for 1 minute. Add the cauliflower rice, black beans, cumin, and a heavy pinch of salt. Sauté for 6 minutes. Remove from the heat and transfer to a bowl. Add the cilantro and lime juice and toss to combine.

2. Prepare the fish: Put the paprika, cumin, garlic powder, onion powder, and salt in a small bowl and stir to combine. Pat the fish dry with a paper towel and sprinkle both sides of the fish with the spice mixture.

3. Heat the olive oil in a large skillet over medium-high heat. Add the fish and cook for 2 to 3 minutes on each side, until the internal temperature is 145°F.

4. Make the sauce: Place all of the ingredients in a small bowl or measuring cup and blend with an immersion blender until smooth. (You can also use a countertop blender or food processor.)

5. Assemble the bowls: Divide the rice and beans evenly among four serving bowls or plates. Top each bowl with one-quarter of the cooked fish, 1 cup of cabbage, ½ sliced avocado, and 1 tablespoon of toasted pumpkin seeds. Drizzle the sauce on top and serve with lime slices.

CURRIED SALMON SALAD

SERVES 4

PREP TIME 5 minutes (not including time to cook salmon if not using canned)

I'm a big fan of protein "salads." Egg, chicken, and tuna are my usual go-tos, but lately I've been mixing it up with salmon to sneak in anti-inflammatory omega-3 fats in addition to protein. I love this refreshing combination of crunchy bell pepper, earthy curry powder, and satiating salmon to top a bed of leafy greens or pair with a piece of Paleo toast. It makes a great lunch to prep for the week when you know you have a few busy days ahead of you.

1 pound cooked and shredded salmon, or 3 (6-ounce) cans salmon (see note)

1 bell pepper (any color), diced

¼ cup avocado oil mayonnaise or organic olive oil–based mayo

¼ cup diced red onions

¼ cup chopped fresh cilantro

2 teaspoons curry powder

Juice of 1 lime (about 2 tablespoons)

Salt

1. Place the salmon, bell pepper, mayo, red onions, cilantro, curry powder, and lime juice in a bowl and stir to combine. Season with salt to taste.

2. Store leftovers in a glass jar or container in the fridge for up to 4 days.

Note To prepare raw salmon for use in this recipe, first remove any skin, then lightly brush the fish with olive oil and sprinkle with salt on both sides. Place the salmon on a parchment paper–lined sheet pan and bake in a preheated oven at 400°F for 12 to 15 minutes, until the internal temperature reaches 145°F.

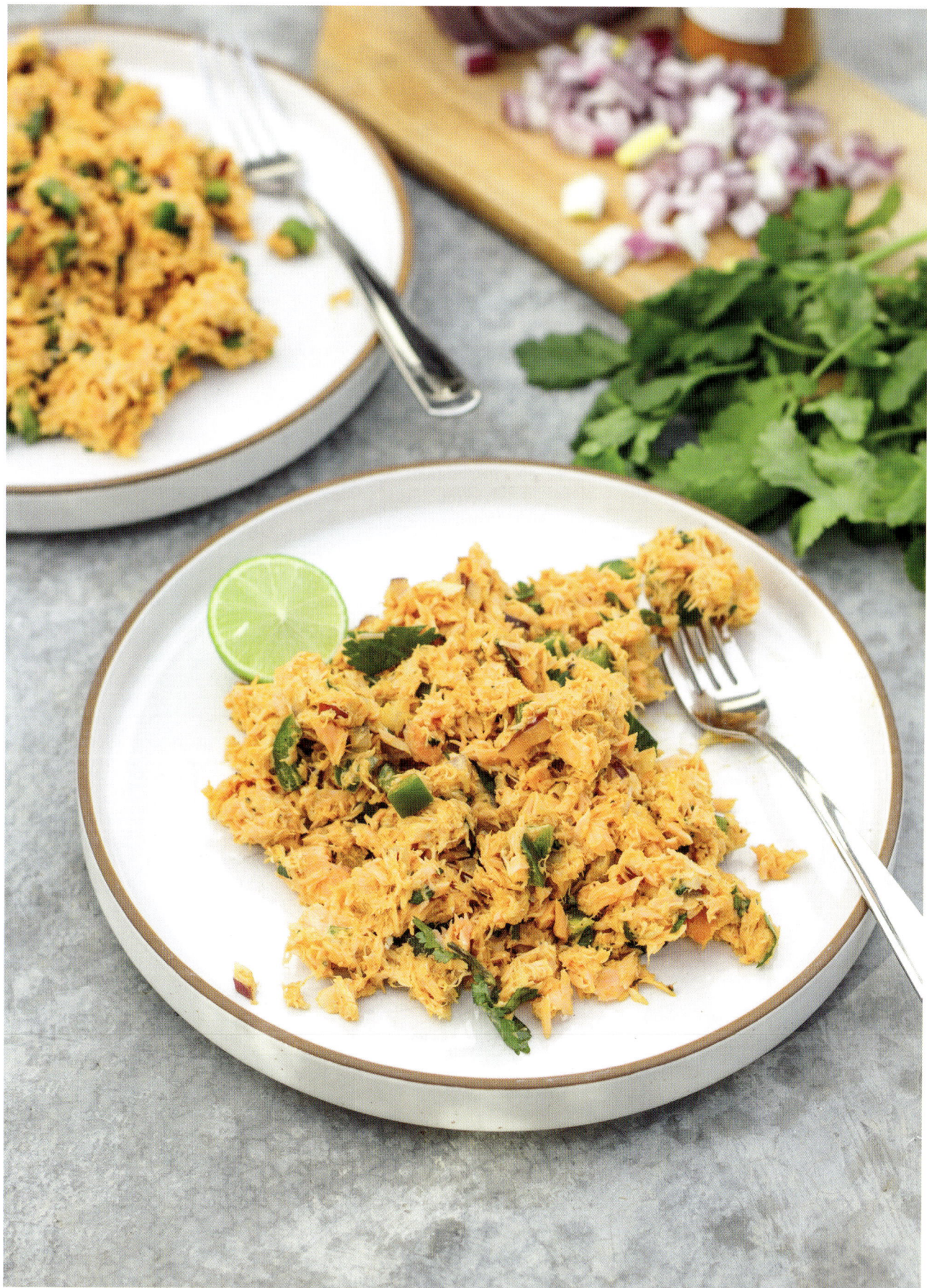

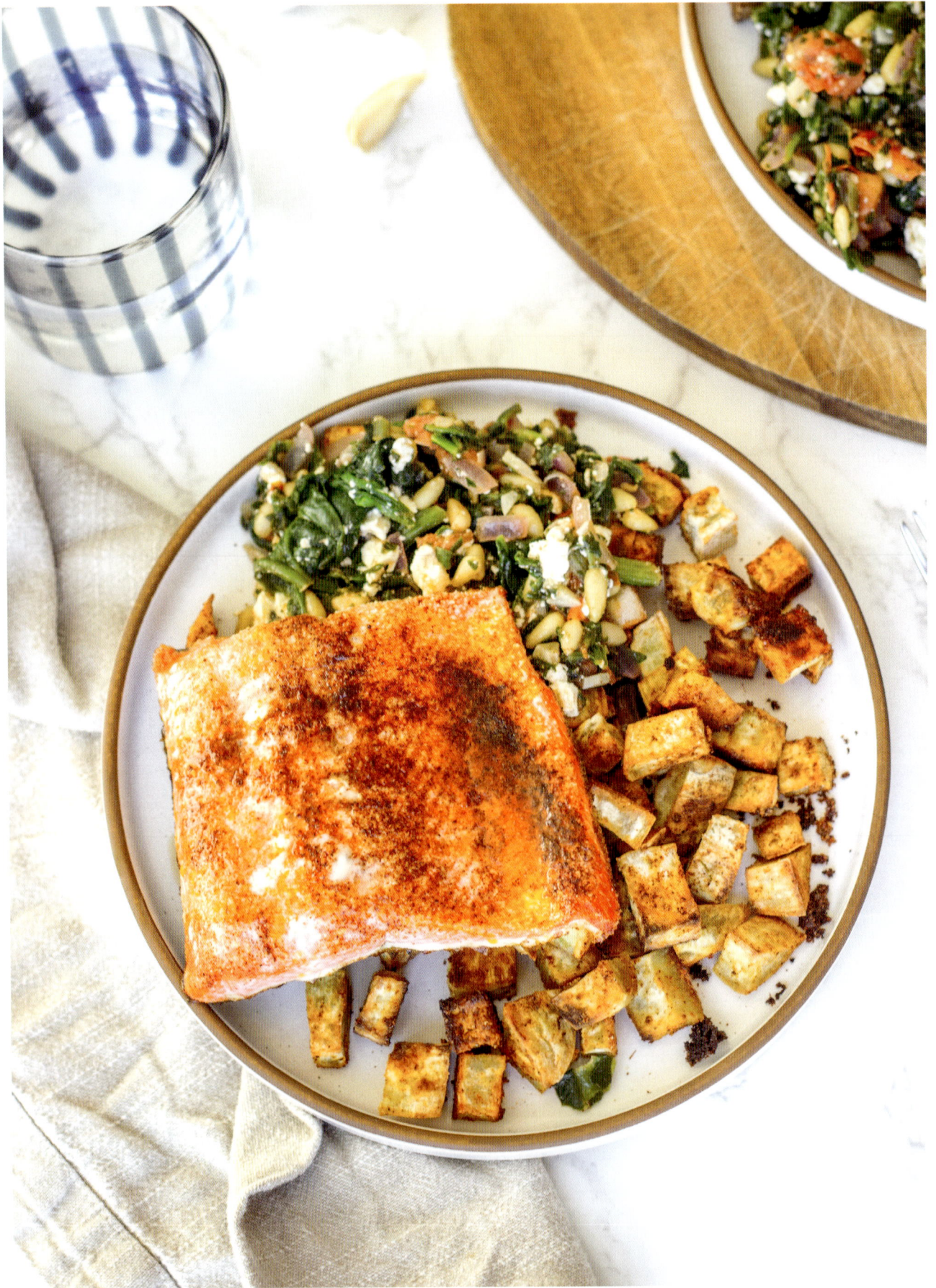

SALMON TRAY BAKE
WITH GARLICKY SPINACH

SERVES 4

PREP TIME 5 minutes

COOK TIME 30 minutes

For a quick, nutrient-packed weeknight meal, this recipe should be a new addition to your rotation. I use frozen spinach because it's easy to always have stowed away in the freezer when you need it. Plus, frozen food is nearly as nutrient dense as fresh, and it lasts a lot longer. The garlicky spinach in this recipe not only provides low–glycemic load veggies but also acts as a sauce for the salmon and sweet potatoes.

2 medium sweet potatoes, peeled and cut into small cubes

2 teaspoons garlic powder

2 teaspoons onion powder

2 teaspoons paprika

Salt

2 tablespoons olive oil, divided, plus extra for drizzling

4 (6-ounce) skin-on salmon fillets

4 cloves garlic, minced

½ cup diced red onions

1 medium tomato, diced

1 (10-ounce) bag frozen spinach

¼ cup crumbled feta cheese

3 tablespoons pine nuts

1. Preheat the oven to 425°F. Line a sheet pan with parchment paper.

2. Spread the sweet potatoes on one half of the prepared pan, making sure none of the pieces overlap. Combine the garlic powder, onion powder, paprika, and 1 teaspoon of salt in a small bowl. Sprinkle half of the seasoning mixture and 1 tablespoon of the olive oil over the sweet potatoes and toss. Put the pan in the oven and set a timer for 20 minutes.

3. Prep the salmon: Place the salmon on a plate and drizzle each fillet with olive oil, ensuring a thin coating on each slice. Sprinkle the remaining seasoning mixture over the salmon. After the oven timer goes off, arrange the salmon on the other half of the pan with the sweet potatoes, put the pan back in the oven, and set a new timer for 10 minutes. After 10 minutes, check to see if the internal temperature of the fish has reached 145°F. If not, place the pan back in the oven for a few more minutes, until the temperature hits 145°F.

4. While the salmon bakes, make the garlicky spinach: Heat the remaining tablespoon of olive oil in a large skillet over medium heat. Add the garlic and onions and sauté for 1 to 2 minutes, until fragrant. Add the tomato and sauté for 3 to 5 minutes, until the tomato has softened. Finally, add the spinach and a heavy pinch of salt. Sauté until the spinach is warmed through and mixed well with the other ingredients, 3 to 5 minutes. Remove the skillet from the heat and stir in the feta and pine nuts.

5. Serve the salmon with the garlicky spinach and roasted sweet potatoes.

TUNA AVOCADO TOAST

SERVES 1

PREP TIME 10 minutes (not including time to make guacamole)

Tuna salad is a forever staple for me because it's so fast and easy. Sometimes I'm in such a rush that I only have time to whip up the "salad" portion and eat it straight out of the bowl. But when I have an extra few minutes, I like to make it more of a meal, and boy, are those few extra minutes worth it! I love combining classic avocado toast with tuna salad and a sprinkle of paprika for a flavor-packed meal that's loaded with protein, fat, and fiber.

2 slices Ezekiel or Paleo bread (see note)

1 (5-ounce) can tuna, drained

2 tablespoons diced red onions

1 tablespoon avocado oil mayonnaise or organic olive oil–based mayo

1 teaspoon Dijon mustard

½ cup Guacamole (page 237)

Paprika, for garnish

1. Toast the bread in a toaster.

2. In a small bowl, stir the tuna, onions, mayo, and mustard with a fork until very well combined.

3. Spread the guacamole on both slices of toast and top with the tuna salad. Sprinkle with paprika before serving.

Note Ezekiel bread contains some complete protein due to the combination of sprouted beans, lentils, and seeds. It also has a low glycemic load, making it one of the better bread options out there. However, if you are particularly carb sensitive, you can opt for a whole food–based Paleo-style bread. My favorite brand is Base Culture, and it can be found in the freezer aisle.

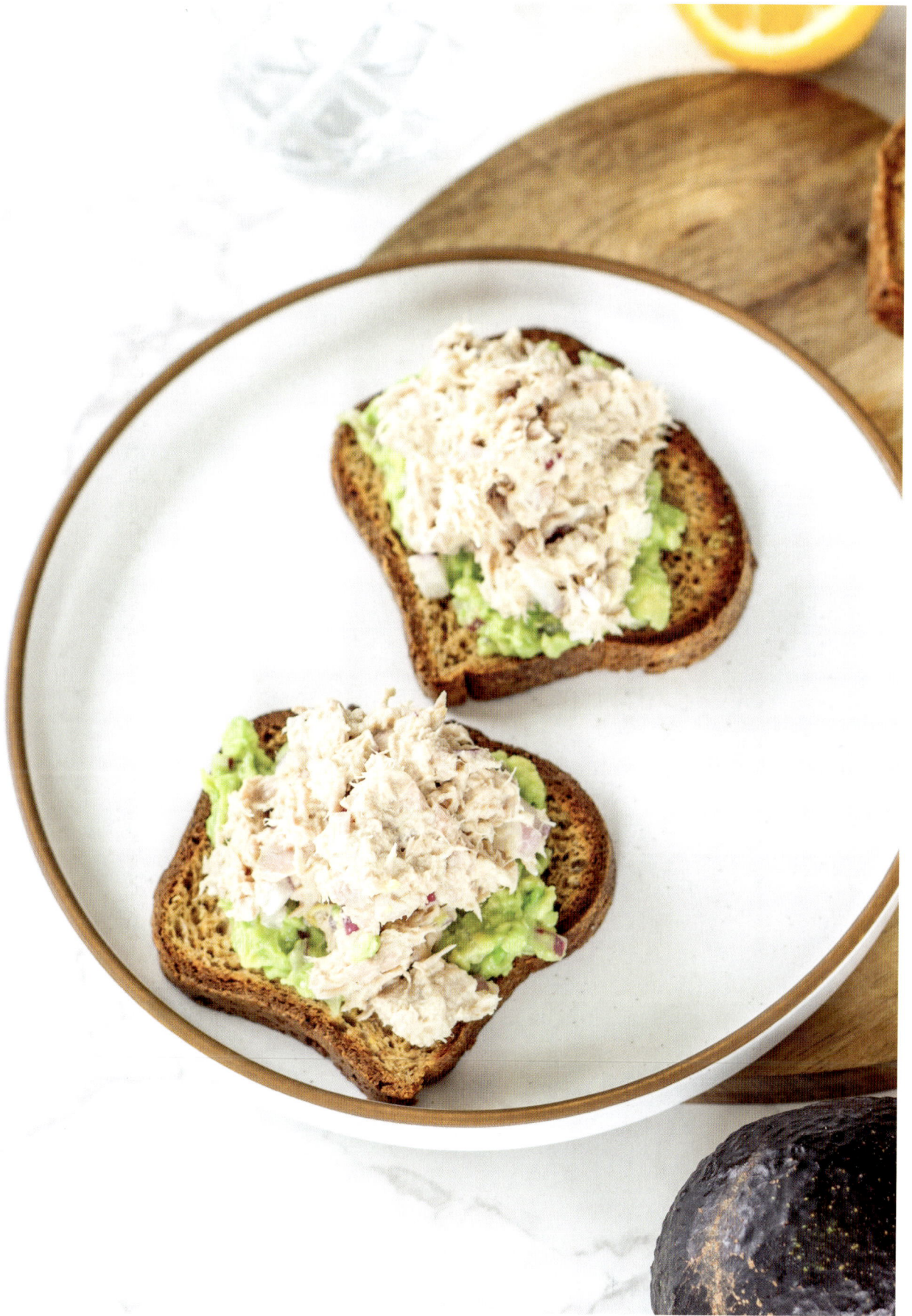

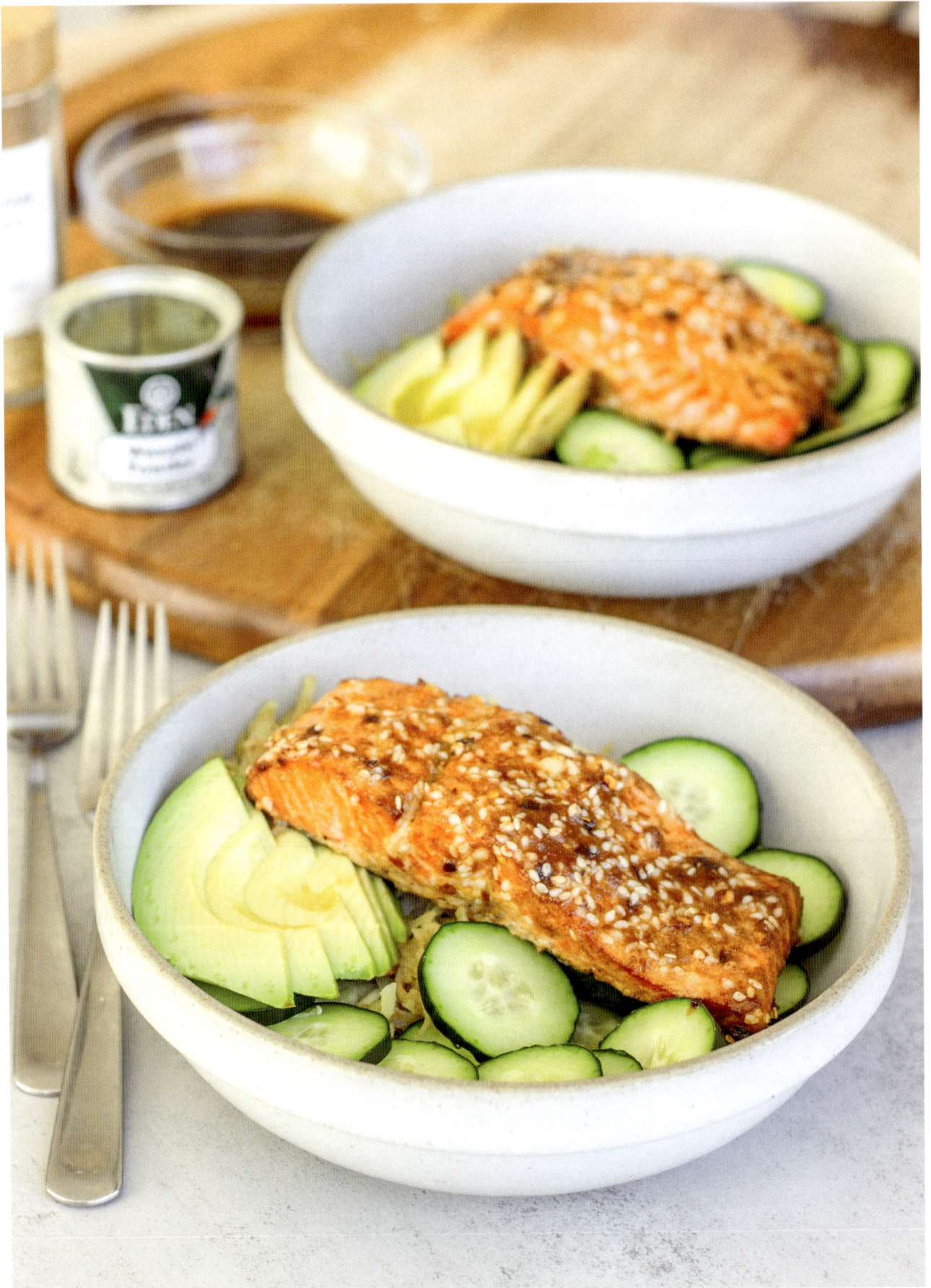

SPICY SALMON AND SWEET POTATO "RICE" BOWL

SERVES 4

PREP TIME 10 minutes

COOK TIME 15 minutes

This bowl is reminiscent of a salmon sushi bowl. But instead of high-glycemic load white rice, I've opted for shredded sweet potatoes. It's surprisingly packed with flavor and, in my opinion, tastes significantly better than the standard white rice option. Wasabi powder can be found in the specialty foods aisle at nearly any health food store. It's a powder, so it lasts a long time and is well worth having in the pantry to spice up a meal.

4 tablespoons olive oil, divided

6 tablespoons tamari, divided

1 tablespoon white sesame seeds

2 teaspoons garlic powder, divided

¾ teaspoon ground ginger

⅛ to ¼ teaspoon red pepper flakes, according to taste

4 (6-ounce) skin-on salmon fillets

2 medium white-fleshed sweet potatoes, peeled

Salt

2 teaspoons wasabi powder

1 medium cucumber, thinly sliced

2 avocados, peeled and sliced

1. In a large bowl, whisk together 3 tablespoons of the olive oil, 2 tablespoons of the tamari, the sesame seeds, 1 teaspoon of the garlic powder, the ginger, and red pepper flakes. Lay the salmon in the sauce mixture and flip it over a few times to ensure that it's thoroughly coated. Set aside.

2. Preheat the oven to 400°F and line a sheet pan with parchment paper.

3. Put the salmon on the prepared pan and pour any leftover sauce over the fillets. Bake for 12 to 15 minutes, until the internal temperature is 145°F.

4. While the salmon bakes, prepare the sweet potato "rice": Using a cheese grater, grate the sweet potatoes. In a large skillet or wok over medium heat, heat the remaining tablespoon of olive oil. Once the pan is hot, add the grated sweet potatoes, remaining teaspoon of garlic powder, and a heavy pinch of salt. Sauté for 5 to 8 minutes, until the potatoes are tender and lightly browned. Divide the sweet potato rice among four bowls.

5. In a small bowl, rehydrate the wasabi powder with a splash of warm water (½ teaspoon should be more than enough). Whisk until it forms a paste. Add the remaining 4 tablespoons of tamari and whisk to combine. There will be some chunks of wasabi, and that's okay.

6. Place the cooked salmon on top of the sweet potato rice. Top the bowl with the sliced cucumber and ½ sliced avocado per serving. Serve with the wasabi-tamari mixture to pour on top.

SALMON PATTIES
WITH BASIL AIOLI

SERVES 4

PREP TIME 15 minutes

COOK TIME 10 minutes

In the past, I didn't like salmon. It was recipes like this that hid salmon within super flavorful patties that helped me learn to love it. If you already have cooked salmon (or canned salmon) on hand, then this is a fast and easy weeknight dinner. It also makes an impressive high-protein meal to serve at a dinner party. These patties are great to make in bulk and have as lunches throughout the week; they'll keep in the fridge for up to 4 days.

SALMON PATTIES

1 pound cooked and shredded salmon, or 3 (6-ounce) cans salmon

2 large eggs

½ cup almond flour

½ cup finely chopped yellow onions

Grated zest and juice of ½ lemon (1 to 1½ tablespoons)

1 teaspoon garlic powder

1 teaspoon paprika

Salt

2 tablespoons avocado oil or other high-heat-tolerant oil

BASIL AIOLI

½ cup avocado oil mayonnaise or organic olive oil–based mayo

1 cup chopped fresh basil

3 cloves garlic, chopped

Juice of ½ lemon (1 to 1½ tablespoons)

FOR SERVING

8 cups mixed leafy greens

Special equipment: immersion blender or food processor

1. Crumble the salmon into a mixing bowl, making sure to remove any bones. Add the eggs, almond flour, onions, lemon zest and juice, garlic powder, paprika, and a heavy pinch of salt. Stir with a fork until the ingredients are very well combined and the mixture resembles tuna salad.

2. Heat the oil in a large skillet over medium heat. Form the salmon mixture into eight 1-inch-thick patties and place in the pan. You may have to work in batches so as not to overcrowd the pan. Cook for 5 minutes, then flip and cook for another 5 minutes, until the patties are lightly golden brown on both sides.

3. Make the aioli: Put all of the ingredients in a glass measuring cup and blend with an immersion blender until smooth. (You can use a food processor if you don't have an immersion blender.)

4. Serve the salmon patties on top of the mixed greens, with the aioli on the side to drizzle on top as desired.

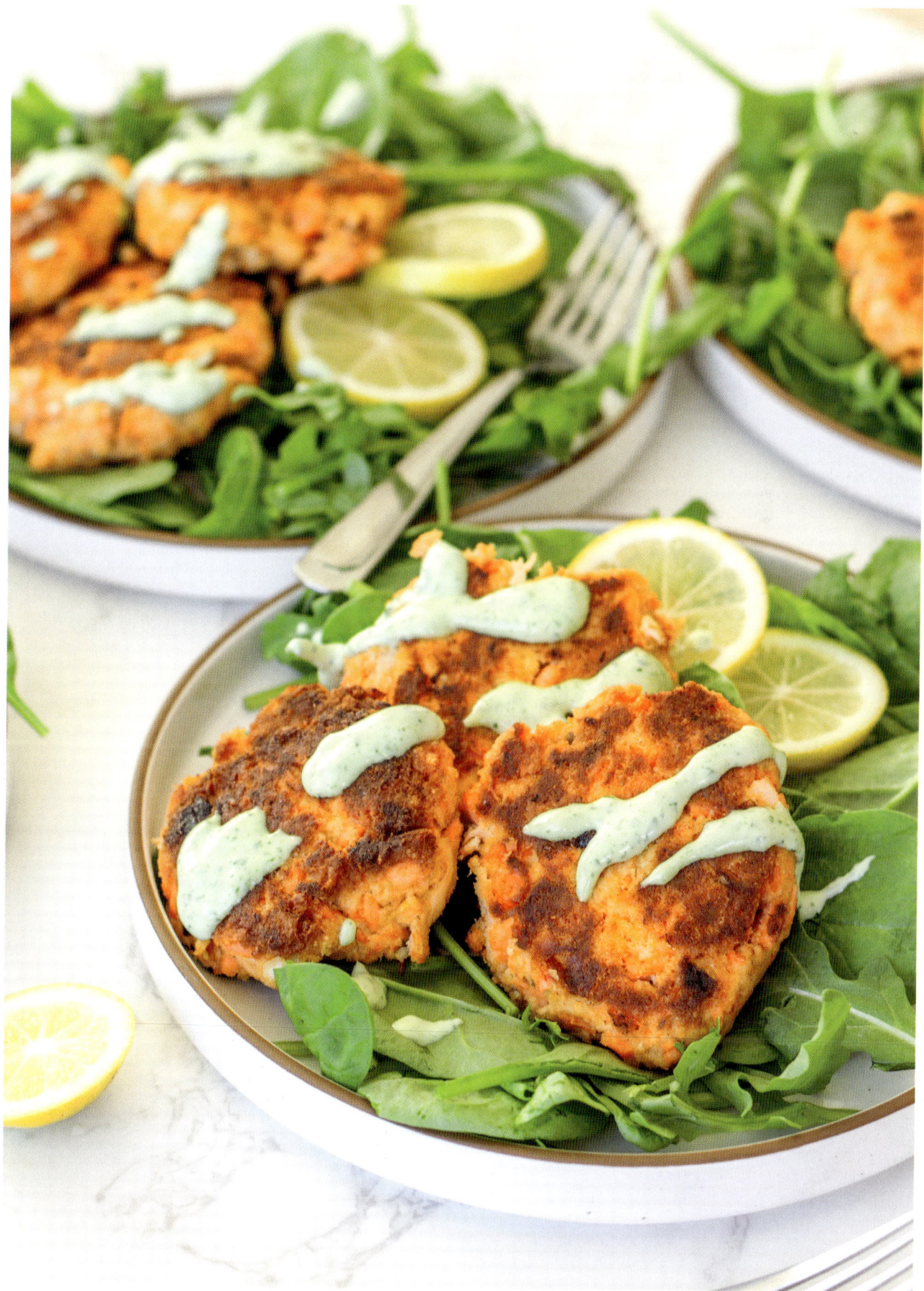

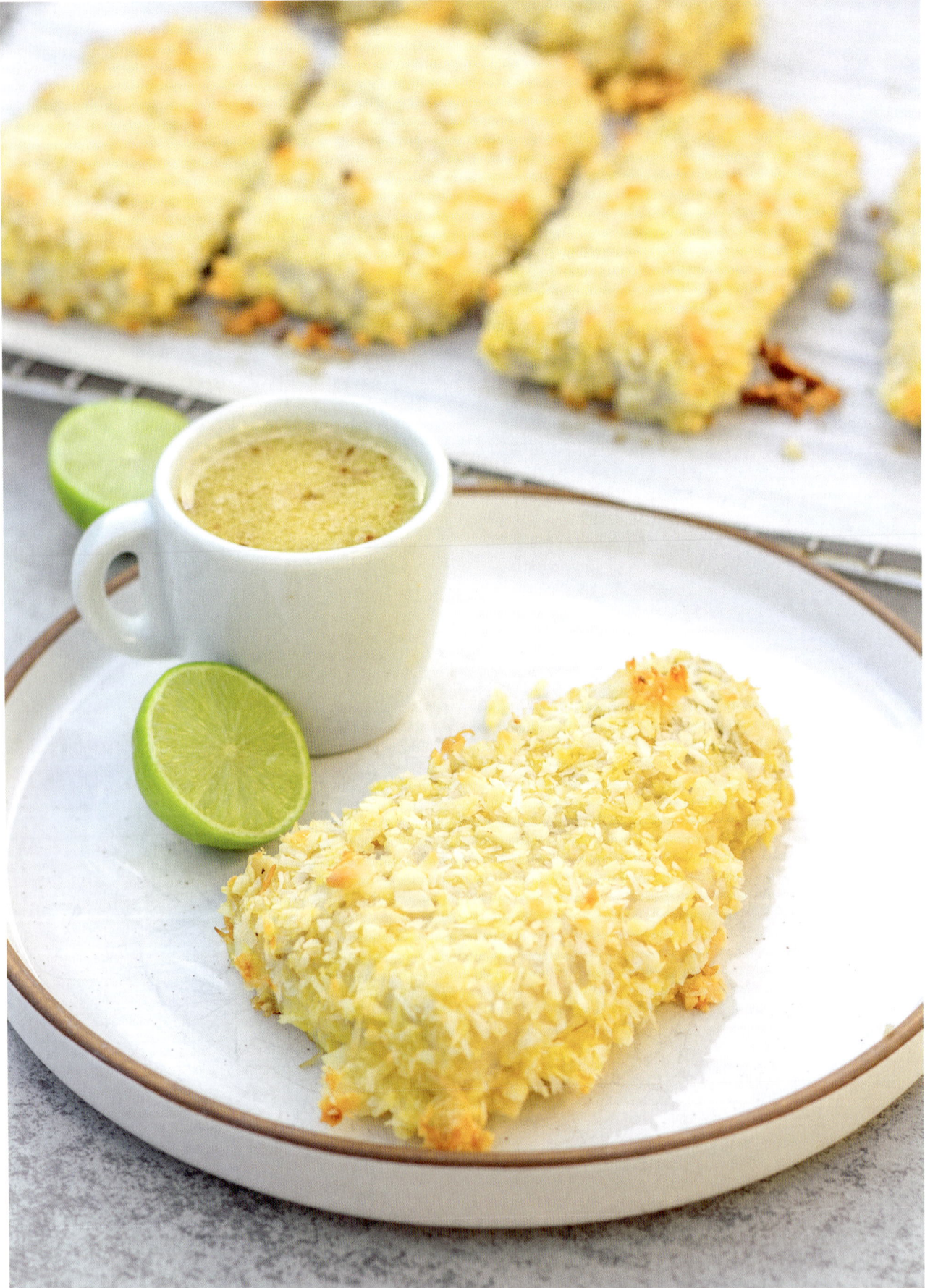

MACADAMIA NUT–CRUSTED MAHI MAHI
WITH COCONUT LIME SAUCE

SERVES 4

PREP TIME 15 minutes

COOK TIME 10 minutes

Every year, we like to go on some type of tropical vacation during the winter months to get some sunshine and escape the rain. Without fail, one of my favorite meals to eat while on these trips is a macadamia nut–crusted mahi mahi. It's so tender and flaky and feels decadent while being outrageously good for you. When I feel like I need a little dose of those tropical vibes, I like to whip up this meal as a reminder of those relaxed, beachy days.

CRUSTED MAHI MAHI

1 large egg

½ cup raw macadamia nuts, finely chopped

½ cup unsweetened coconut flakes

1 (1¼-pound) mahi mahi or other white fish fillet, such as cod, halibut, or tilapia, cut into 4 equal servings

Salt

1 tablespoon olive oil

COCONUT LIME SAUCE

1 teaspoon olive oil

1 medium shallot, finely diced

2 cloves garlic, minced

1 teaspoon grated ginger

¼ teaspoon red pepper flakes

1 cup canned full-fat coconut milk

Juice of 1 lime (about 2 tablespoons)

FOR GARNISH

Fresh cilantro leaves

1. Preheat the oven to 400°F and line a sheet pan with parchment paper.

2. In a shallow bowl, whisk the egg. In a second shallow bowl, combine the macadamia nuts and coconut flakes.

3. Pat the fish dry with a paper towel and season both sides with salt. Dip each piece of fish into the egg, shaking off the excess. Then dip each side of the fish in the nut mixture, gently pressing to make sure it sticks. Place the fish on the prepared pan.

4. Drizzle the olive oil over the fish and bake for 10 minutes, or until the internal temperature reaches 145°F.

5. While the fish bakes, prepare the sauce: Heat the olive oil in a medium-sized skillet over medium-high heat. Add the shallot and sauté for 5 minutes, or until softened. Add the garlic, ginger, and red pepper flakes and sauté for 1 minute. Pour in the coconut milk and whisk to combine. Reduce the heat and simmer for 2 to 3 minutes, until the sauce has reduced and thickened slightly. Squeeze in the lime juice and stir to combine before removing the pan from the heat.

6. Serve the mahi mahi with a drizzle of coconut lime sauce and garnish with cilantro.

GRILLED SHRIMP TOSTADAS WITH SPICY SLAW

SERVES 4

PREP TIME 15 minutes

COOK TIME 12 minutes

Here in Santa Barbara, summer heat peaks in September. One year it hit 104°F, which made cooking inside over a hot stove or using the oven unbearable. On days like these, easy dinners that don't rely on the stove or oven are a must. Here, I've adapted typical fried or baked tostada shells to be made outside on the grill for a no-fuss—and oven-free—weeknight dinner. Topped with protein-packed ingredients like Greek yogurt and shrimp, these tostadas also help stabilize blood sugar and keep you feeling full for longer.

SLAW

2 cups thinly sliced green cabbage

2 cups thinly sliced purple cabbage

1 cup chopped fresh cilantro

½ cup diced red onions

1 jalapeño pepper, diced (remove membranes and seeds if you prefer less heat)

2 tablespoons rice vinegar

1 tablespoon olive oil

Salt

TOSTADAS

12 (6-inch) corn tortillas, store-bought or homemade (page 77)

1 tablespoon avocado oil

Salt

1 canned chipotle chili pepper in adobo sauce

3 tablespoons adobo sauce (from the can)

1½ pounds large shrimp, peeled and deveined

¾ cup plain whole milk Greek yogurt, store-bought or homemade (page 81)

2 avocados, peeled and sliced

Special equipment:
4 (16-inch) metal skewers

1. Prepare the slaw: In a large bowl, combine the green and purple cabbage, cilantro, onions, jalapeño, vinegar, and olive oil. Season with a heavy pinch of salt and toss to combine. Taste and add more salt as needed.

2. Make the tostada shells: Preheat a grill to medium-high heat (425°F to 450°F). Lay the tortillas on a sheet pan and brush both sides with the avocado oil. Sprinkle each tortilla with salt. Place on the grill and cook for 2 minutes, then flip and cook for another 2 minutes, until the tortillas are slightly charred. Don't worry if the tortillas aren't very crispy when you pull them off the grill; they will continue to crisp up as they cool.

3. Prepare the shrimp: In a medium-sized mixing bowl, combine the chipotle pepper and adobo sauce, using your hands to break up the chipotle pepper into rough chunks. Add the shrimp and ½ teaspoon of salt to the bowl. Use your hands to coat the shrimp in the sauce mixture.

4. Thread the shrimp onto the skewers. Grill for 4 minutes, then flip and cook for another 4 minutes, or until the shrimp are bright pink with a few grill marks.

5. To assemble the tostadas, spread 1 tablespoon of yogurt on each grilled tortilla. Top each with some slaw, avocado slices, and three or four shrimp.

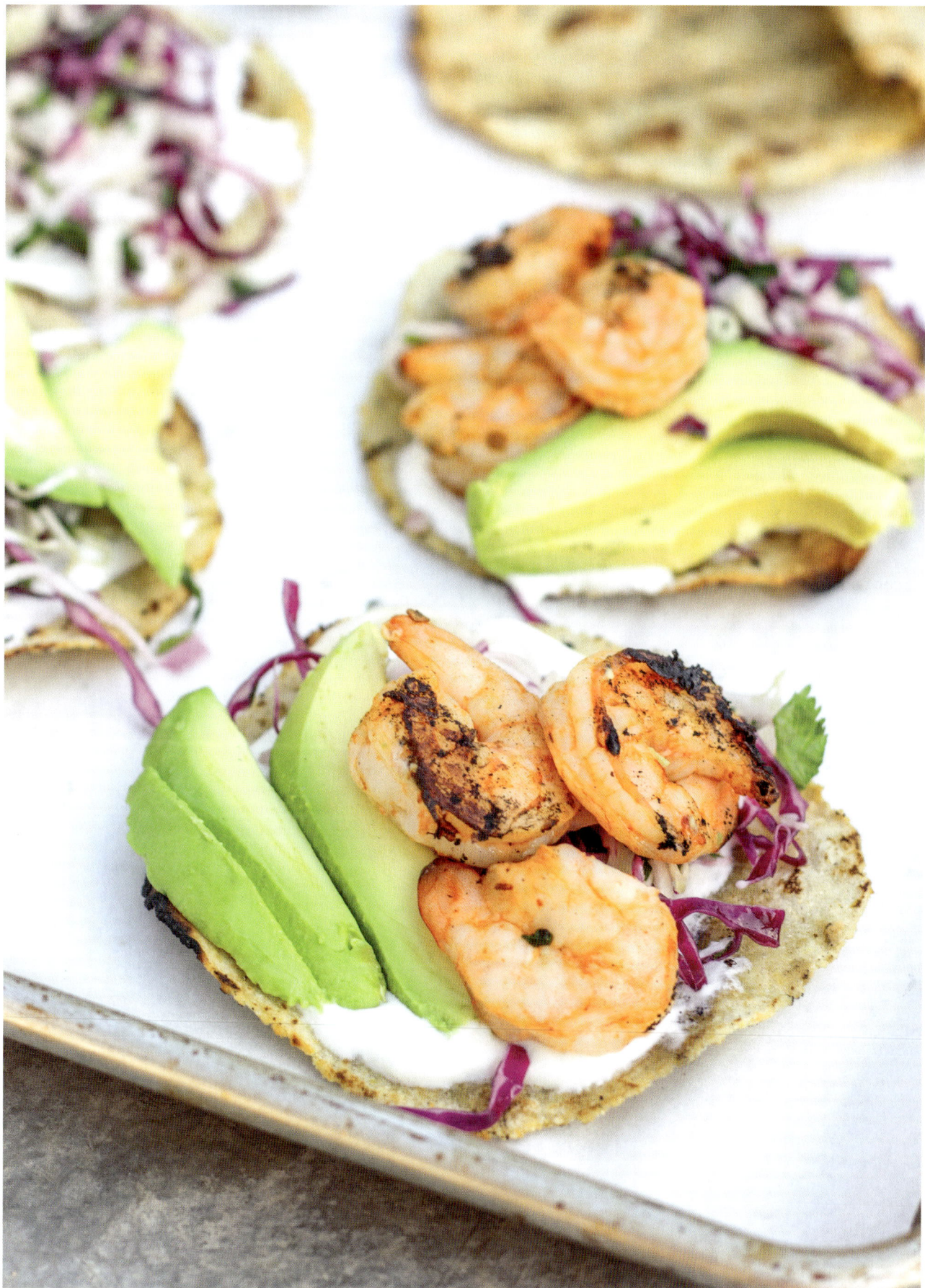

VEGETARIAN MAINS

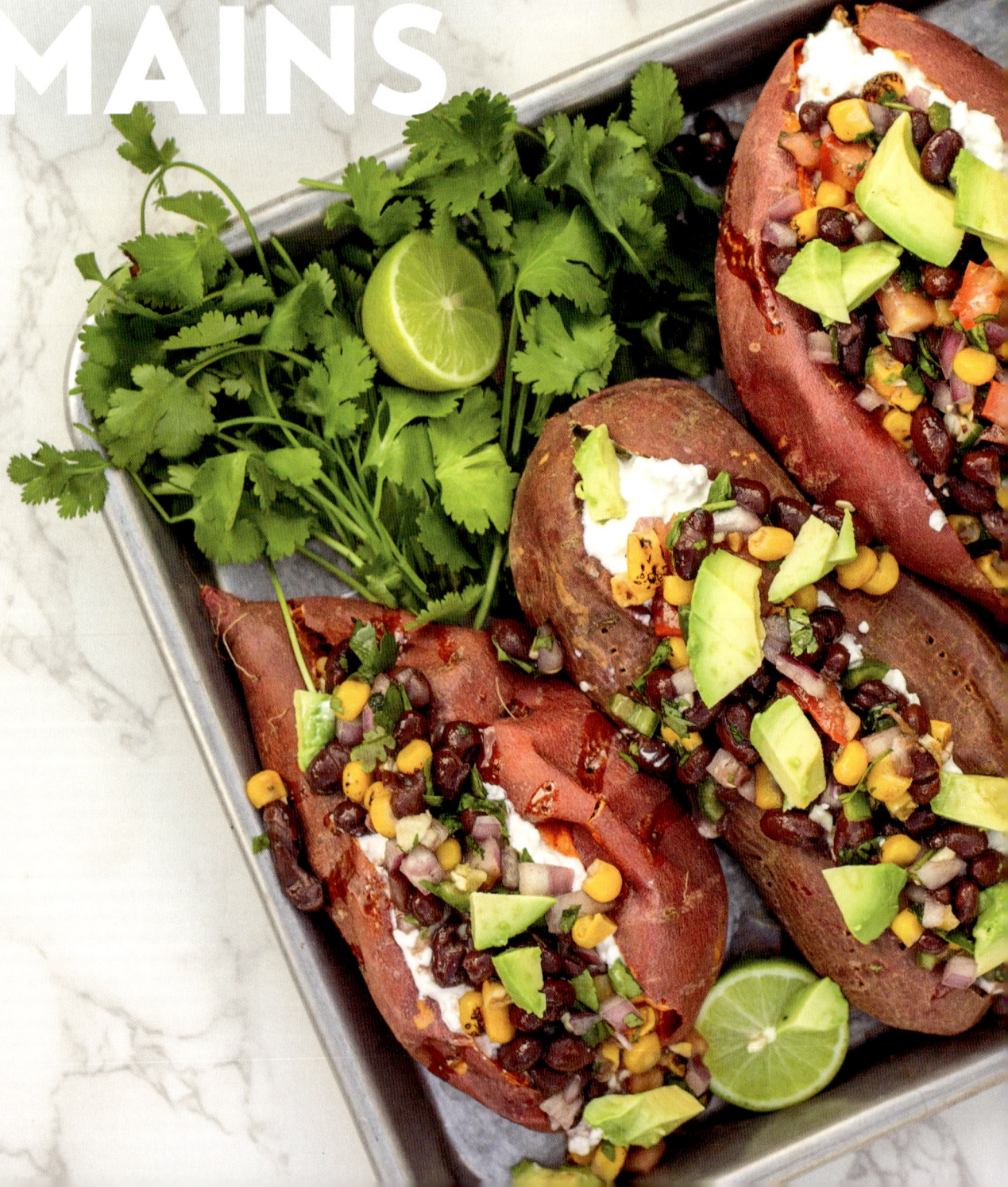

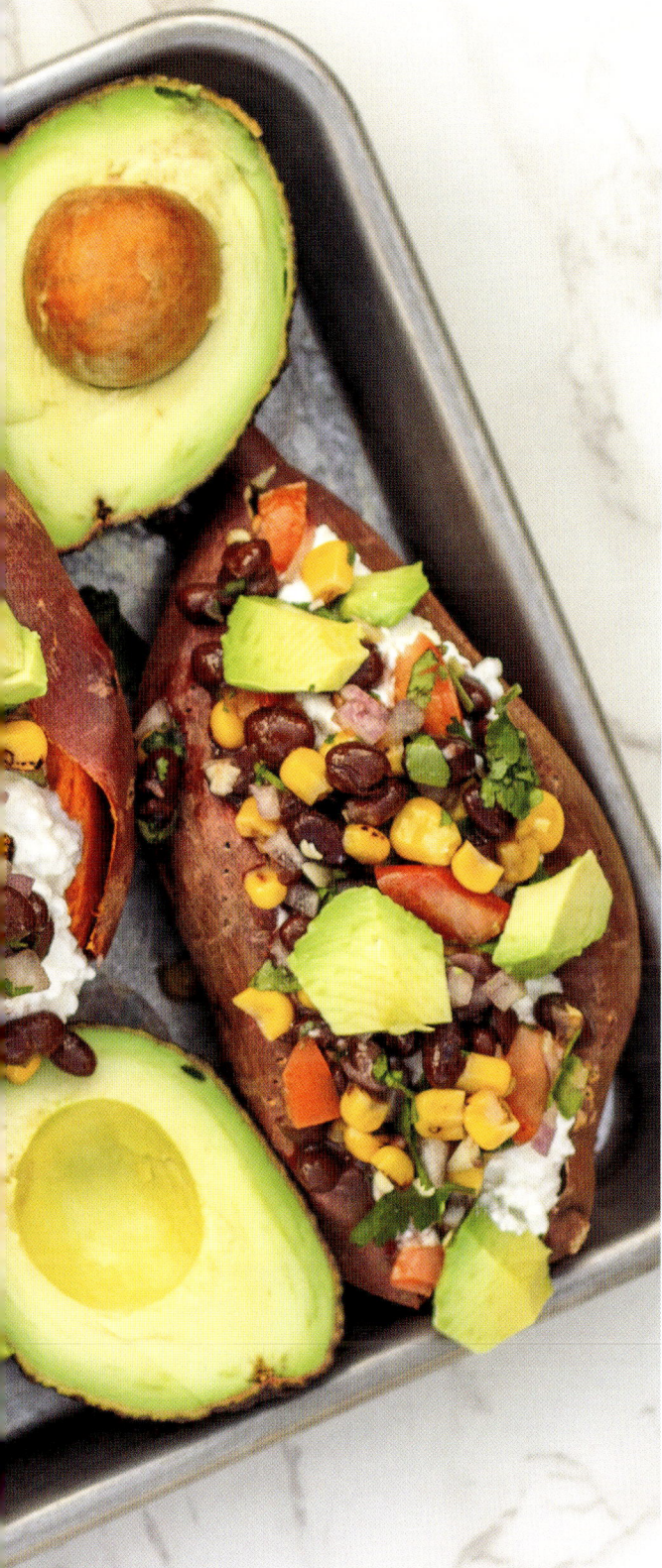

HIGH-PROTEIN MUSHROOM KALE FRITTATA WITH TOMATOES

SERVES 4

PREP TIME 10 minutes

COOK TIME 40 minutes

Most frittatas aren't as high in protein as they might seem because eggs are fairly low in protein; each egg only has 5 to 7 grams of protein. So it's important to add other protein-rich ingredients to bring this number up. Cottage cheese and Parmesan both provide fluffy goodness here while significantly boosting the protein content from vegetarian sources. This meal is also nutrient dense, with excellent levels of choline, B vitamins, vitamins K1 and K2, selenium, and calcium. Serve it with Zucchini Sweet Potato Hash (page 222) for an ultra-satisfying meal.

FRITTATA

1 tablespoon salted butter

½ medium red onion, diced

2 cups sliced mushrooms (any type)

4 cups finely chopped curly kale

3 cloves garlic, minced

1 teaspoon dried thyme leaves

Salt

12 large eggs

1 cup cottage cheese

½ cup grated Parmesan cheese

TOMATOES

4 tomatoes, sliced

Olive oil, for drizzling

Balsamic vinegar, for drizzling

Salt

1. Preheat the oven to 350°F and grease a 9 by 13-inch glass or ceramic baking dish.

2. Melt the butter in a large skillet over medium heat. Add the onion, mushrooms, kale, garlic, thyme, and a heavy pinch of salt. Sauté until the veggies are softened, about 8 minutes.

3. Evenly spread the cooked veggies in the greased baking dish.

4. Crack the eggs into a large bowl and whisk to combine the whites and yolks. Add the cottage cheese, Parmesan, and a pinch of salt and give it another whisk. Pour the egg mixture over the cooked veggies. Bake for 30 minutes, or until a knife comes out clean when poked through the center.

5. While the frittata bakes, place the tomato slices on individual serving plates. Lightly drizzle olive oil and balsamic vinegar over the tomatoes and sprinkle with salt. Leave the oil and vinegar on the table in case more is needed when serving.

6. Remove the frittata from the oven and allow to cool for 5 to 10 minutes before slicing and serving on top of the tomatoes.

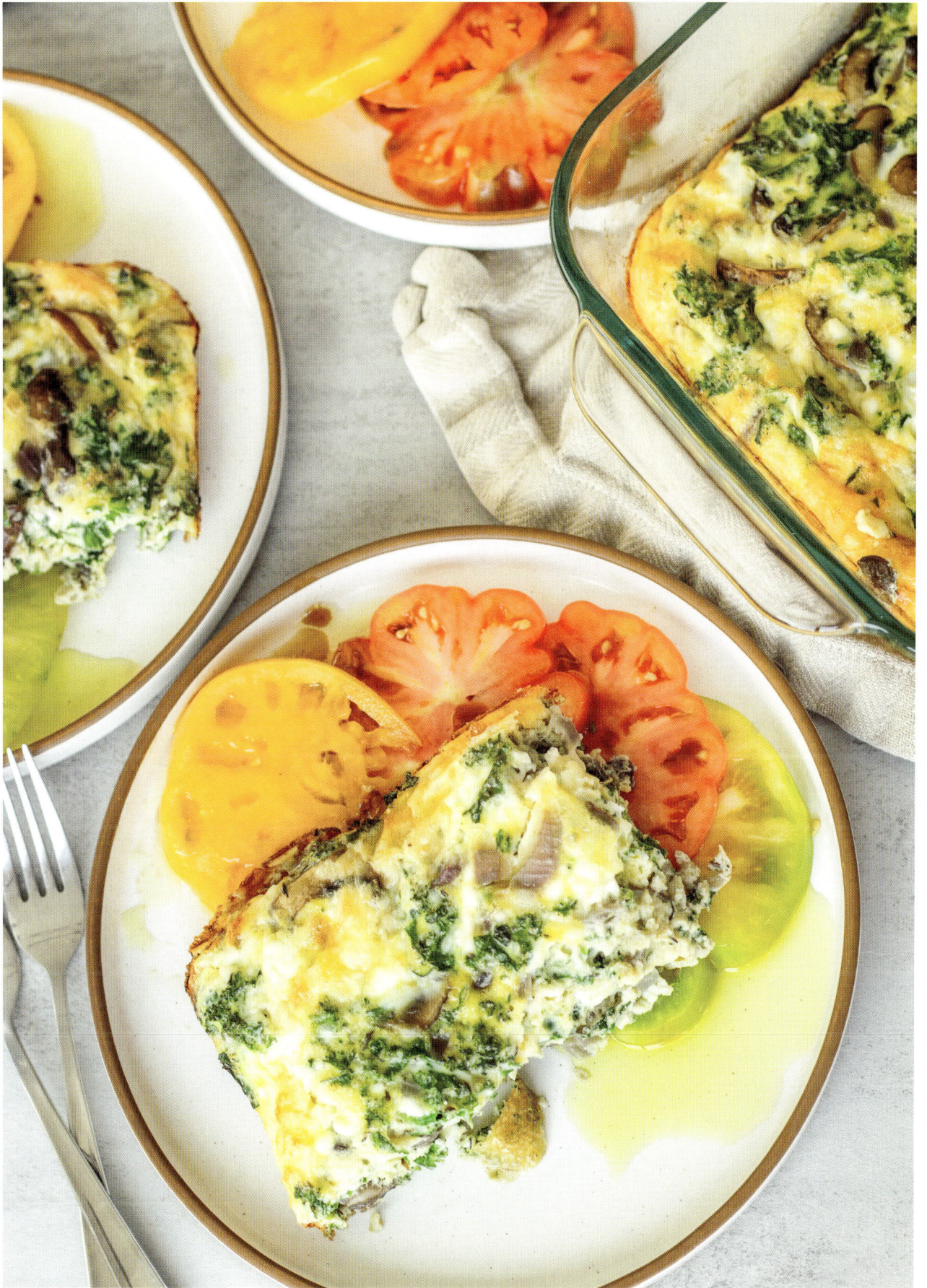

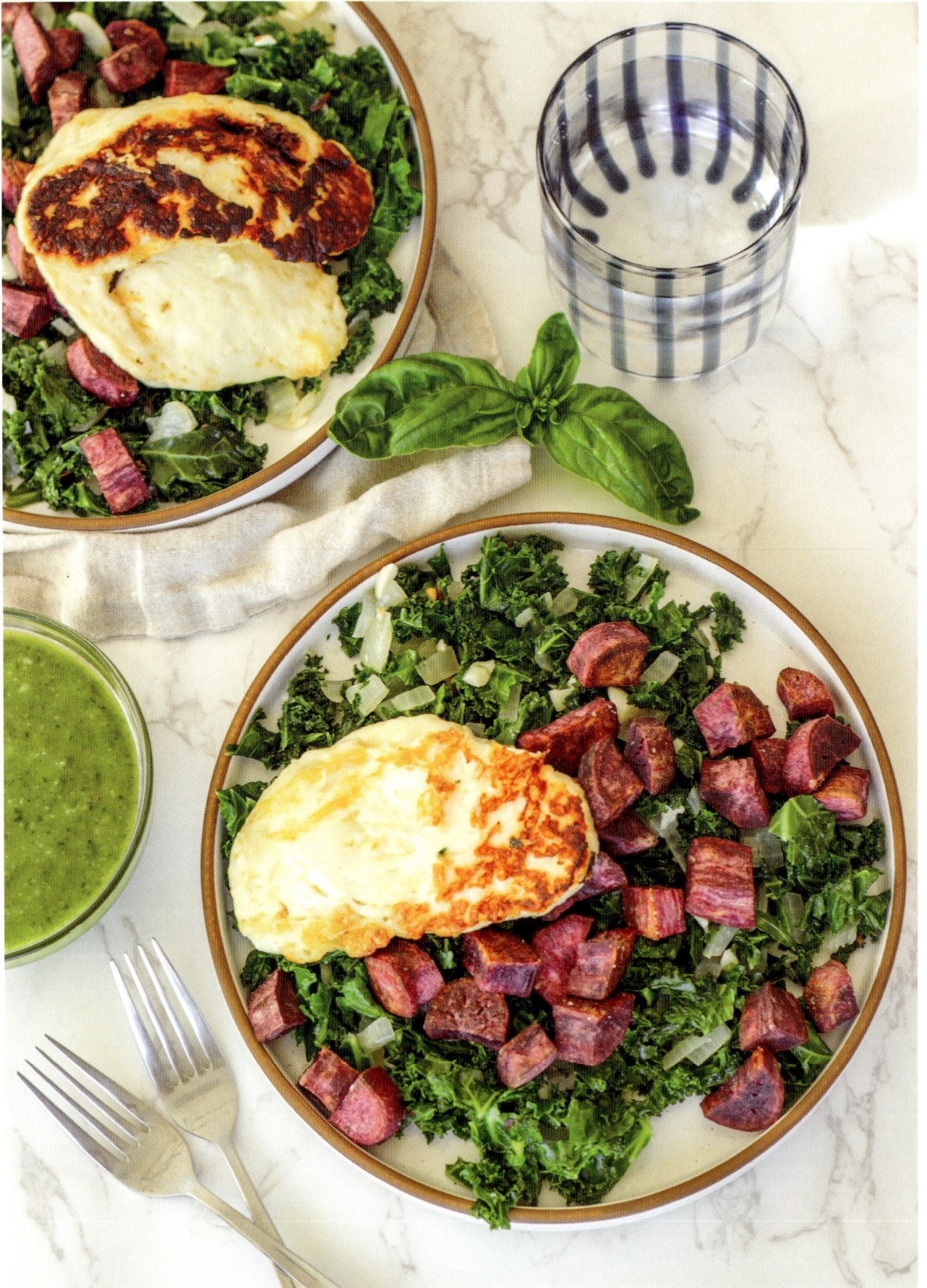

CRISPY HALLOUMI BOWL
WITH PESTO

SERVES 4

PREP TIME 10 minutes

COOK TIME 25 minutes

Halloumi is an excellent vegetarian protein that can be used in place of meat, chicken, or fish in many dishes. You can eat it on its own, but this semi-hard cheese really shines when it's lightly seared. Because halloumi is high in fat as well as protein, I have paired it with lighter ingredients like kale and a small portion of roasted purple sweet potato.

1 medium purple sweet potato, peeled and diced

2 tablespoons olive oil, divided

Salt

½ cup diced yellow onions

5 cloves garlic, minced

1 bunch curly kale, stems removed and leaves finely chopped

½ teaspoon red pepper flakes

1 pound halloumi cheese, cut horizontally across the middle into 4 thin strips

¼ cup pesto, for drizzling

1. Preheat the oven to 425°F and line a sheet pan with parchment paper.

2. Place the sweet potato on the prepared sheet pan and drizzle 1 tablespoon of the olive oil over it. Sprinkle with a heavy pinch of salt and toss to combine. Bake for 25 minutes.

3. Meanwhile, heat 2 teaspoons of the olive oil in a large skillet over medium heat. Add the onions, garlic, and a pinch of salt and sauté until fragrant, about 2 minutes. Add the kale, red pepper flakes, and another heavy pinch of salt. Sauté for 5 to 8 minutes, until the kale has wilted. Divide the kale mixture among four serving bowls.

4. Pour the remaining teaspoon of olive oil into the skillet and increase the heat to medium-high. Once the pan is hot, add the strips of halloumi. Sear for 2 to 3 minutes on each side. They should be lightly browned and crispy once flipped.

5. Top each bowl with one-quarter of the seared halloumi, followed by one-quarter of the roasted sweet potato and a 1-tablespoon drizzle of pesto.

SOUTHWEST STUFFED SWEET POTATOES

SERVES 4

PREP TIME 10 minutes

COOK TIME 1 hour

One of the best sources of vegetarian protein is cottage cheese. It naturally goes with a baked white potato, but I made this recipe lower glycemic load by swapping in sweet potatoes (I used purple ones, but feel free to opt for typical orange sweet potatoes if you prefer). It's also loaded with flavor from the red onions, jalapeño, and lime juice.

4 medium sweet potatoes

½ cup cooked black beans, canned or homemade (page 85)

½ cup fresh corn kernels or thawed frozen corn

1 jalapeño pepper, diced (remove membranes and seeds if you prefer less heat)

½ cup chopped fresh cilantro

¼ cup diced red onions

1 clove garlic, minced

Juice of 1 lime (about 2 tablespoons)

Salt

5 cups cottage cheese

1 avocado, peeled and diced

1. Preheat the oven to 400°F and line a sheet pan with parchment paper.

2. Using a fork, poke each sweet potato 4 or 5 times. Place on the prepared sheet pan and bake for 45 minutes to 1 hour, until fork-tender.

3. In a bowl, toss the beans, corn, jalapeño, cilantro, onions, garlic, lime juice, and a heavy pinch of salt.

4. Remove the sweet potatoes from the oven and place one on each plate. Cut each potato in half lengthwise and top with 1¼ cups of cottage cheese, one-quarter of the black bean mixture, and ¼ avocado, then serve.

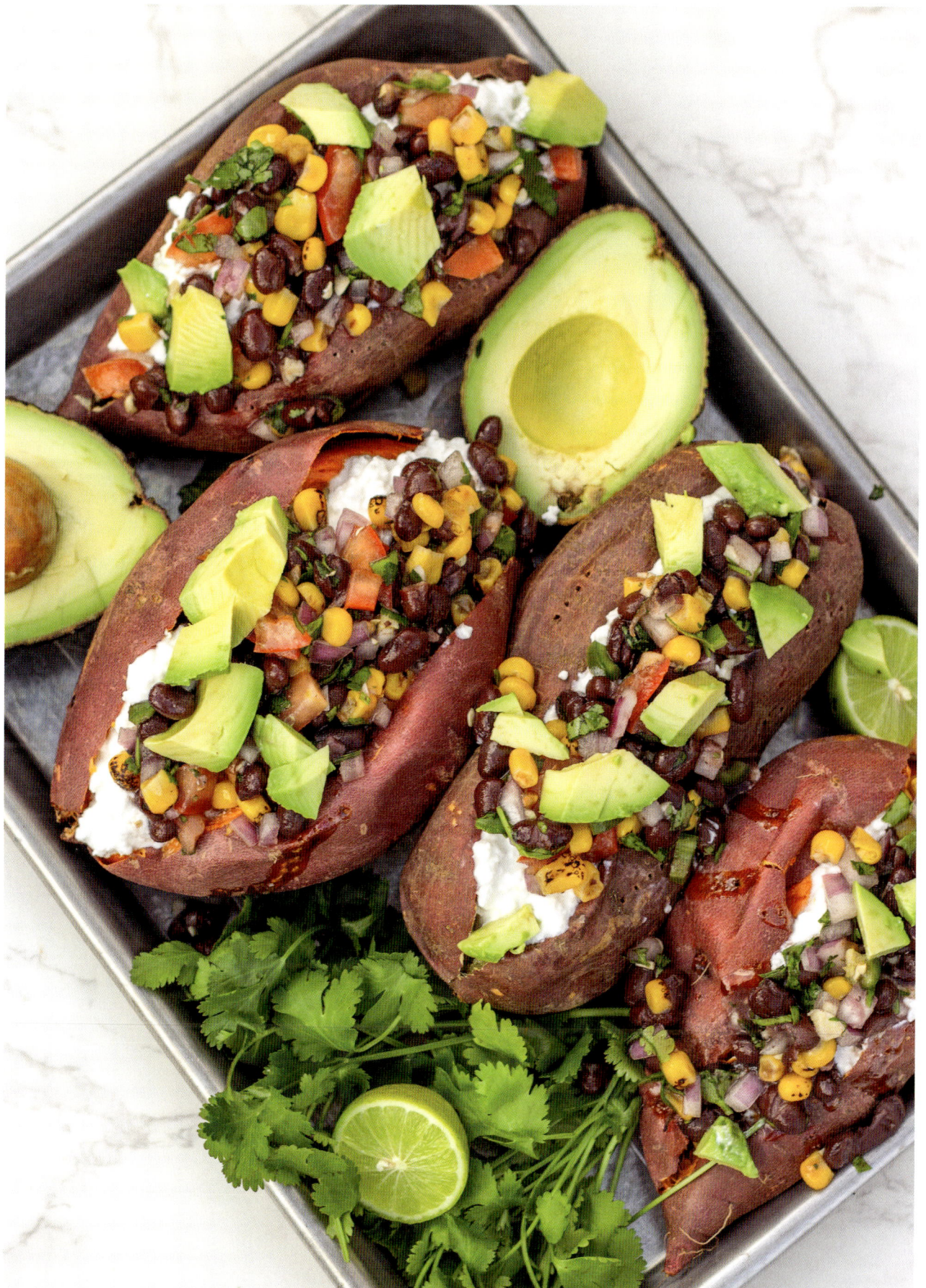

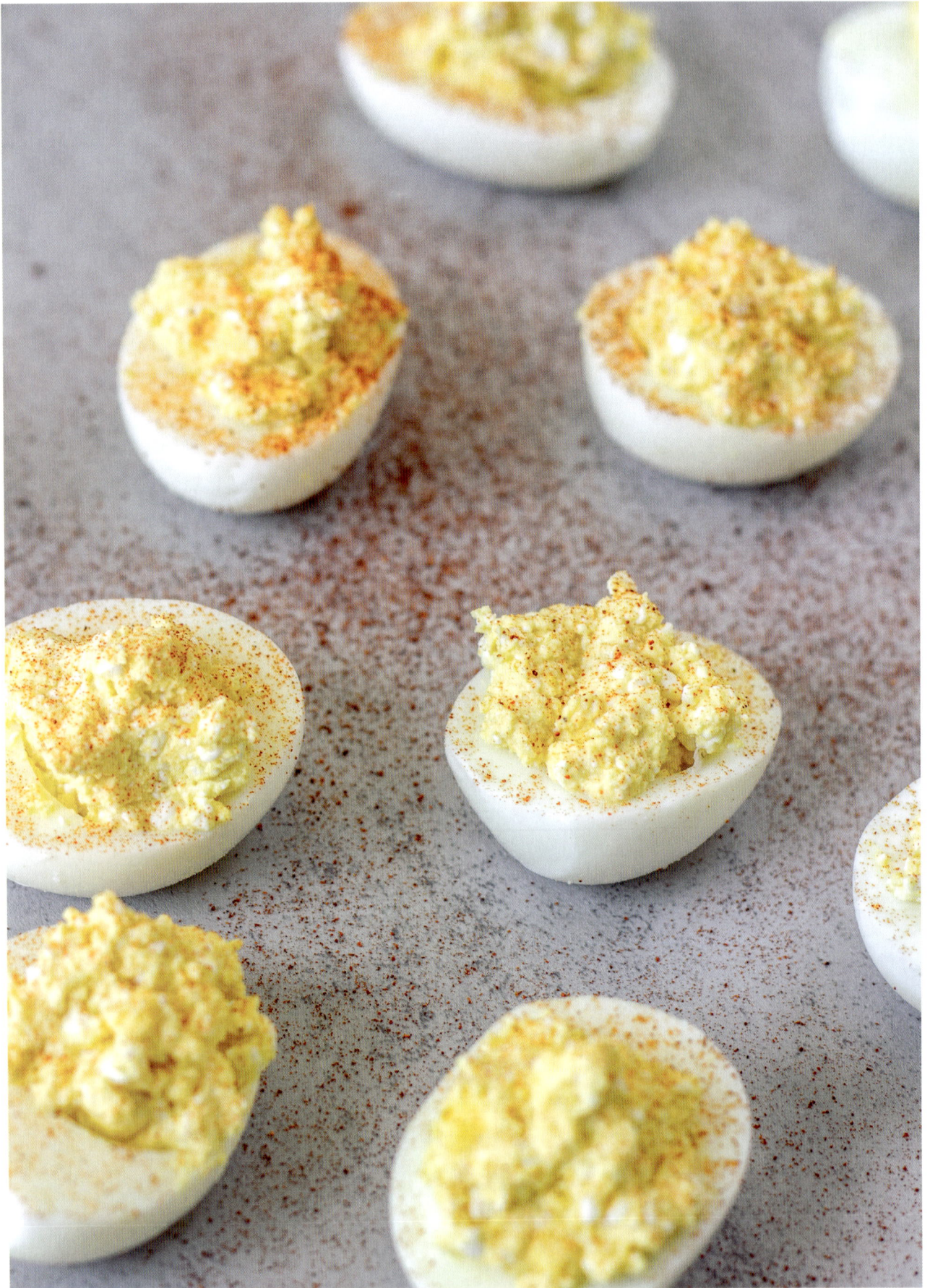

COTTAGE CHEESE DEVILED EGGS

SERVES 2

PREP TIME 10 minutes (not including time to hard-boil eggs)

Who says deviled eggs are just an appetizer? Although eggs on their own aren't super high in protein, mixing cottage cheese into the yolks ups the protein content significantly. I like to pair these deviled eggs with an ounce of sharp cheddar cheese to hit a total of 30 grams of complete protein and a leafy green salad for a boost of fiber.

6 hard-boiled eggs, peeled and sliced in half through the center

½ cup cottage cheese

2 teaspoons Dijon mustard

Salt

Smoked paprika, for garnish

1. Carefully scoop the cooked egg yolks into a small bowl. Add the cottage cheese, mustard, and a heavy pinch of salt. Mash with a fork until smooth and creamy.

2. Spoon the yolk mixture into the egg white halves. Garnish with a sprinkle of smoked paprika.

TEMPEH BLT

SERVES 1

PREP TIME 5 minutes

COOK TIME 8 minutes

This recipe is inspired by a sandwich I used to order all the time in college at our local food co-op. Tempeh is the one of the best plant-based sources of protein because the soy has been fermented to help reduce antinutrients. Tempeh bacon is pretty easy to find at nearly any grocery store. The brand I usually grab is called Light Life. To keep this meal lower in carbs, you could swap out the bread and use more lettuce as a wrap. However, both Ezekiel bread and real fermented whole-wheat sourdough are good lower-glycemic options for a "true" sandwich experience.

1 teaspoon olive oil

8 slices tempeh bacon, cut in half crosswise

2 slices Ezekiel bread or fermented whole-wheat sourdough

1 tablespoon avocado oil mayonnaise or organic olive oil–based mayo

2 leaves crunchy lettuce, such as romaine

2 slices tomato

¼ avocado, sliced

Salt and pepper

1. Heat the olive oil in a large skillet over medium-high heat. Add the tempeh bacon and fry for 3 to 4 minutes per side, until golden brown.

2. Toast the bread in a toaster, then spread the mayonnaise on one side of each slice.

3. Assemble the sandwich: Top a piece of bread with the lettuce, tomato, tempeh bacon, and avocado. Sprinkle the avocado with salt and pepper and top with the second piece of bread.

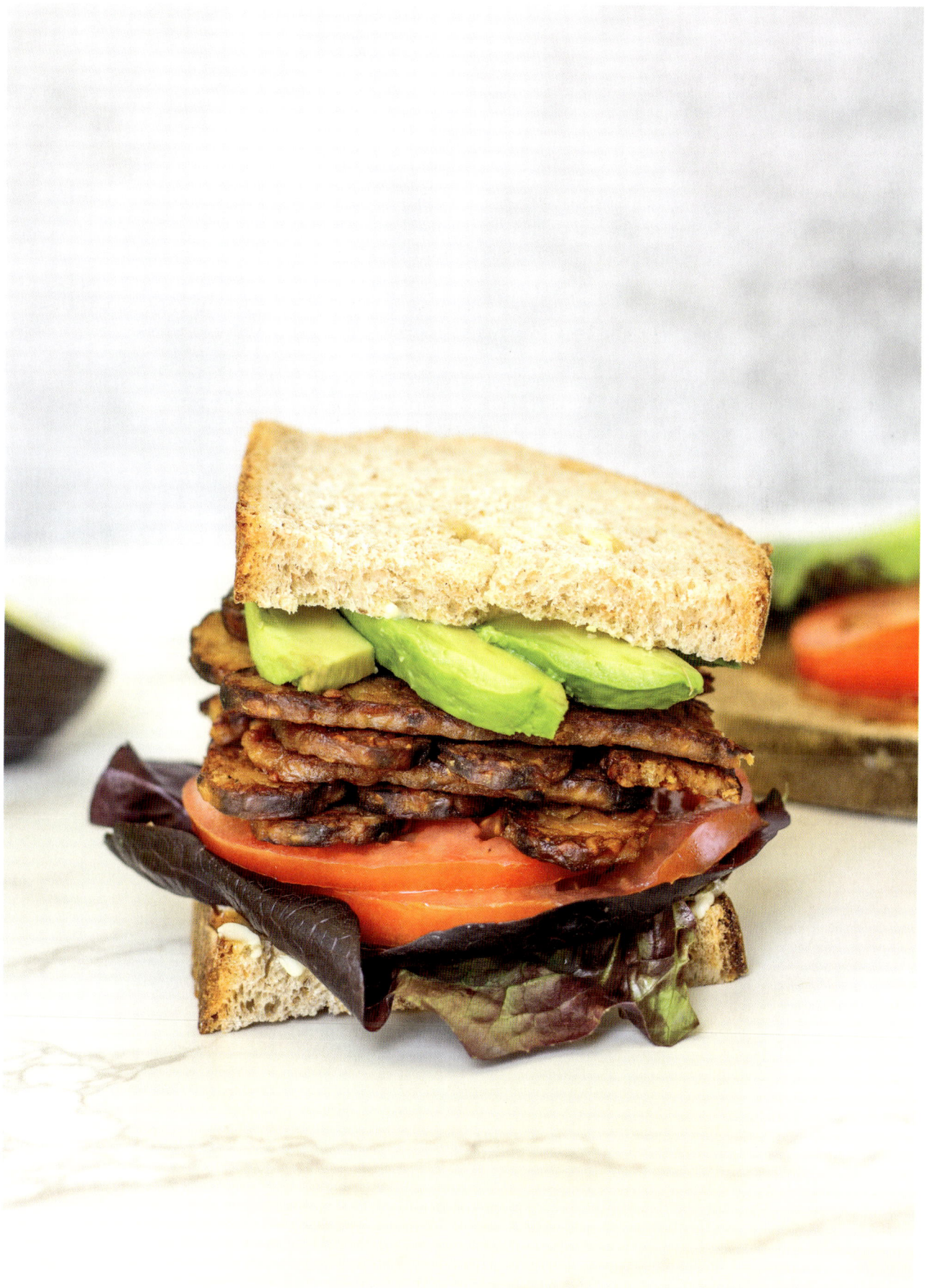

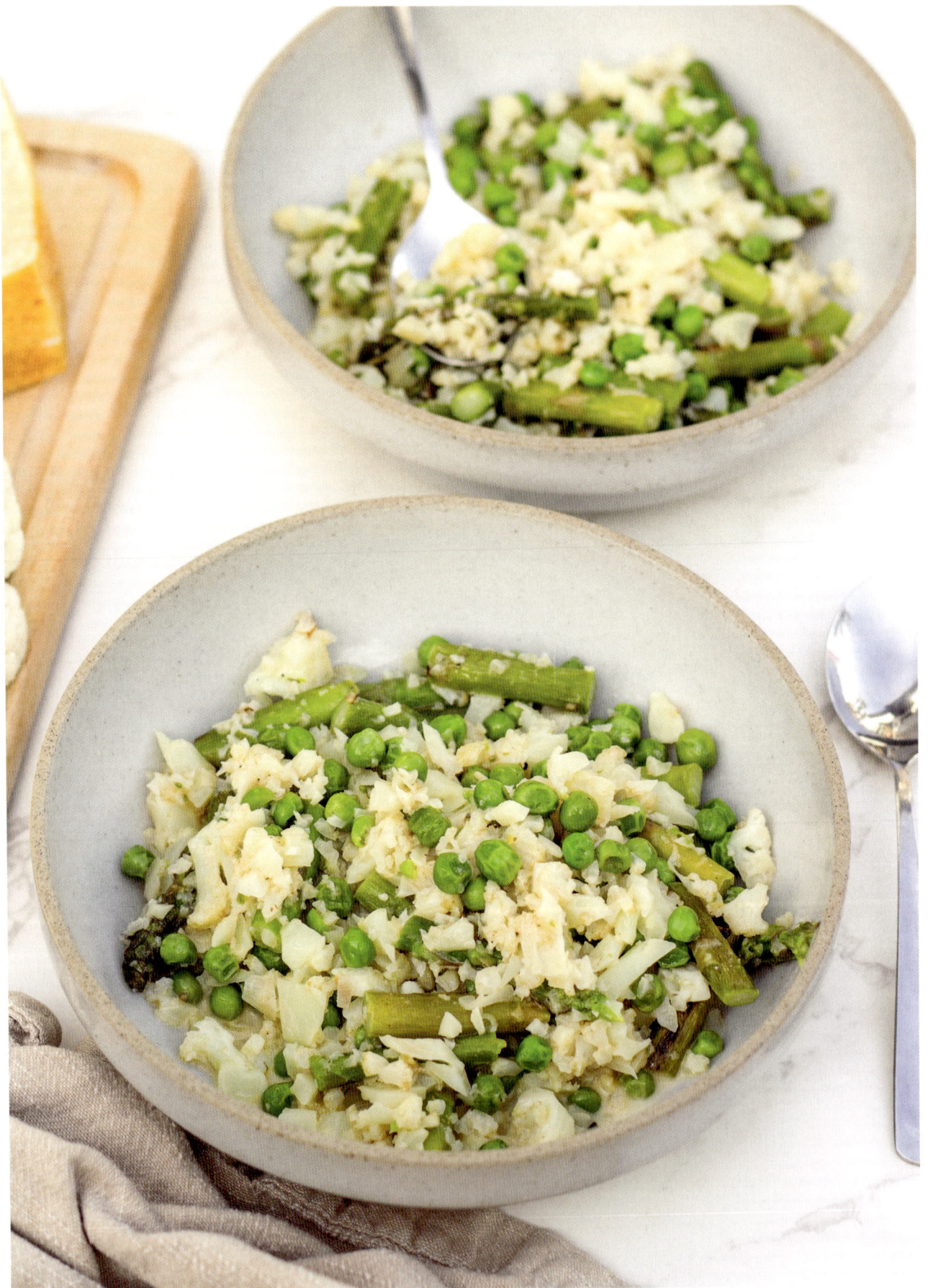

SUPER CHEESY SPRING "RISOTTO"

You're getting a *lot* of veggie action in this meal! To keep it vegetarian but still packed with protein, I focused on two main ingredients: Parmesan and peas. Each serving of "risotto" has nearly 30 grams of protein and 12 grams of fiber. By swapping out rice, we're also able to make a typically high–glycemic load meal into a low–glycemic load one.

2 tablespoons salted butter

1 medium shallot, diced

2 cloves garlic, minced

Salt

1 cup roughly chopped asparagus

4 cups cauliflower rice

2 cups frozen peas

1 cup grated Parmesan cheese

¼ cup heavy cream

1. Melt the butter in a large skillet over medium heat. Add the shallot, garlic, and a heavy pinch of salt and sauté until softened, about 2 minutes.

2. Add the asparagus and a pinch of salt and sauté for 5 minutes, until the asparagus has just started to soften but is still fairly firm.

3. Add the cauliflower rice and another heavy pinch of salt. Sauté for 5 to 7 minutes, until the asparagus is fork-tender and the cauliflower is softened.

4. Add the peas, Parmesan, and heavy cream. Cook for a few more minutes, stirring frequently, until most of the liquid has evaporated. Serve immediately.

SIDES and DIPS

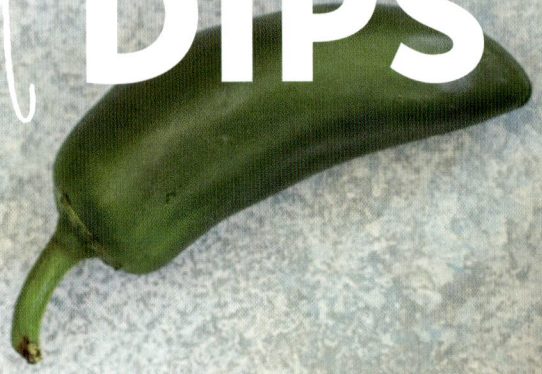

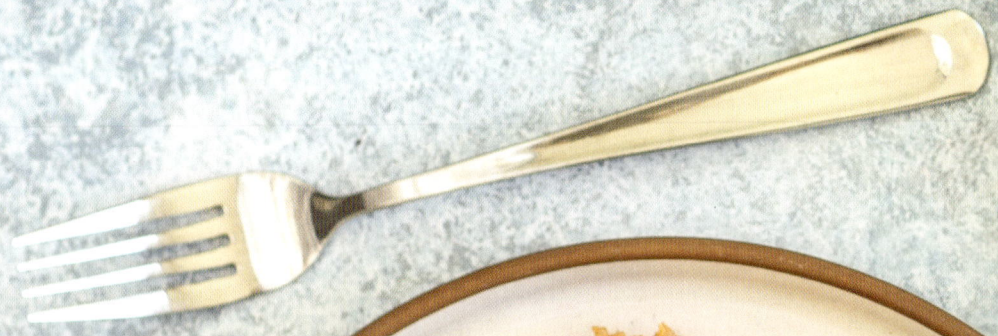

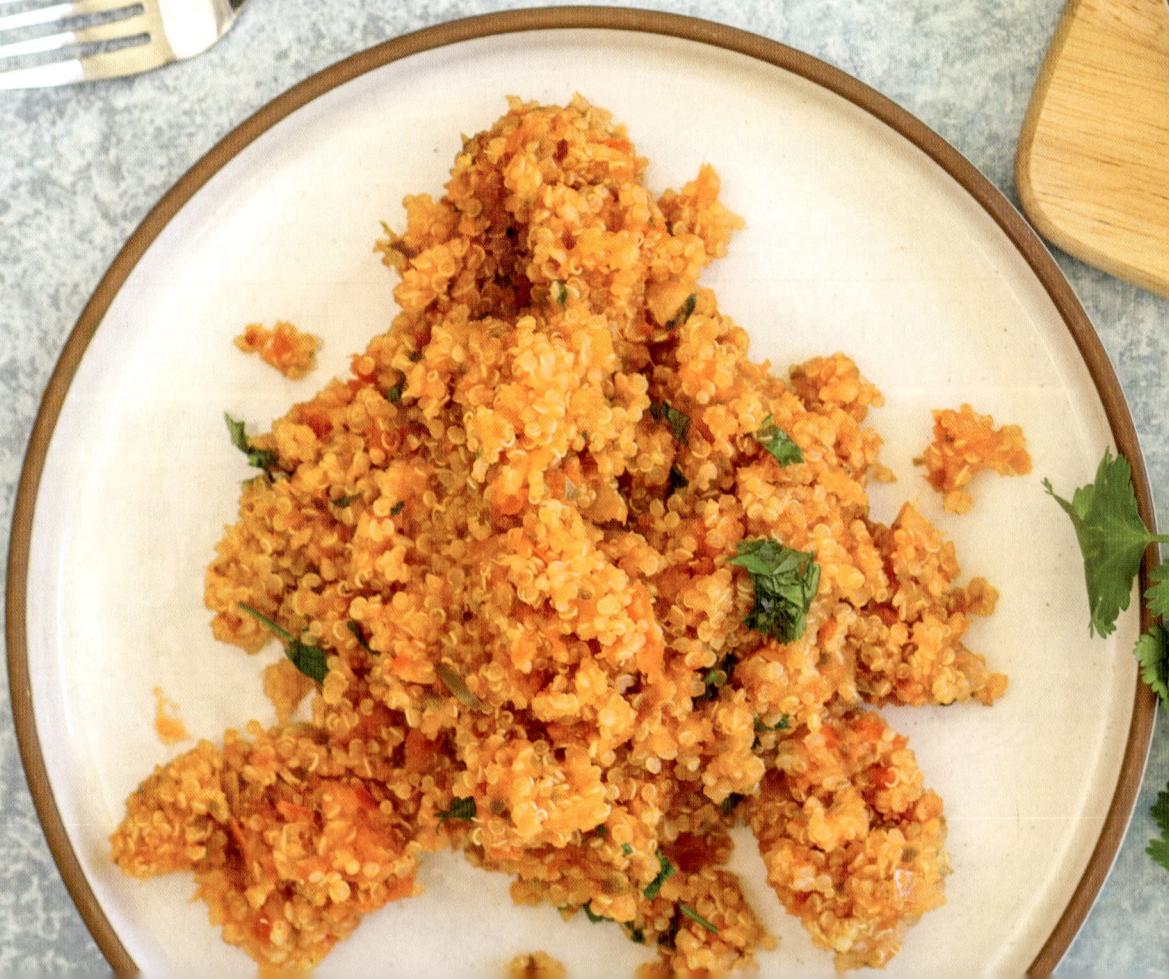

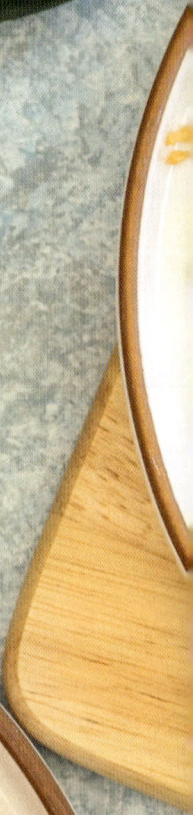

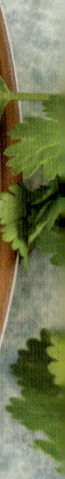

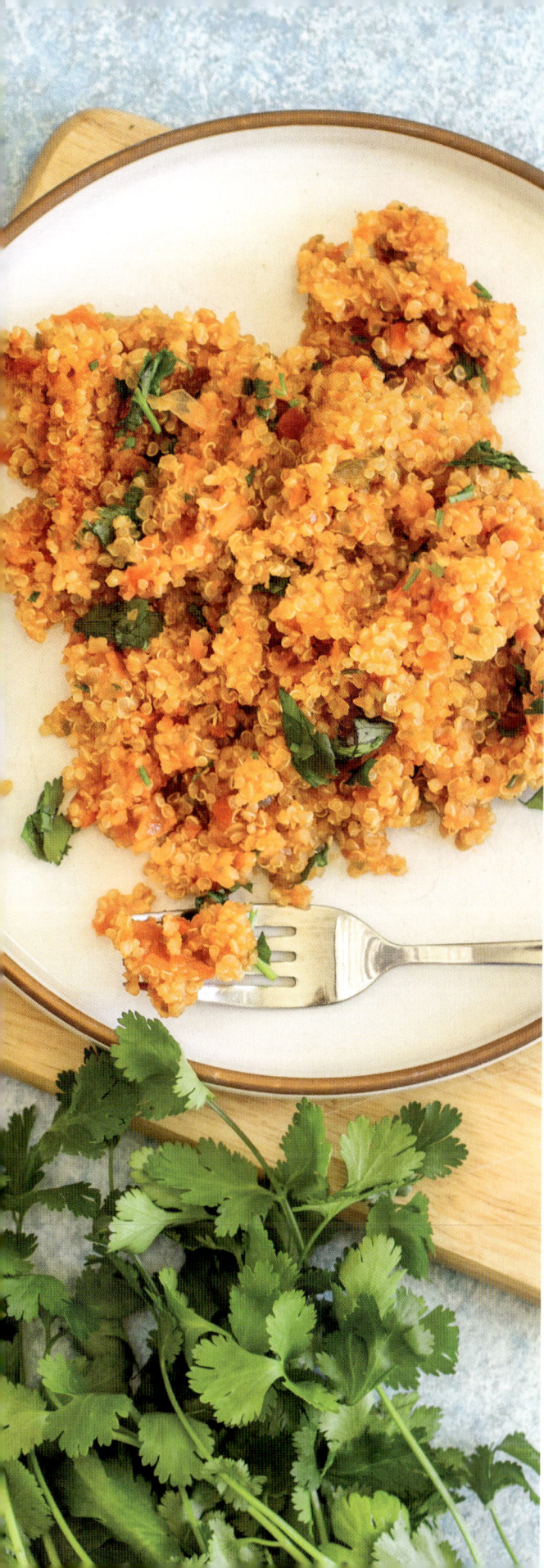

CRISPY BROCCOLINI

SERVES 4

PREP TIME 5 minutes

COOK TIME 15 minutes

Broccolini is similar to regular broccoli, but its stalks are longer and more tender, making it much tastier to eat the entire thing. Even though this recipe is incredibly simple, it's always a crowd-pleaser, especially when paired with Grilled Flank Steak with Chimichurri (page 143). This dish is an excellent way to get a boost of nutrient-dense carbohydrates with a low glycemic load.

1 pound broccolini

1 tablespoon olive oil

Salt

½ lemon

1. Preheat the oven to 400°F. Line a sheet pan with parchment paper.

2. Place the broccolini pieces on the prepared pan. Drizzle with the olive oil and sprinkle with a heavy pinch of salt; toss the broccolini to evenly coat. Spread it out so that no pieces are overlapping.

3. Roast for 15 minutes, or until the broccolini is crispy on the edges but has some tenderness in the middle.

4. Squeeze the lemon over the broccolini and serve.

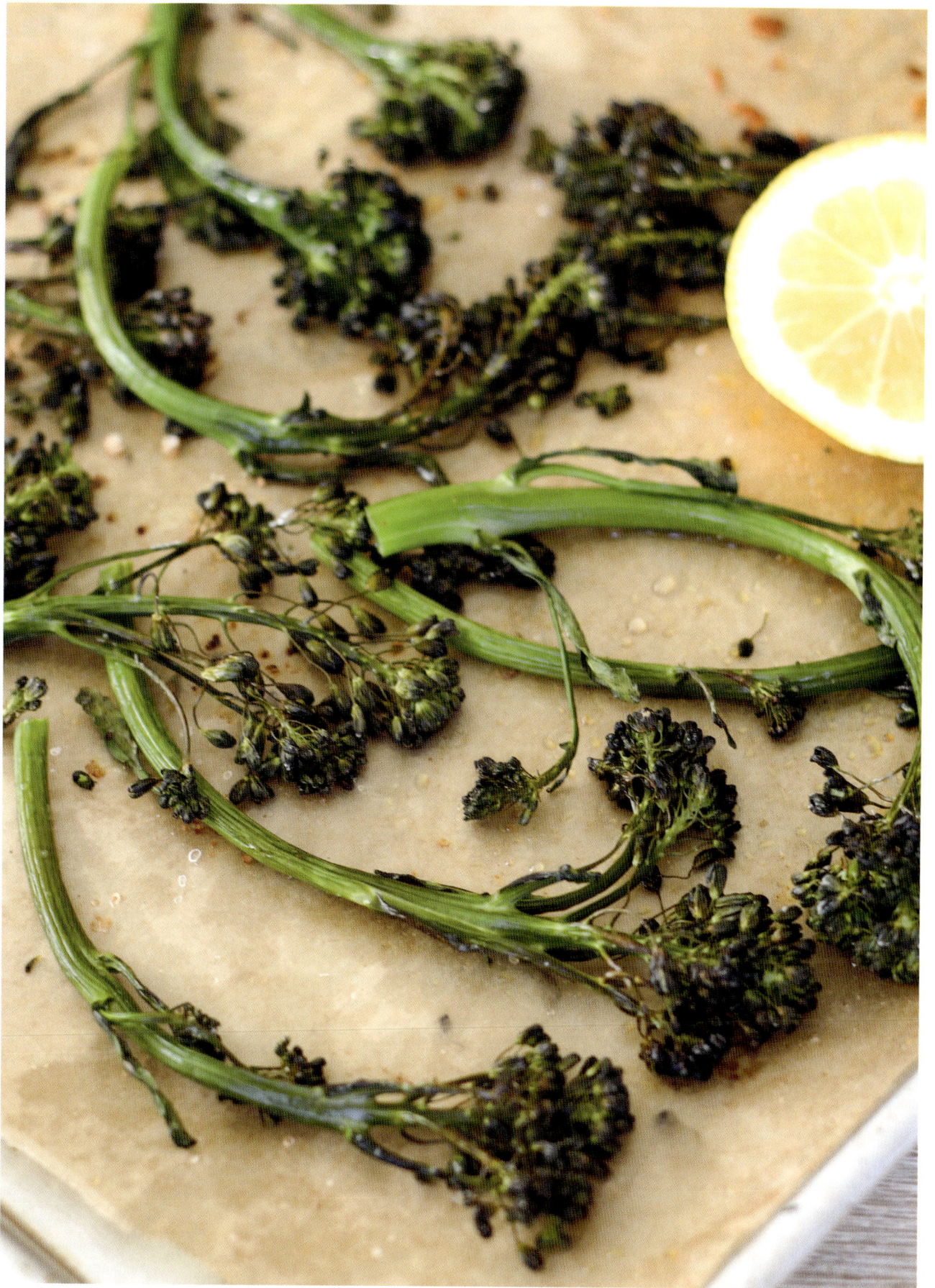

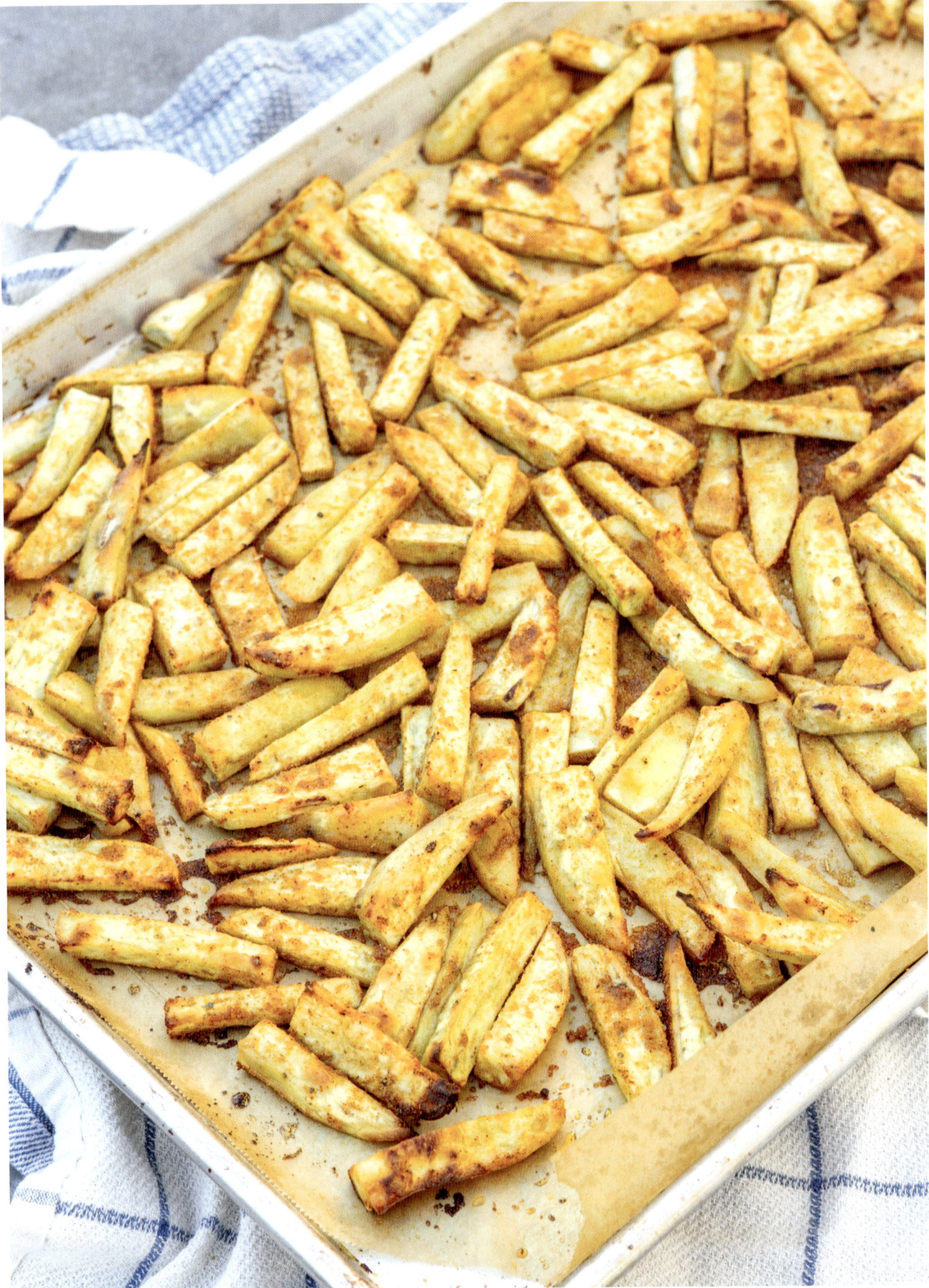

OVEN-ROASTED SWEET POTATO FRIES

SERVES 4

PREP TIME 5 minutes

COOK TIME 30 minutes

This is a staple side dish in our household. Our daughter, Sage, loves these fries and would eat them at every meal if we allowed it! Sweet potatoes come in a ton of varieties, so feel free to experiment with different options—this cooking method can be applied to all of them. I personally love Japanese and purple sweet potatoes. However, if you are carb sensitive, you can swap out the sweet potatoes for 1 pound of carrots. These fries are great served with my Swiss Smash Burgers (page 144).

SEASONING BLEND

1 teaspoon salt

1 teaspoon garlic powder

1 teaspoon onion powder

1 teaspoon paprika

¼ teaspoon cayenne pepper

¼ teaspoon dried oregano leaves

FRIES

2 large sweet potatoes (about 1 pound), peeled and cut into french fry strips

1 tablespoon olive oil

1. Preheat the oven to 425°F. Line a sheet pan with parchment paper.

2. In a small bowl, combine the ingredients for the seasoning blend.

3. Put the sweet potato strips on the prepared pan and sprinkle with the seasoning blend and olive oil. Toss to evenly coat, then spread them out into a single layer. Roast for 25 to 30 minutes, until the fries are tender and slightly crispy.

ZUCCHINI SWEET POTATO HASH

SERVES 4

PREP TIME 5 minutes

COOK TIME 15 minutes

This super simple dish is in our regular meal rotation. Whenever we need a fast and filling veggie side to pair with burgers, we usually make this hash! The trick to a perfect hash is to make sure the veggies are even in size and preferably cut to a thickness of about ½ inch. If they are any thicker, the outsides will burn before the insides have a chance to cook. You can use any type of sweet potato or yam here, but I love purple sweet potatoes for their bright color.

1 tablespoon olive oil

½ medium yellow onion, diced

1 large zucchini, diced

1 large sweet potato, peeled and diced

2 teaspoons paprika

1 teaspoon dried oregano leaves

1 teaspoon garlic powder

1 teaspoon onion powder

1 teaspoon salt

1. Heat the olive oil in a large skillet over medium heat. Add the onion and sauté until softened, 2 to 3 minutes.

2. Bring the heat up to medium-high. Add the zucchini, sweet potato, paprika, oregano, garlic powder, onion powder, and salt. Cover and cook for 7 to 10 minutes, until the zucchini and sweet potato pieces are slightly browned and easily pierced with a fork. About halfway through the cooking time, give the veggies a stir to prevent them from sticking and burning, then re-cover the pan for the remainder of the cooking time.

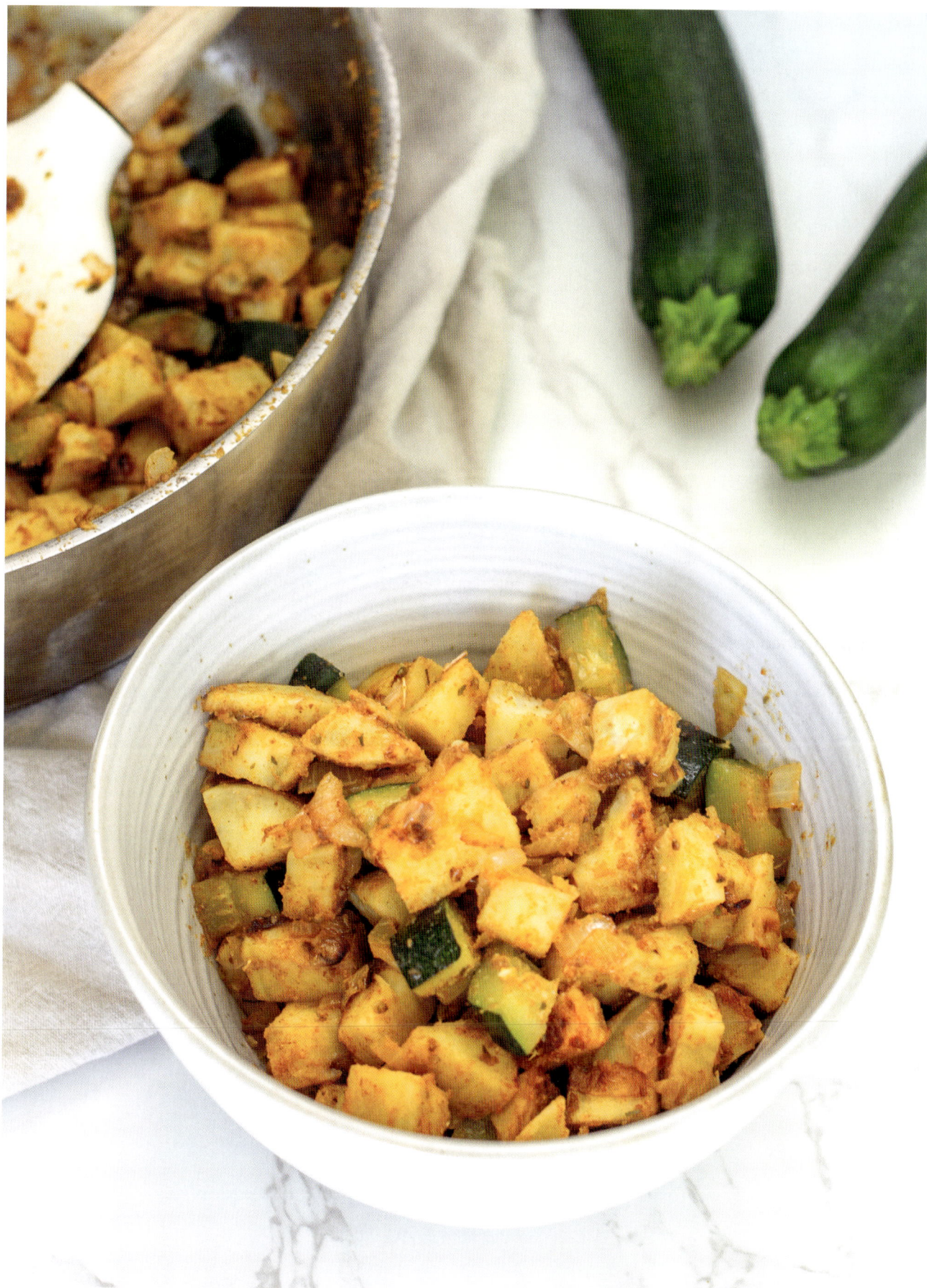

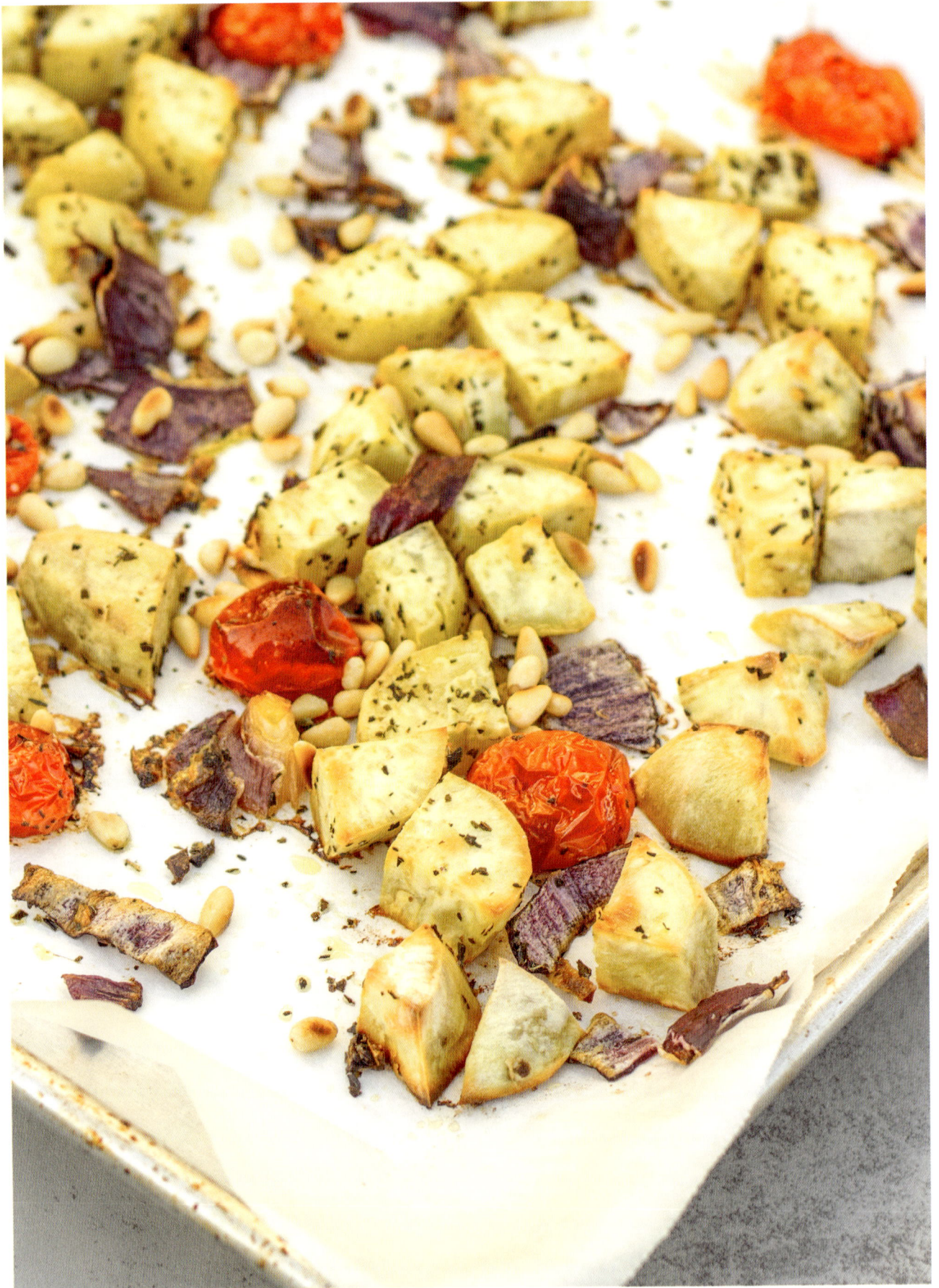

SUMMER SWEET POTATO AND TOMATO TRAY BAKE

SERVES 4

PREP TIME 10 minutes

COOK TIME 35 minutes

During the summer, the only thing I want to eat is tomatoes. We love to go to our local Sunday farmers market, where each stall is packed to the brim with a variety of flavorful tomatoes. One way I like to make use of this seasonal harvest is by making a quick and flavorful tray bake. Even though basil is in season at the same time, I prefer dried basil in this recipe, as it withstands the higher-temperature baking a lot better than fresh basil. If you're particularly carb sensitive, you can swap out the sweet potatoes for four chopped carrots. To make this a complete meal, I like to pair it with my Balsamic Grilled Chicken (page 168) or Lamb Burgers (page 156).

2 medium sweet potatoes, peeled and cubed

1 pound grape or cherry tomatoes

1 medium red onion, roughly chopped

5 cloves garlic, minced

1 tablespoon olive oil

2 teaspoons dried basil leaves

Salt

¼ cup pine nuts

1. Preheat the oven to 425°F and line a sheet pan with parchment paper.

2. Place the sweet potatoes, tomatoes, onion, and garlic on the prepared pan. Drizzle with the olive oil and sprinkle with the basil and a heavy pinch of salt. Use your hands to toss all of the ingredients until evenly coated.

3. Bake for 30 to 35 minutes, until the sweet potatoes are easily pierced with a fork and the tomatoes are blistered.

4. Meanwhile, toast the pine nuts: Preheat a small skillet over medium-high heat. Pour in the pine nuts and toast, shaking the pan every 20 seconds or so to prevent burning. When the pine nuts are lightly browned, remove the pan from the heat and pour the nuts into a small bowl.

5. Top the roasted veggies with the toasted pine nuts before serving.

PINTO BEANS AND VEGGIES

SERVES 4

PREP TIME 5 minutes

COOK TIME 15 minutes

I love bulking up beans with low–glycemic load veggies to make a side that goes well with nearly any meat-based meal. If you have the time to make homemade beans, it makes a big difference to the overall taste and texture of this simple dish. Try pairing it with Weeknight Ground Beef Tacos (page 151) or Balsamic Grilled Chicken (page 168). It also makes great leftovers for lunch!

1 tablespoon olive oil

½ medium yellow onion, diced

4 cloves garlic, minced

Salt

2 medium zucchini, chopped

1 teaspoon paprika

1 cup cooked pinto beans, canned or homemade (page 85)

1. Heat the olive oil in a medium-sized skillet over medium-high heat. Add the onion, garlic, and a heavy pinch of salt. Sauté for 3 to 5 minutes, until the onion is softened and the garlic is fragrant.

2. Add the zucchini and paprika and sauté for 5 to 7 minutes, until the zucchini is slightly browned and tender but not mushy.

3. Add the beans and another pinch of salt. Sauté for 3 more minutes, or until the beans are warmed through and incorporated into the other ingredients.

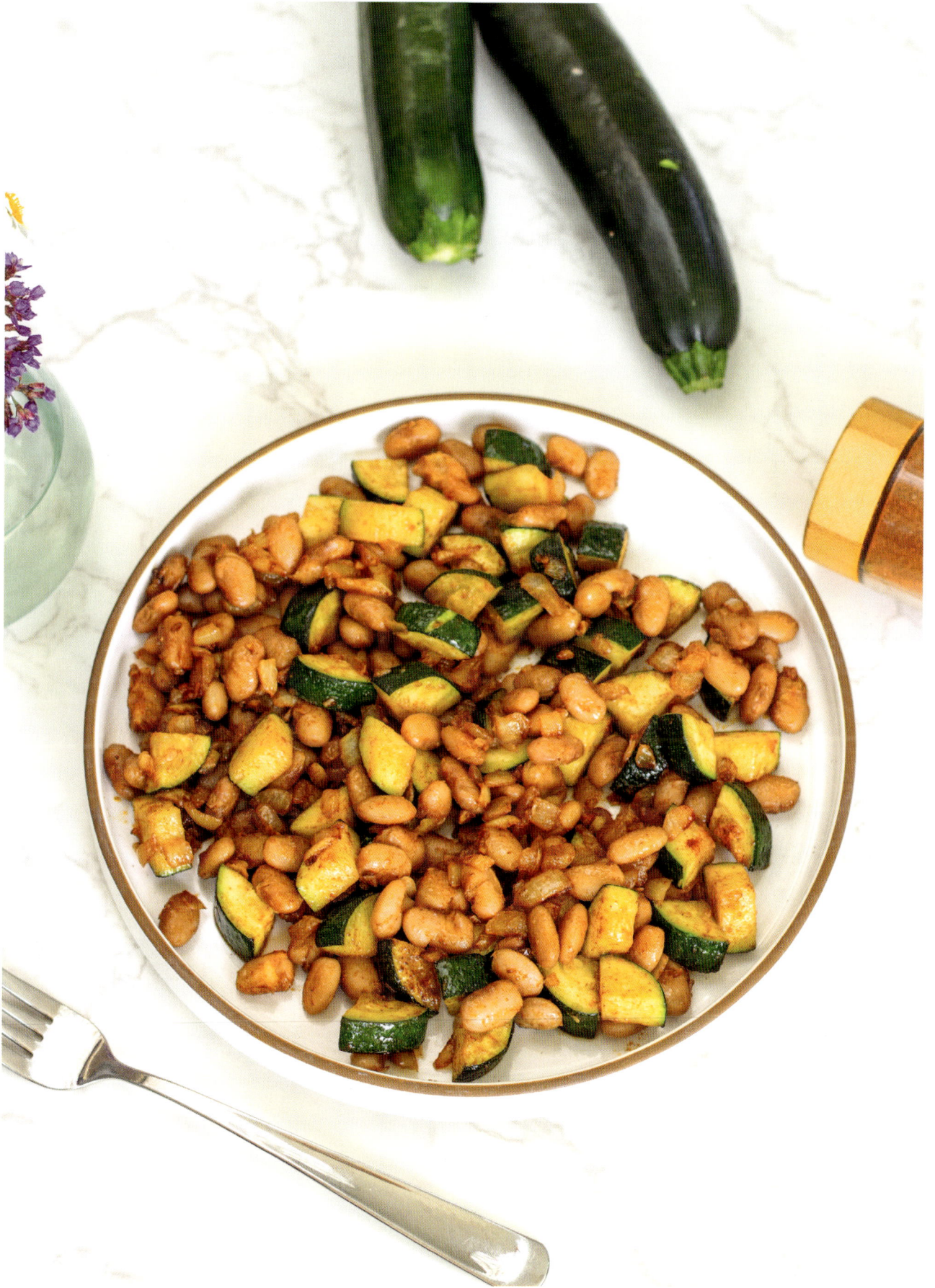

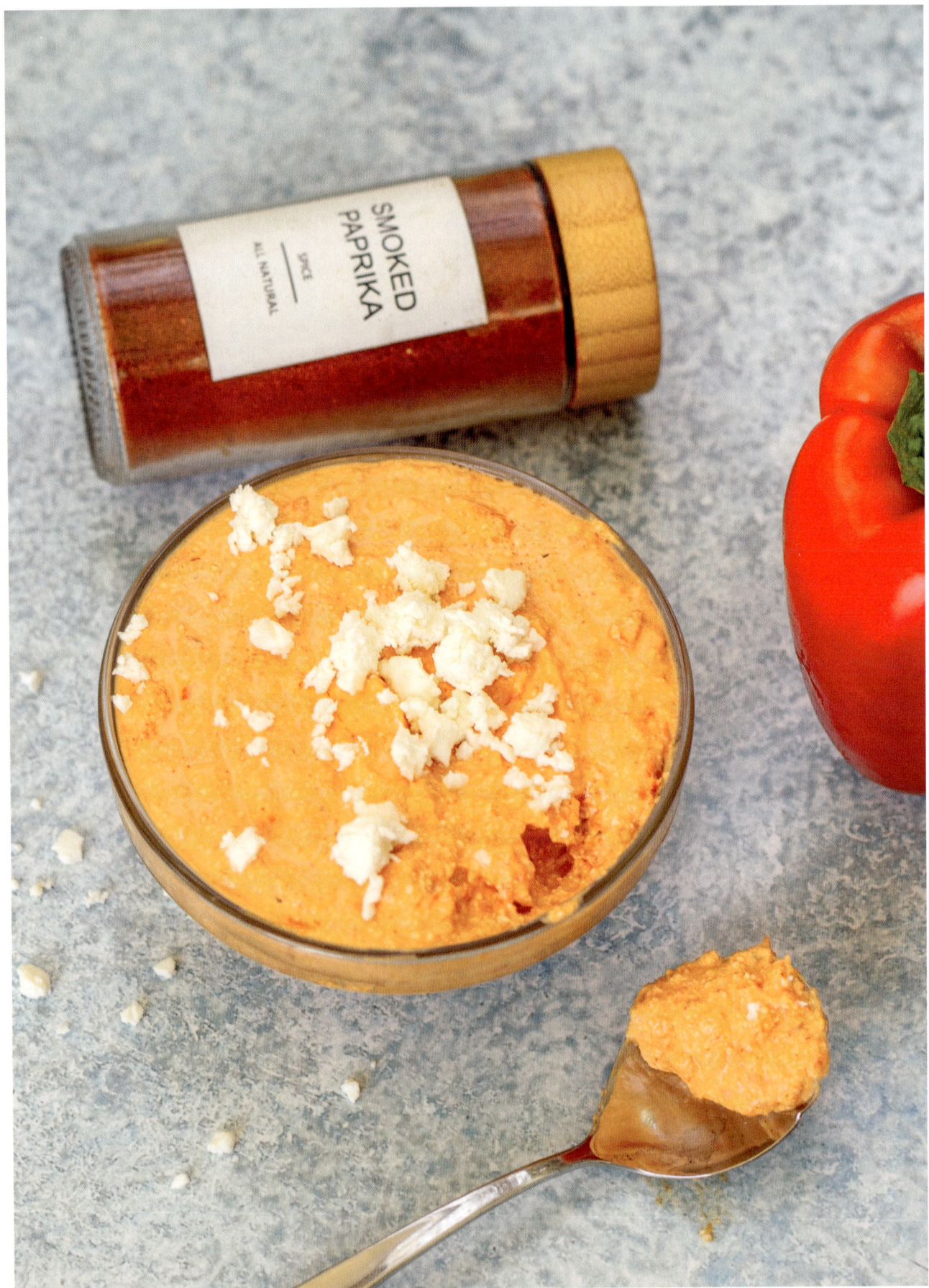

ROASTED RED PEPPER DIP

MAKES 1 cup

PREP TIME 5 minutes

COOK TIME 10 minutes

This veggie and cheese dip provides some fat, protein, a dash of fiber, and a whole lot of flavor! I love making a batch and having it for the week to top salads, dip veggies into, spread on a wrap, or eat with scrambled eggs. This dip also tastes delicious with my Lamb Kefta with Grilled Zucchini (page 152).

1 red bell pepper, sliced in half lengthwise, ribs, seeds, and stem removed

8 ounces feta cheese

2 tablespoons olive oil

Juice of ½ lemon (1 to 1½ tablespoons)

½ teaspoon smoked or sweet paprika

⅛ teaspoon cayenne pepper

1. Set the oven to broil and line a sheet pan with aluminum foil.

2. Place the bell pepper halves cut side down on the prepared pan. Broil for 7 to 10 minutes, until the pepper is lightly charred. Remove from the oven and fold the foil around the pepper to allow it to steam while you prepare the rest of the ingredients.

3. Put the feta, olive oil, lemon juice, paprika, and cayenne in a food processor or blender. Carefully add the roasted bell pepper halves. Cover and blend until smooth.

4. Store leftovers in a sealed container in the fridge for up to 5 days.

SPICED CAULIFLOWER RICE

SERVES 4

PREP TIME 5 minutes

COOK TIME 20 minutes

While working with clients, I realized that a lot of people were preparing cauliflower rice in a way that made it soggy and bland. Cauliflower as an ingredient can take on nearly any flavor and therefore should be an excellent side dish to most meals, but to taste great, it needs to have flavor added to it and be cooked properly. I've found that baking cauliflower rice after tossing it with seasonings helps eliminate the sogginess that can occur when it's sautéed or steamed. If using this rice as the base for my Fish Taco Bowls (page 187), you'll want to make it serve two rather than four to allow for enough bulk for the meal. Also note that cauliflower rice does not store very well, so if you don't think you can eat a whole batch, consider halving this recipe.

4 cups cauliflower rice

2 teaspoons paprika

2 teaspoons garlic powder

1 teaspoon onion powder

¼ teaspoon cayenne pepper

Salt

1 tablespoon olive oil

1. Preheat the oven to 425°F and line a sheet pan with parchment paper.

2. Pour the cauliflower rice onto the prepared sheet pan. Sprinkle with the paprika, garlic powder, onion powder, cayenne, and a heavy pinch of salt. Drizzle with the olive oil and use your hands to toss until the cauliflower rice is evenly coated with the seasonings. Bake for 20 minutes, or until lightly browned and tender.

3. Serve immediately.

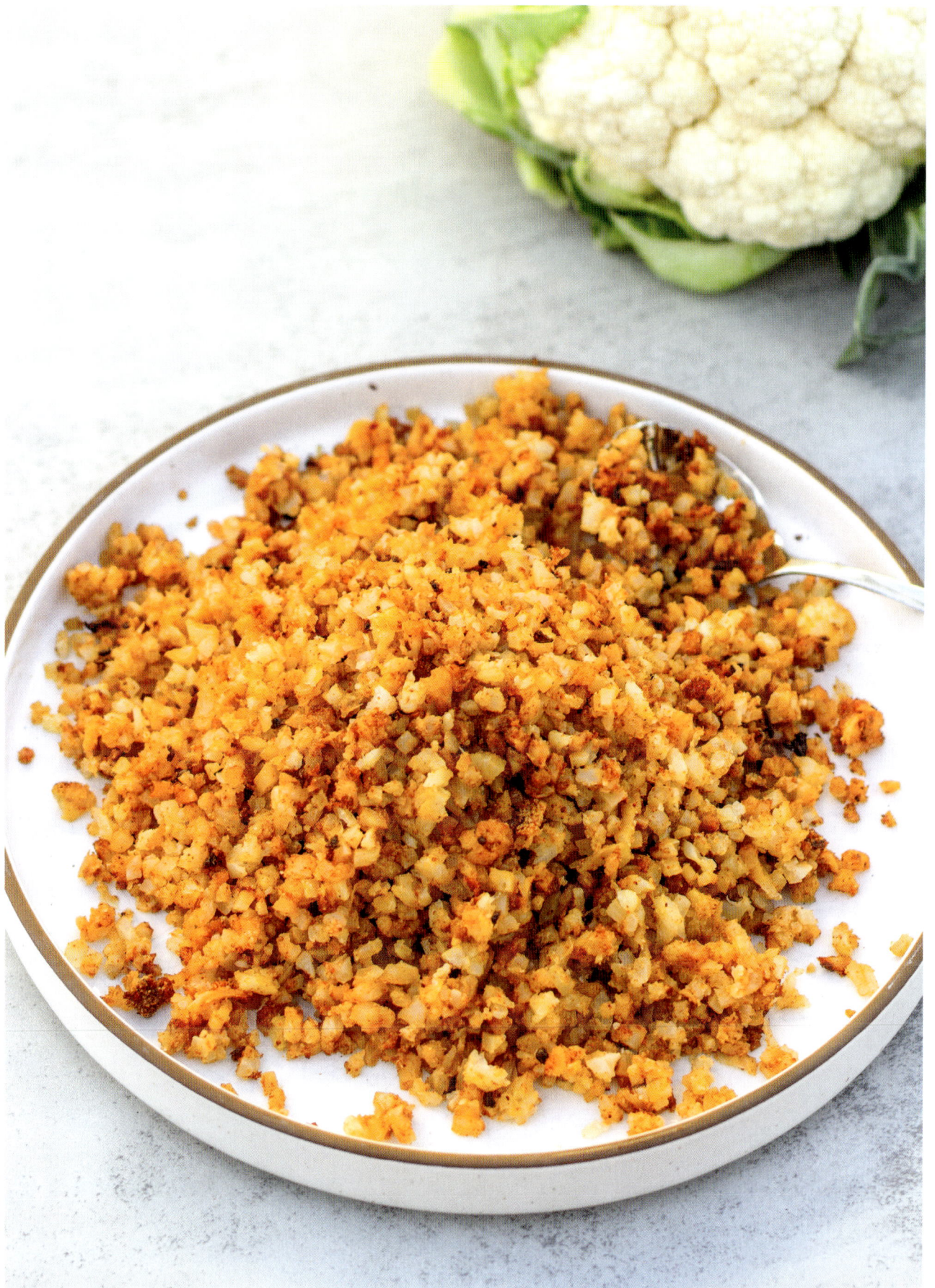

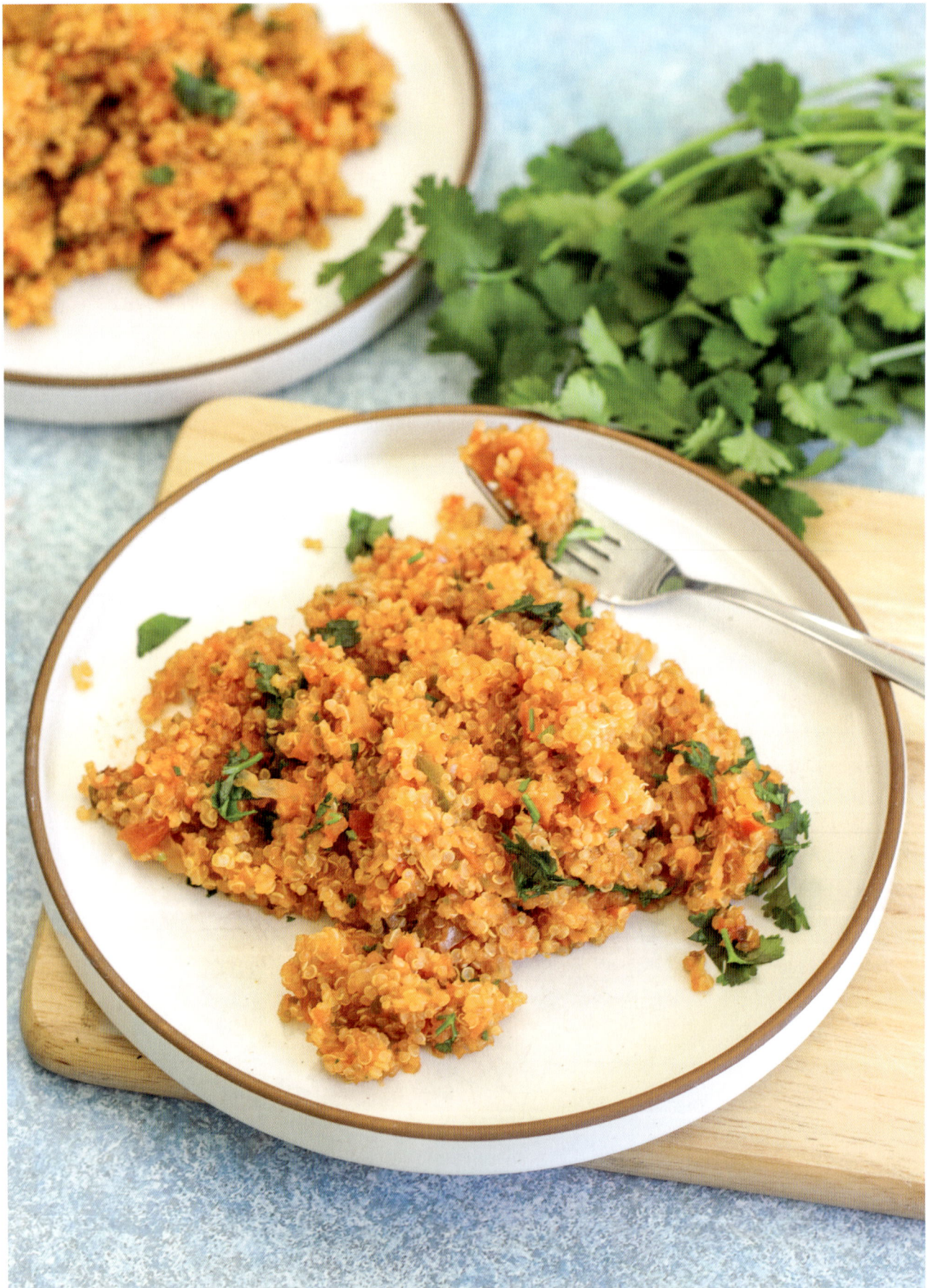

MEXICAN-STYLE QUINOA

SERVES 4

PREP TIME 10 minutes

COOK TIME 20 minutes

With this recipe, I've adapted traditional Mexican rice to use quinoa, which is a medium–glycemic load grain alternative to white rice that is much more blood sugar stabilizing. Although quinoa is better than rice, it is still a medium- to high-GL food, depending on the amount you eat. For this reason, it's best consumed during weight maintenance or when pursuing a fitness goal. I love pairing this dish with grilled steak and sautéed bell pepper and onions for a fajita-style bowl.

2 medium tomatoes, quartered

½ medium yellow onion, chopped

4 cloves garlic

2 jalapeño peppers, chopped (remove membranes and seeds if you prefer less heat)

2 tablespoons olive oil

¾ cup quinoa, rinsed

1¼ cups beef or chicken bone broth or water

1 tablespoon tomato paste

1 teaspoon ground cumin

1 teaspoon salt

¼ cup chopped fresh cilantro

Special equipment: food processor

1. Put the tomatoes, onion, garlic, and jalapeños in a food processor and pulse until pureed.

2. Heat the olive oil in a Dutch oven over medium heat. Add the quinoa and sauté for 2 minutes, or until lightly toasted.

3. Add the pureed tomato mixture, broth, tomato paste, cumin, and salt. Bring to a boil, then reduce to a simmer, cover, and cook for 15 minutes, until the quinoa is fluffy.

4. Remove the pan from the heat and stir in the cilantro before serving.

CAULIFLOWER AVOCADO TABBOULEH

SERVES 4

PREP TIME 10 minutes

Tabbouleh is a refreshing herby side dish that pairs well with Middle Eastern–style meals. Typically, tabbouleh is made with bulgur, which is a wheat-based product that is a bit high glycemic load. Here, I've swapped it for fresh cauliflower rice to give a similar experience without the blood sugar spike. I also add avocado and feta to bump up the overall satiety. Try this dish with any of your favorite grilled meats (it's great with my Lamb Burgers on page 156) and some hummus. It is also used in my Lebanese-Style Brekky Bowl recipe (page 102).

4 cups fresh cauliflower rice, store-bought or homemade (see note)

1 bunch fresh parsley, minced

1 medium tomato, diced

½ avocado, peeled and diced

½ cup sliced green onions

¼ cup chopped fresh mint

Juice of 1 lemon (2 to 3 tablespoons)

2 tablespoons crumbled feta cheese

1 tablespoon olive oil

1 teaspoon garlic powder

Salt to taste

1. Put all of the ingredients in a bowl and toss to combine.
2. Eat immediately or store in a glass container in the fridge for up to 4 days.

Note: For this recipe, you need the crunch of fresh cauliflower rice; the frozen kind won't cut it here. To make your own fresh cauliflower rice, start by removing the green leaves from a large head of cauliflower. Wash the cauliflower and pat it completely dry. Then grate the entire head (including the stalk as well as the florets) using the large holes on a cheese grater. This will yield 2 to 4 cups of cauliflower rice, depending on the exact size of the head. Use the rice immediately or store it in a zip-top plastic bag in the fridge for up to 3 days. You can also freeze it for up to 6 months, although frozen cauliflower rice should only be used for cooked recipes, such as my Spiced Cauliflower Rice (page 230).

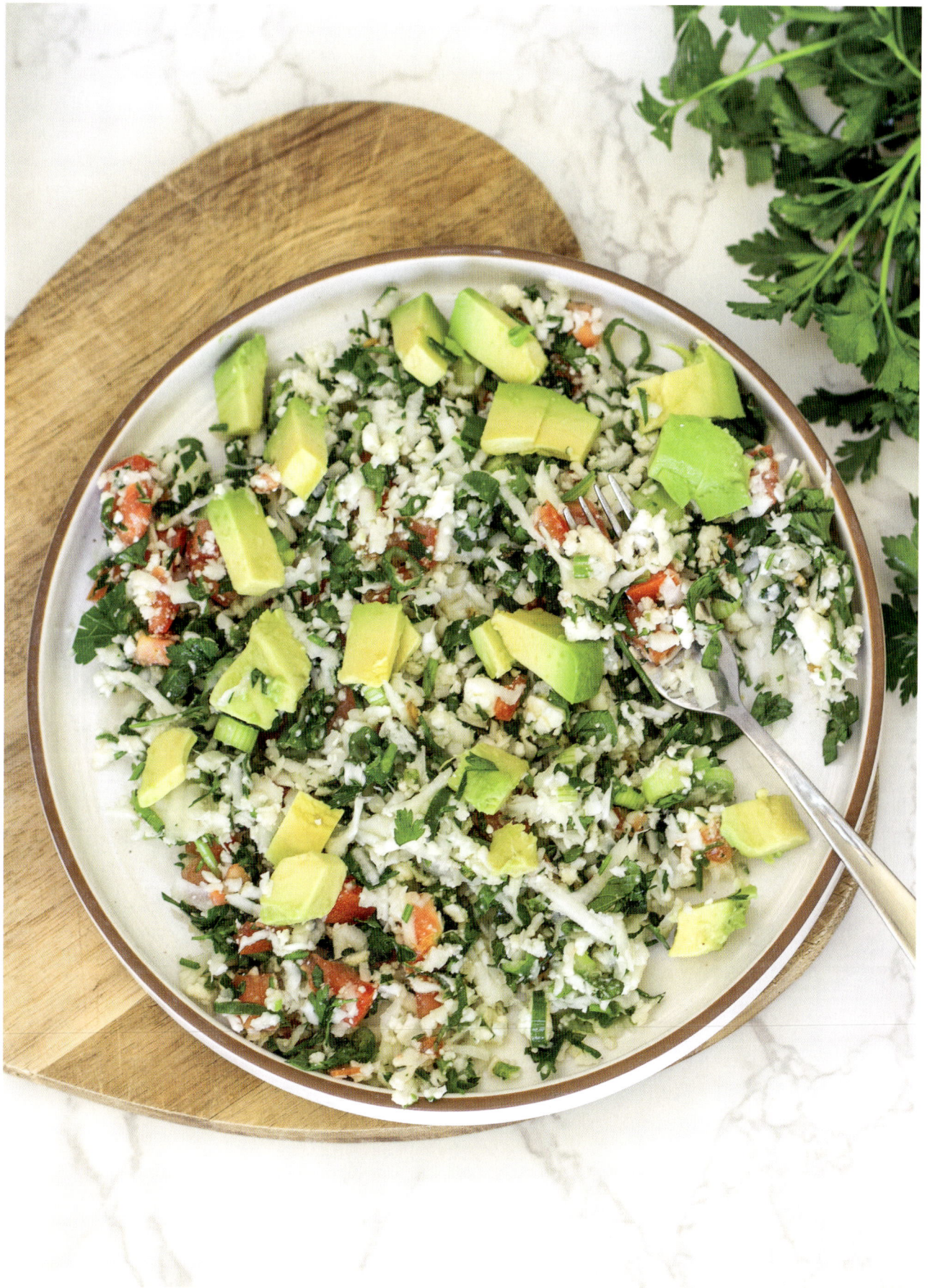

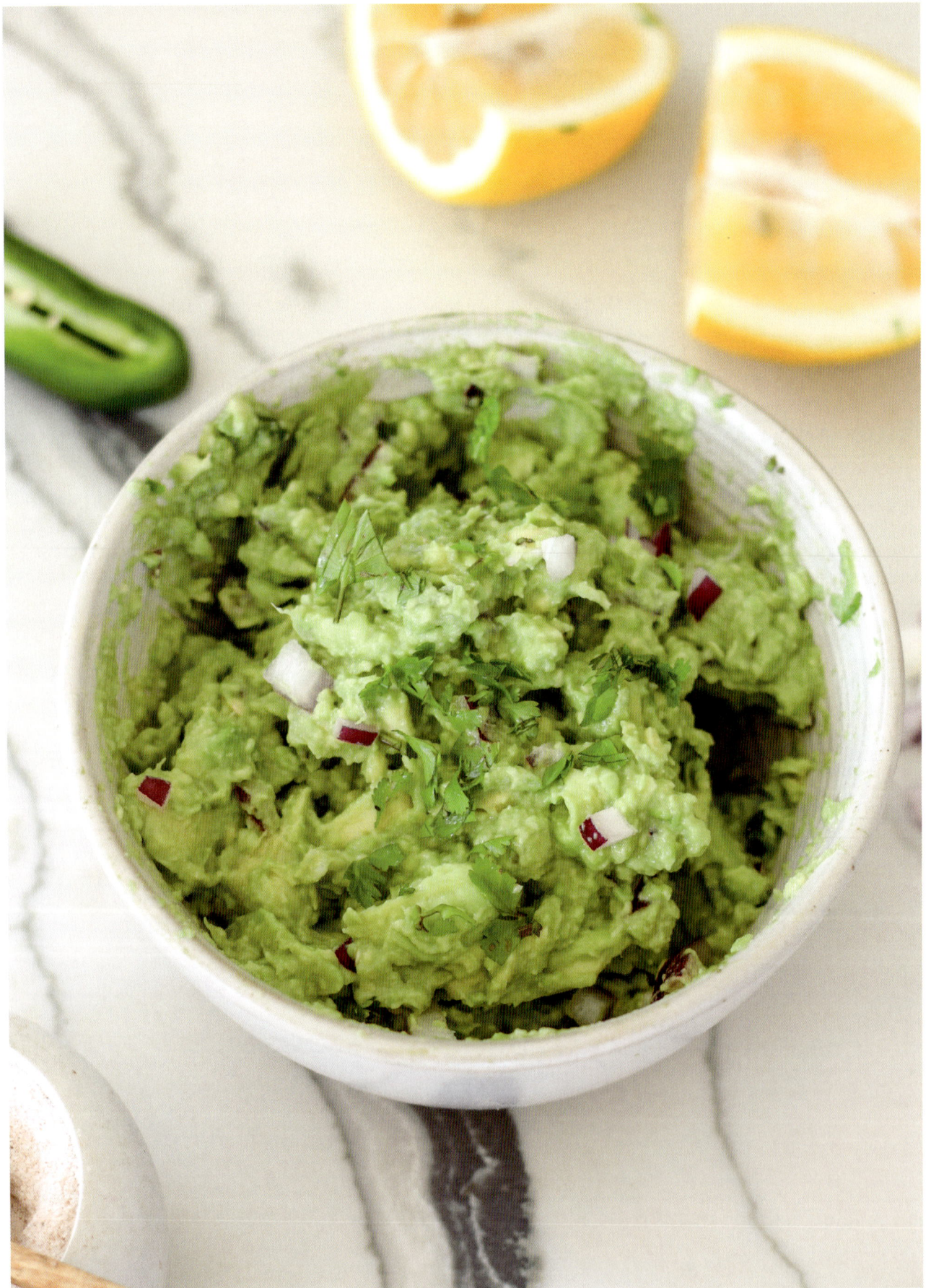

GUACAMOLE

MAKES 2 cups

PREP TIME 5 minutes

Fresh guacamole is a great way to add a high-quality source of fat and fiber to a meal. I prefer to mash my guacamole lightly so that there are still some avocado chunks in it. This gives it a fresh texture that regular store-bought guacamole can't really replicate.

2 large ripe avocados, peeled and pitted

¼ cup chopped fresh cilantro

¼ cup diced red onions

½ jalapeño pepper, finely diced (remove membranes and seeds if you prefer less heat)

Juice of ½ lemon (1 to 1½ tablespoons)

¼ teaspoon salt

1. Put all of the ingredients in a medium-sized mixing bowl. Gently mash with a fork to combine.
2. Taste and add more salt if needed. Enjoy immediately.

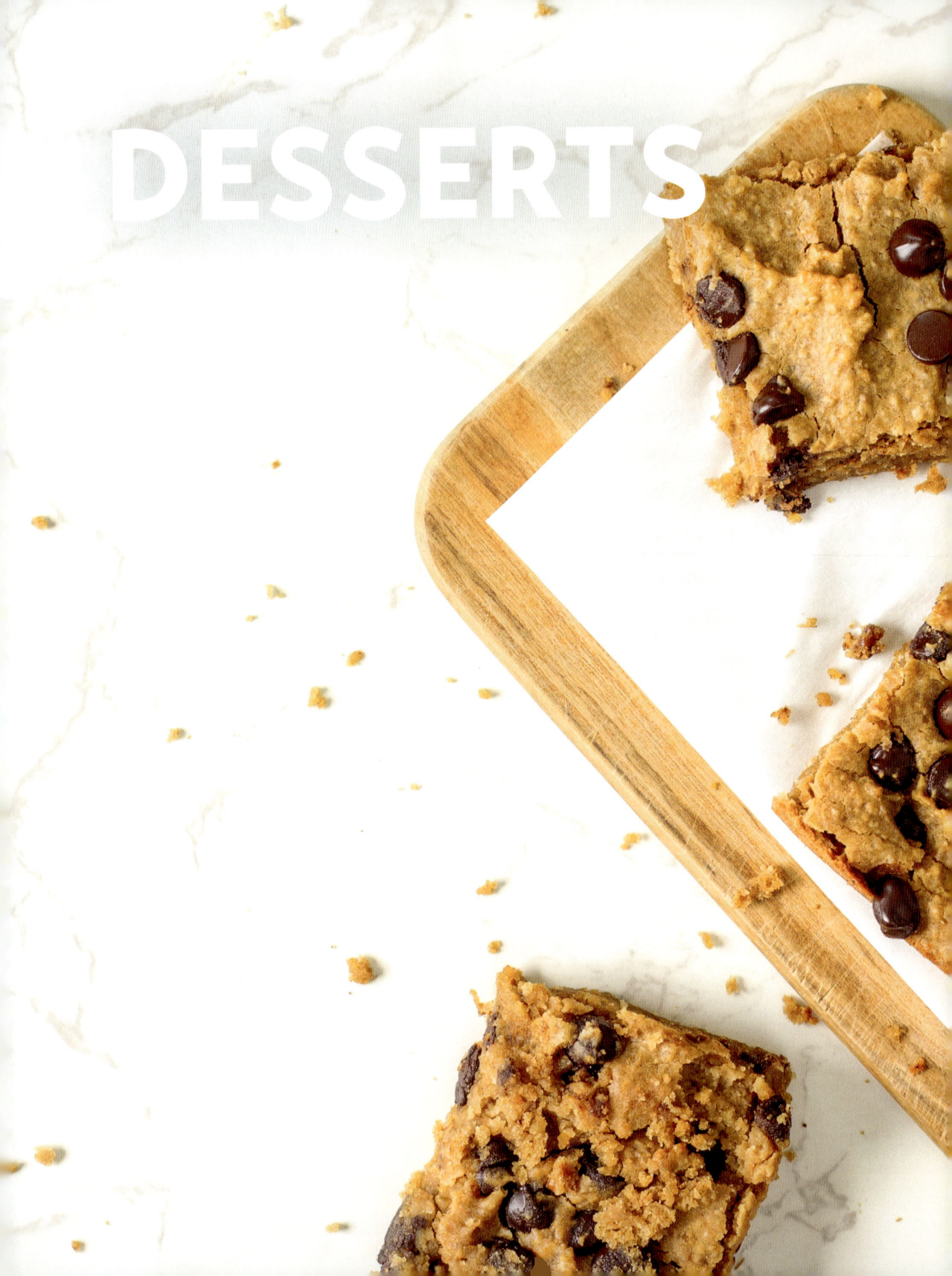

DESSERTS

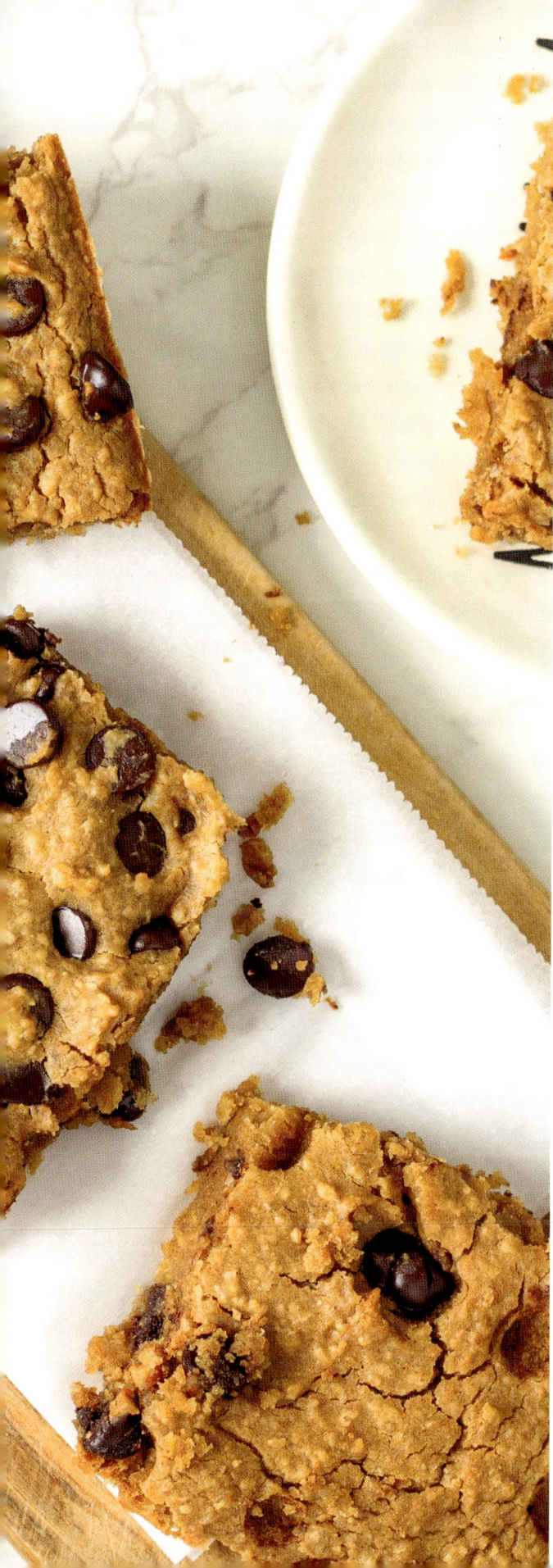

GREEK YOGURT DESSERT BOWL

SERVES 1

PREP TIME 5 minutes

This is my go-to dessert when I'm feeling like something a little sweet after dinner. I love that it satisfies my sweet tooth with minimal added sugar while also giving me a hit of protein—28 grams. Choosing a zero-added-sugar brand of chocolate chips (I like Lily's) can further reduce the total sugar content. Just remember to opt for an unsweetened Greek yogurt! Otherwise, the sugar content starts to add up quite a bit.

¾ cup plain whole milk Greek yogurt, store-bought or homemade (page 81)

1 scoop vanilla protein powder (or ½ serving that equates to 10 grams of protein)

1 cup fresh strawberries, halved

2 tablespoons dark chocolate chips (preferably stevia sweetened)

Scoop the yogurt into a bowl and stir in the protein powder until dissolved. Top with the strawberries and chocolate chips and enjoy!

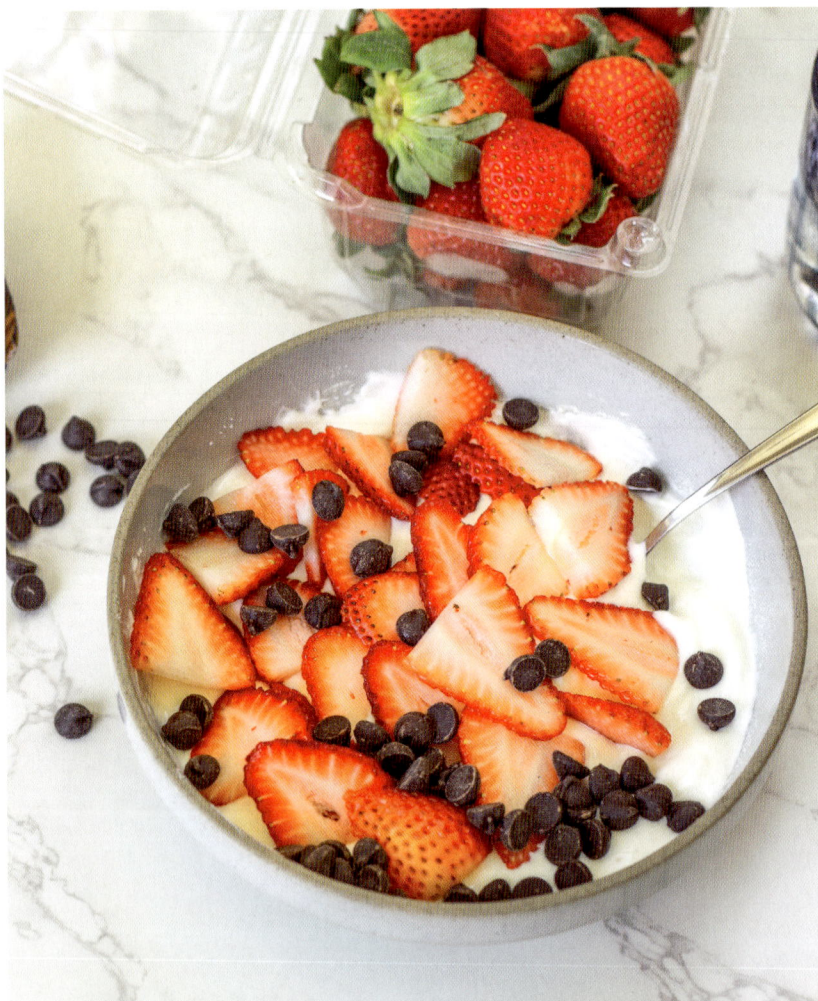

CINNAMON SAUTÉED APPLE

SERVES 1

PREP TIME 5 minutes

COOK TIME 10 minutes

If you're in the cozy fall spirit, then this recipe is for you. Especially after reducing your sugar intake, these sautéed apples will taste like quite the decadent treat. This super simple dessert is perfect on its own, but you can add a tablespoon of pumpkin seeds if you want a little extra crunch. Eat these on their own or use them to top Greek yogurt, cottage cheese, or protein pancakes (see page 97).

1 tablespoon salted butter

1 red apple, peeled and cut into ½-inch slices

1 teaspoon ground cinnamon

¼ teaspoon ground nutmeg

Salt

Melt the butter in a large skillet over medium heat. Add the apple, cinnamon, nutmeg, and a heavy pinch of salt and sauté for 7 minutes, or until the apple is tender. Serve immediately.

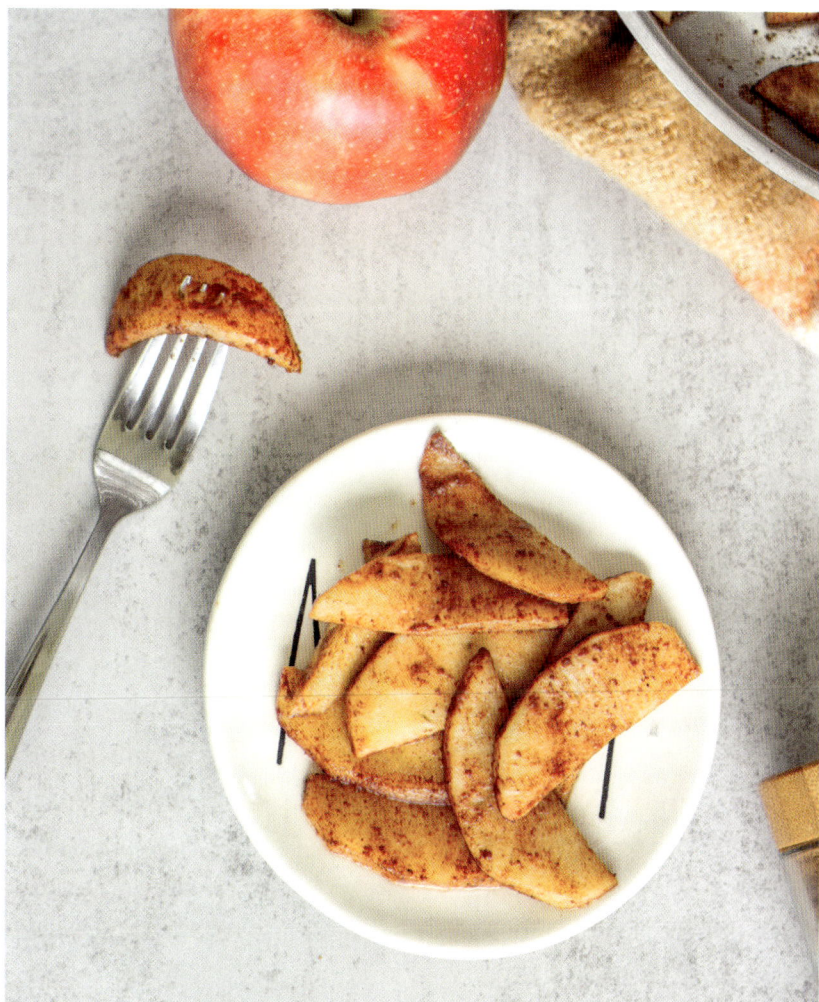

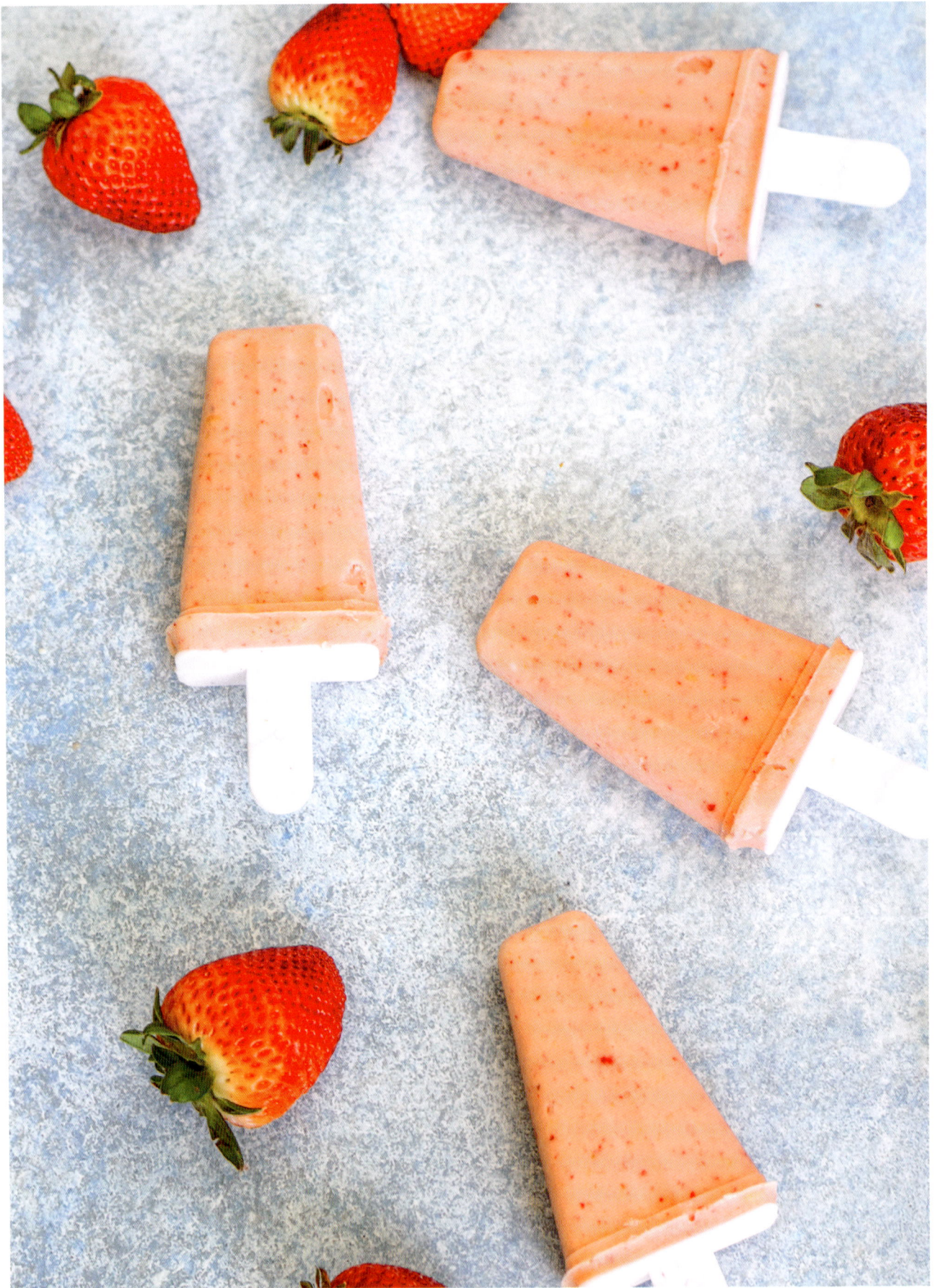

TROPICAL LIME POPSICLES

MAKES 6 popsicles

PREP TIME 5 minutes, plus 4 hours to freeze

Instead of buying sugary popsicles, I like to make homemade zero-added-sugar popsicles. This tropical version uses canned coconut milk for extra creaminess and a boost of satiating fat. Coconut is high in medium-chain triglycerides that help keep you full and satisfied. These treats store well in the freezer for a few months and are great to have on hand, especially if you have kids!

1 cup frozen mango chunks

1 cup frozen strawberries

¾ cup canned full-fat coconut milk

Juice of 1 lime (about 2 tablespoons)

1 scoop vanilla protein powder (or ½ serving that equates to 10 grams of protein)

Special equipment: 3-ounce popsicle mold(s) with at least 6 cavities

1. Put all of the ingredients in a blender and blend until thick and creamy. You might have to stop the blender a time or two and push down the fruit before continuing to blend.

2. Pour the mixture into the popsicle mold(s) and freeze for at least 4 hours or overnight before eating.

PEANUT BUTTER CHOCOLATE CHUNK COOKIES

MAKES 10 cookies

PREP TIME 10 minutes

COOK TIME 10 minutes

This is an all-time community favorite recipe of mine that's featured in my Level Up Program. These flourless cookies only use six ingredients. People are often hesitant to try this recipe at first because they assume that I left off an ingredient or two. But once they try it, they're converts! This is the perfect cookie if you're looking for a healthier treat or something you can give to your kids that has only real, natural ingredients and zero refined sugars.

1 cup unsweetened peanut butter

¼ cup maple syrup or honey

1 large egg

½ teaspoon baking soda

½ teaspoon salt

1 (2-ounce) bar dark chocolate, chopped into chunks

1. Preheat the oven to 350°F and line a cookie sheet with parchment paper.

2. Put the peanut butter, maple syrup, egg, baking soda, and salt in a bowl and stir with a fork until you have a uniform dough. Gently fold in the chocolate pieces.

3. Scoop 2-tablespoon-sized cookies onto the prepared pan, spacing them 2 inches apart to allow for spreading; you should get ten cookies.

4. Bake for 8 to 10 minutes, until the cookies are lightly browned on the edges. You don't want to overbake these, so as soon as you see light browning, pull the pan out of the oven. Transfer the cookies to a wire rack to cool for 10 minutes before eating.

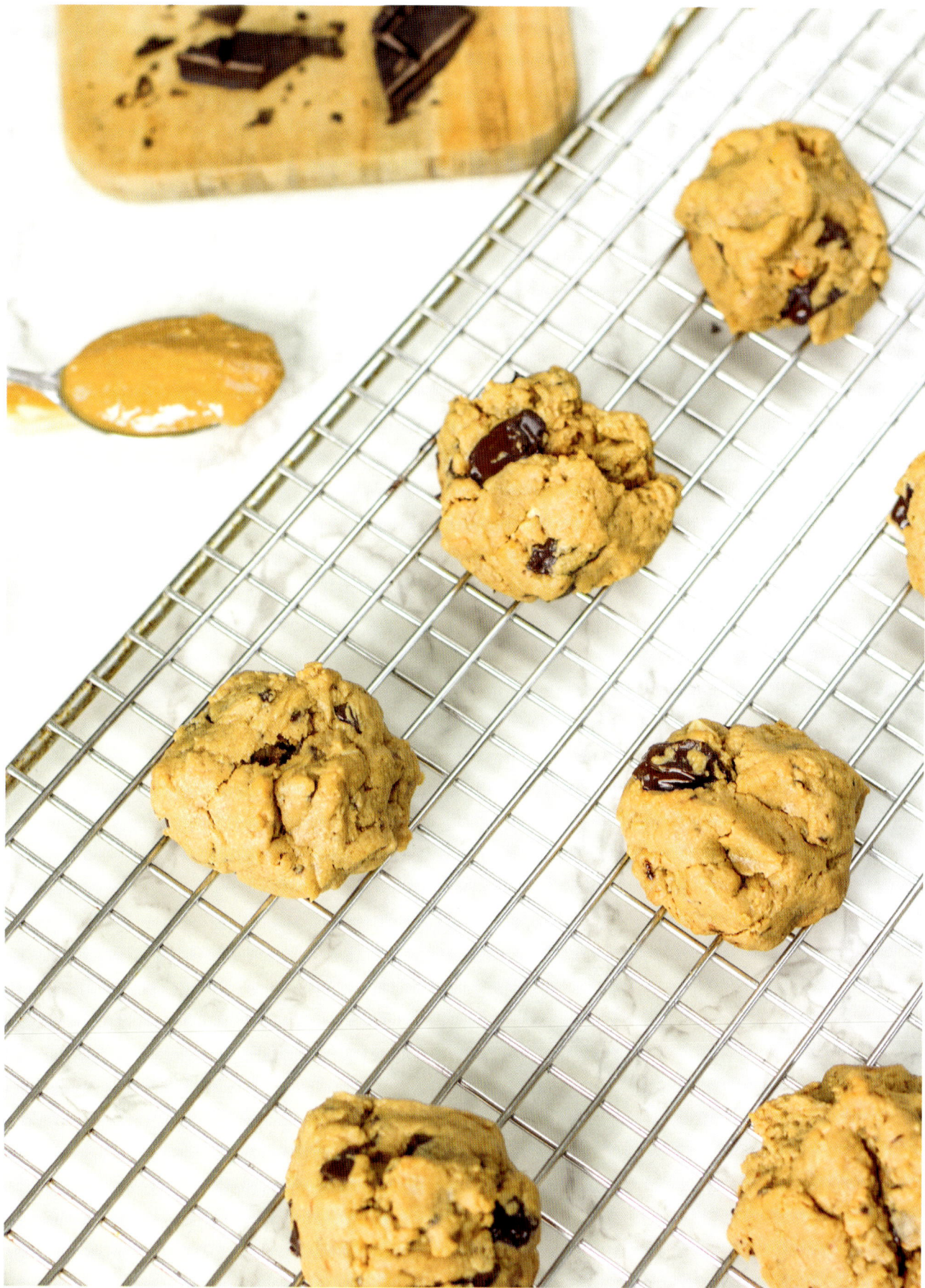

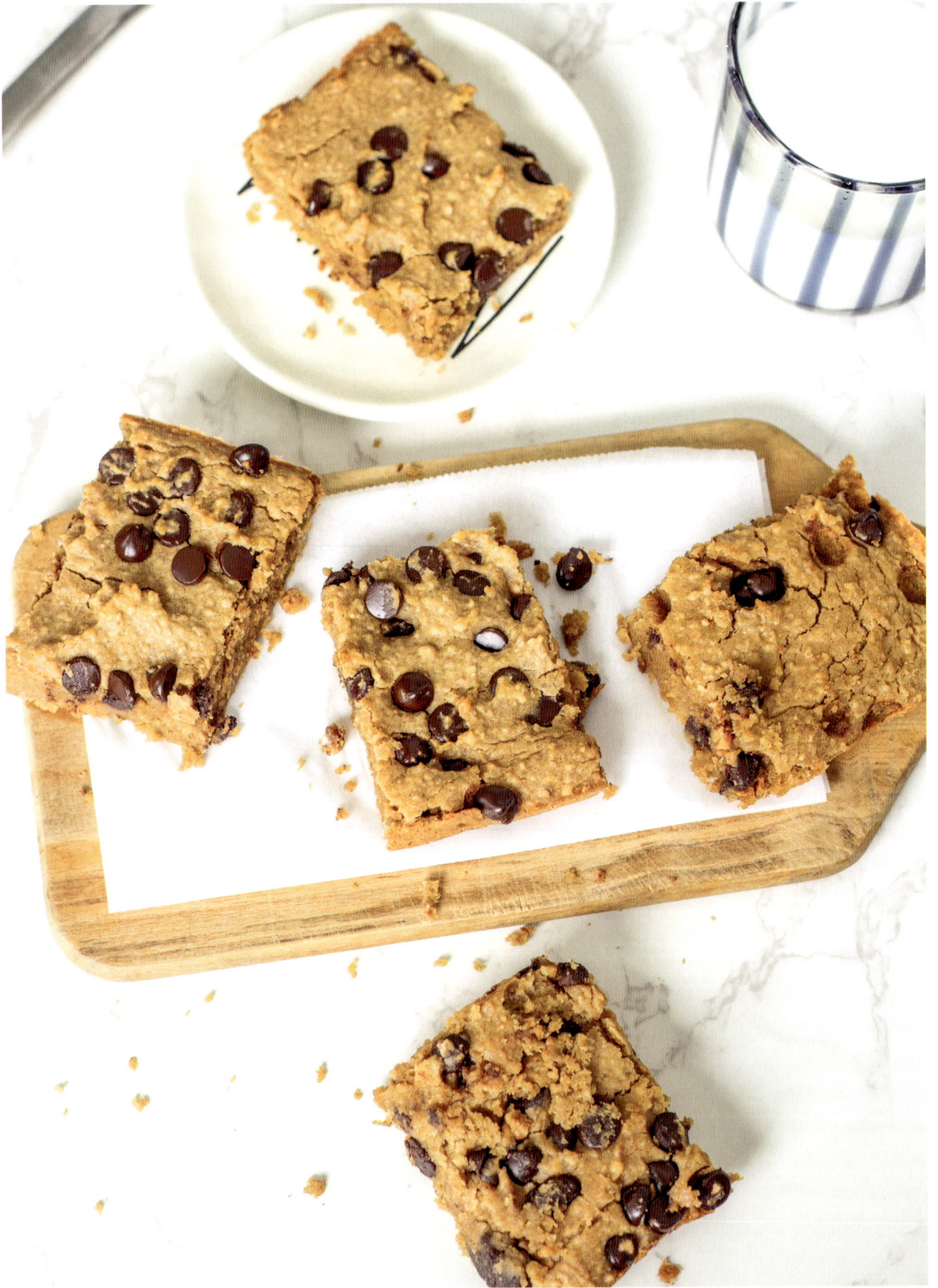

CHOCOLATE CHIP BLONDIE BARS

MAKES 8 bars

PREP TIME 10 minutes, plus 20 minutes to cool

COOK TIME 35 minutes

When I lived in Manhattan Beach, I used to order a similar blondie bar from a local smoothie shop so often that I realized I *needed* to develop my own recipe to better control the ingredient quality (and reel in my spending!). Chickpeas make an incredible base for baked goods. They're fairly high in protein and fiber, making them a low-glycemic swap for regular flour. Plus, chickpeas help keep baked goods moist. I love bringing these bars to baby showers, birthday parties, and playdates, and they're always a hit—even when people don't realize they are enjoying a healthy alternative to the classic version.

1 teaspoon coconut oil, plus extra for greasing

1 (15-ounce) can chickpeas, or 1¾ cups homemade chickpeas (page 85)

½ cup unsweetened peanut butter

¼ cup maple syrup

1 teaspoon ground cinnamon

1 large egg

¼ teaspoon salt

¼ teaspoon baking powder

¼ teaspoon baking soda

¼ cup dark chocolate chips (see note)

Special equipment: food processor

1. Preheat the oven to 350°F. Grease a 9 by 13-inch baking dish with coconut oil.

2. Put all of the ingredients except the chocolate chips in a food processor and process until smooth. Pour the batter into the greased baking dish and sprinkle the chocolate chips on top, then carefully press them into the batter.

3. Bake for 30 to 35 minutes, until a toothpick poked into the center comes out clean. Let cool for at least 20 minutes before slicing into eight bars.

> Note I like to use dark chocolate chips with minimal sugar. You can even find stevia-sweetened ones with zero added sugar!

BLACK BEAN BROWNIE BITES

MAKES 20 to 24 brownie bites

PREP TIME 10 minutes

COOK TIME 30 minutes

As a 1990s child, I have vivid memories of packaged brownie bites. My parents were very health-conscious, so I was never allowed to have them, but I always envied my friends when they brought those little packaged brownies to school. My healthier version uses black beans instead of refined flour to reduce the blood sugar spike and provide important nutrients while still allowing you to enjoy a sweet treat.

½ cup (1 stick) salted butter, melted and cooled, plus extra for greasing (see note)

1 (15-ounce) can black beans, or 1¾ cups homemade black beans (page 85)

2 large eggs

3 tablespoons unsweetened cocoa powder

¼ cup maple syrup

1 tablespoon vanilla extract

Salt

¼ cup dark chocolate chips

Special equipment: food processor and mini muffin tin

1. Preheat the oven to 325°F and grease a mini muffin tin with butter.

2. Put the beans, eggs, butter, cocoa powder, maple syrup, vanilla extract, and a pinch of salt in a food processor and process until the batter is smooth.

3. Pour the batter into the greased mini muffin tin, filling each well about three-quarters of the way. Top each brownie bite with a few chocolate chips. Bake for 25 to 30 minutes, until a toothpick poked into the center of a brownie bite comes out clean. Allow to cool for 5 minutes before removing from the muffin tin.

Note I like to use grass-fed butter, which tends to be higher in a type of fatty acid called butyric acid that has been found to improve gut health.

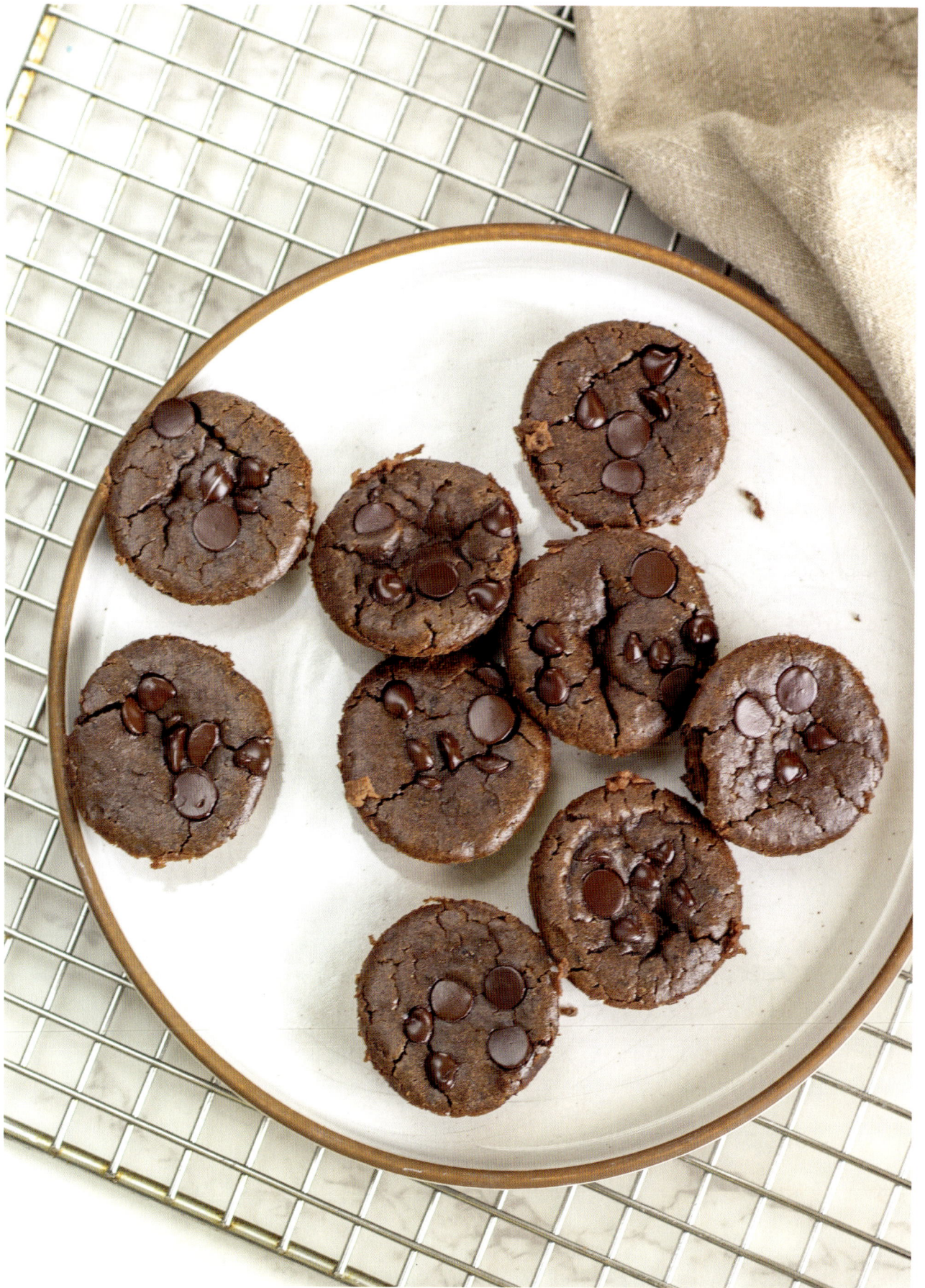

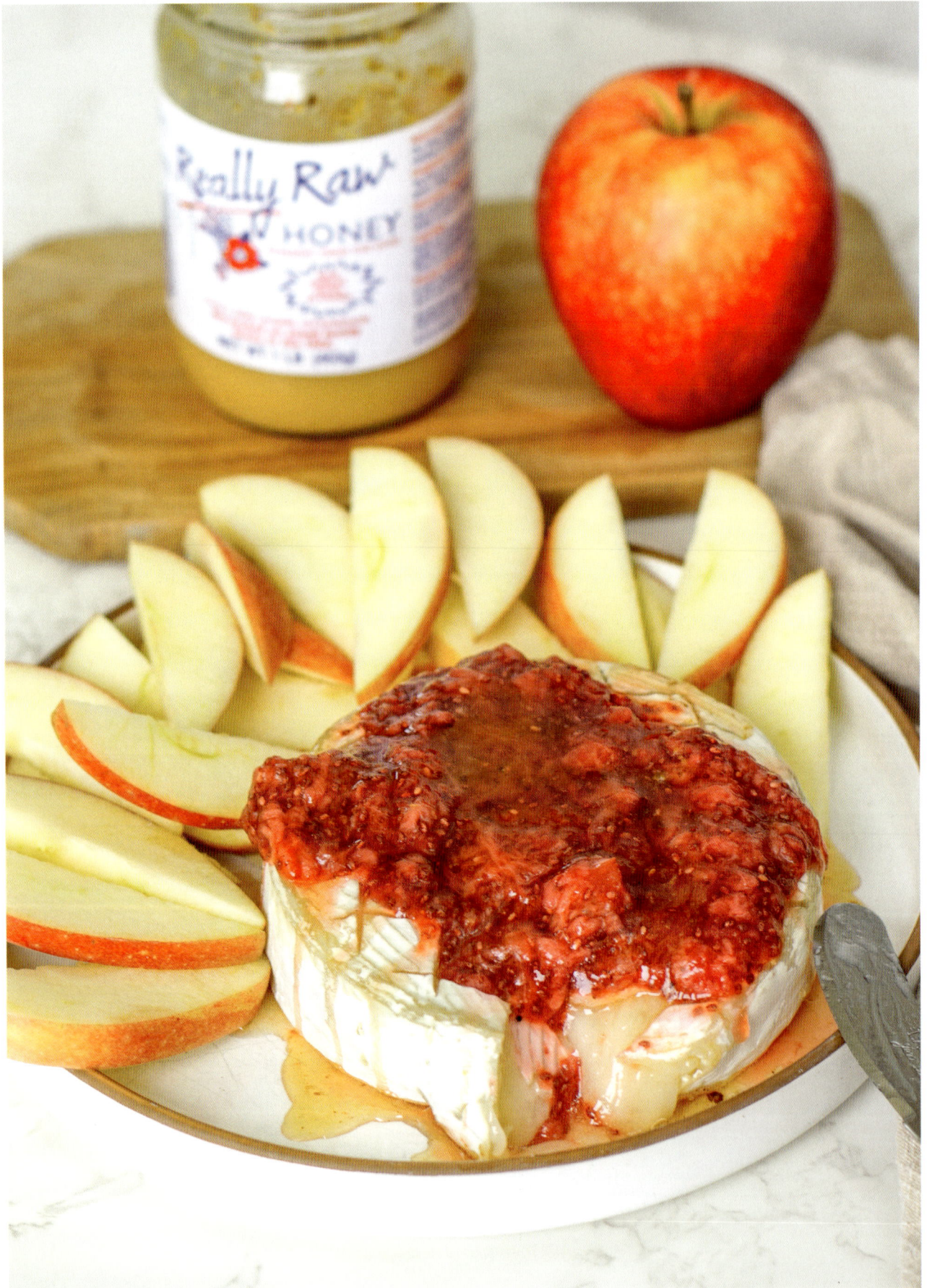

BAKED BRIE
WITH CHIA JAM AND HONEY

SERVES 4 to 6

PREP TIME 5 minutes (not including time to make jam)

COOK TIME 20 minutes

When done right, cheese can absolutely be a dessert. My first "real" job was waitressing at a local restaurant while I was in high school. It was a Mediterranean café that served the tastiest honey-baked Brie I've ever had. Each day, we got to order one thing for free at the end of our shift, and I would *always* get the Brie to go. Although they treated it as an appetizer, I love eating it as a dessert. Unlike many desserts, this one uses simple, wholesome ingredients with minimal added sugar and is a good source of quality protein. If you serve this at a dinner party, absolutely no one will complain about having cheese for dessert.

1 (8- to 10-ounce) wheel Brie cheese

1 apple (any type), for dipping

¼ cup Strawberry Lemon or Blackberry Chia Jam (page 78) (see note)

2 tablespoons honey

1. Preheat the oven to 350°F.

2. Place the Brie in a small baking dish and score the top of the cheese in a crisscross pattern. Bake for 15 to 20 minutes, until the cheese feels soft and gooey when you poke it.

3. While the cheese bakes, thinly slice the apple.

4. Remove the cheese from the oven and immediately spread the jam on top. Drizzle with the honey before serving. Use the apple slices to dip into the Brie like crackers.

Note You can buy premade chia jam to simplify this dessert even further. One great company that I love is Smash Foods. However, they do use a bit of sugar in the form of dates, so if you're looking to keep this dessert as low in sugar as possible (and reduce the cost per serving), opt for my homemade chia jam instead.

BETTER THAN MOVIE THEATER POPCORN

MAKES about 14 cups
(3½ cups per serving)

COOK TIME 10 minutes

I've always loved going to the movies and getting a big bag of popcorn. For me, a movie night isn't a movie night without it. But have you ever looked at the ingredients in movie theater popcorn? It's full of things you wouldn't normally consider edible. This cheesy homemade popcorn recipe uses wholesome ingredients that will make you feel a lot better after your movie.

¼ cup (½ stick) salted butter

½ cup popcorn kernels

½ cup shredded Parmesan cheese

Salt

1. In a large pot over medium heat, combine the butter and popcorn kernels. Cover and allow the kernels to cook, shaking the pan every 30 seconds or so to prevent sticking. You'll start to hear a lot of popping within a few minutes.

2. Once you hear the popping slow down (with only about one pop every couple of seconds), remove the pot from the heat.

3. Pour the popcorn into a large bowl. Top with the Parmesan and a pinch of salt.

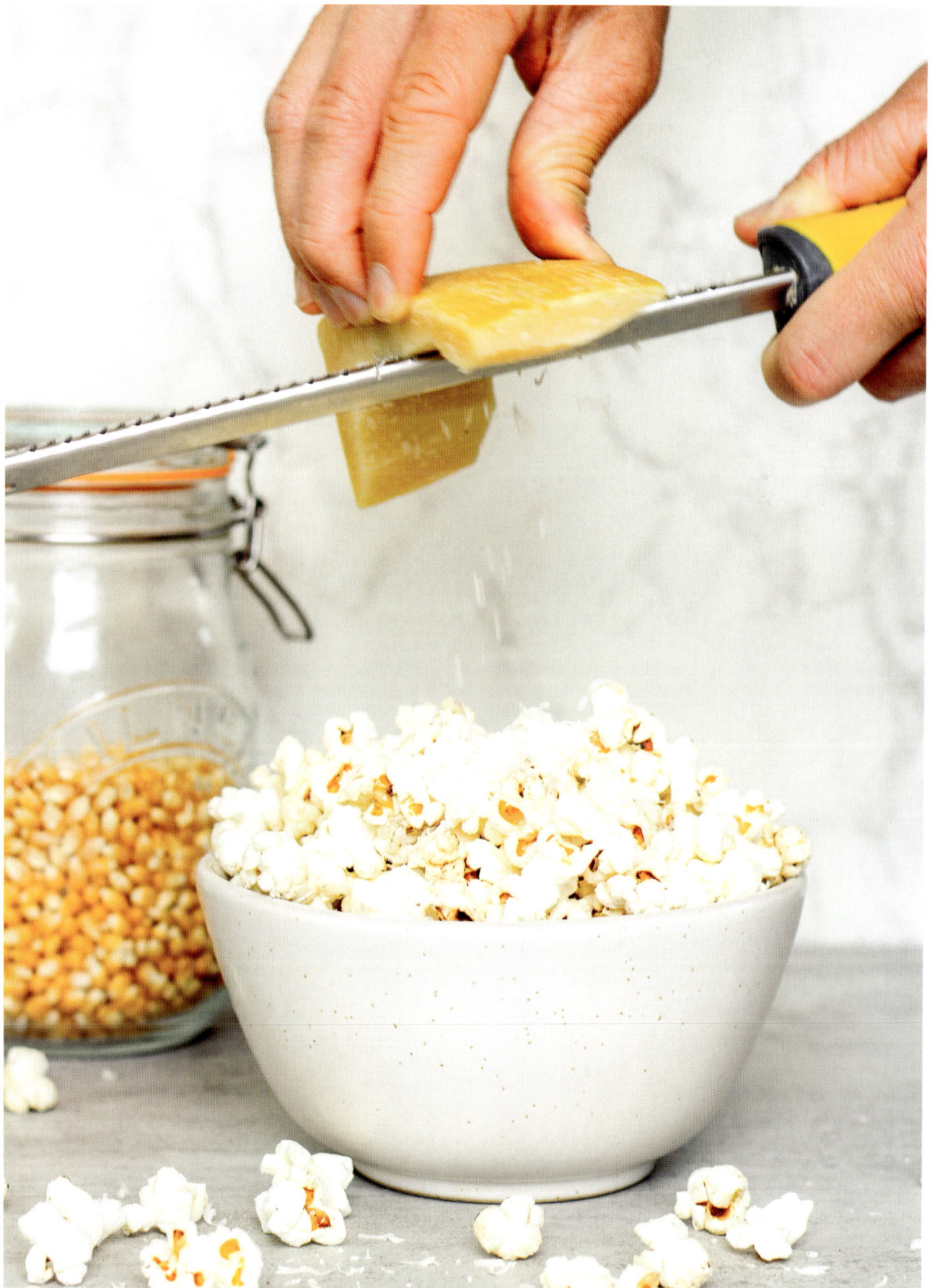

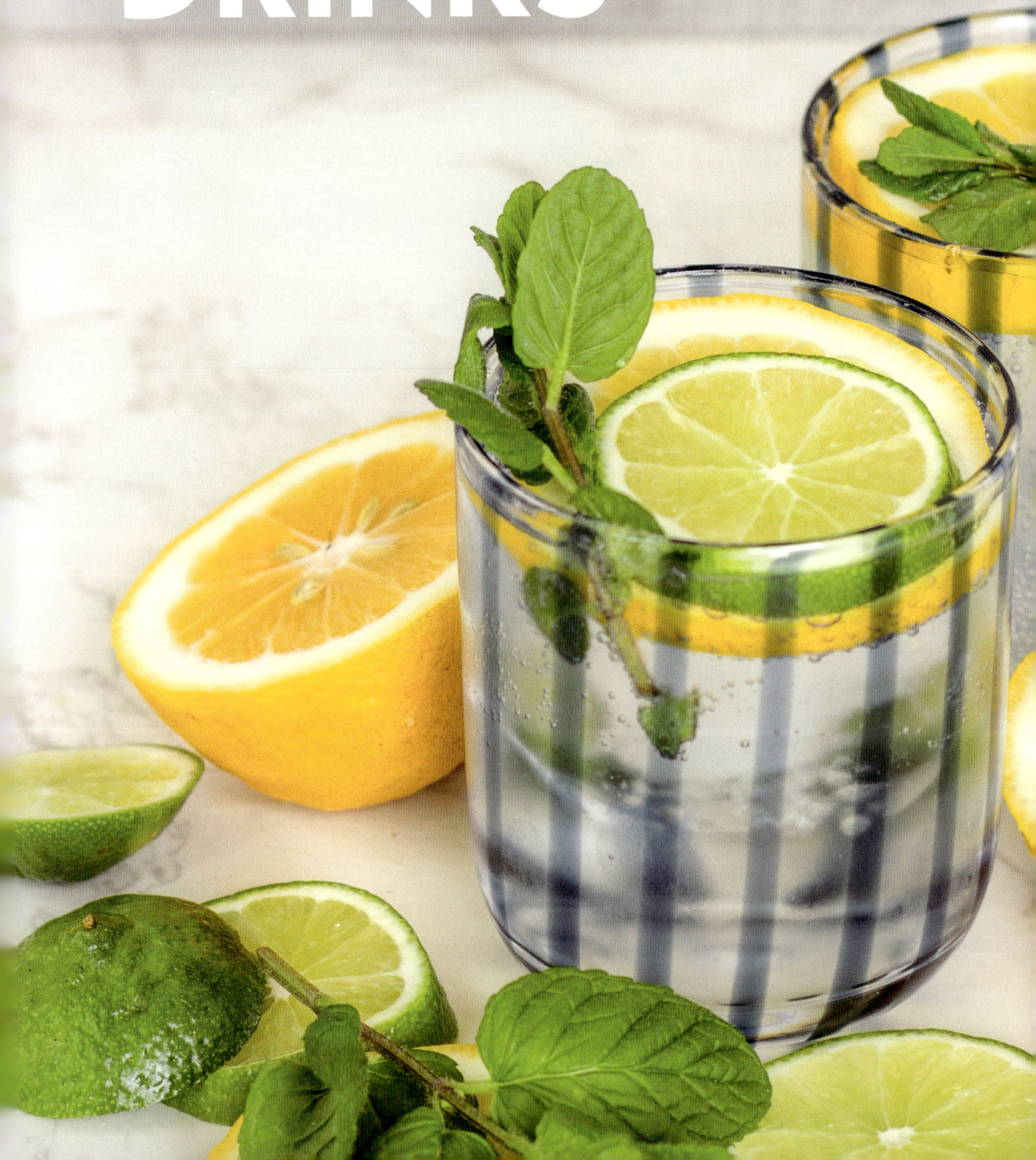

DRINKS

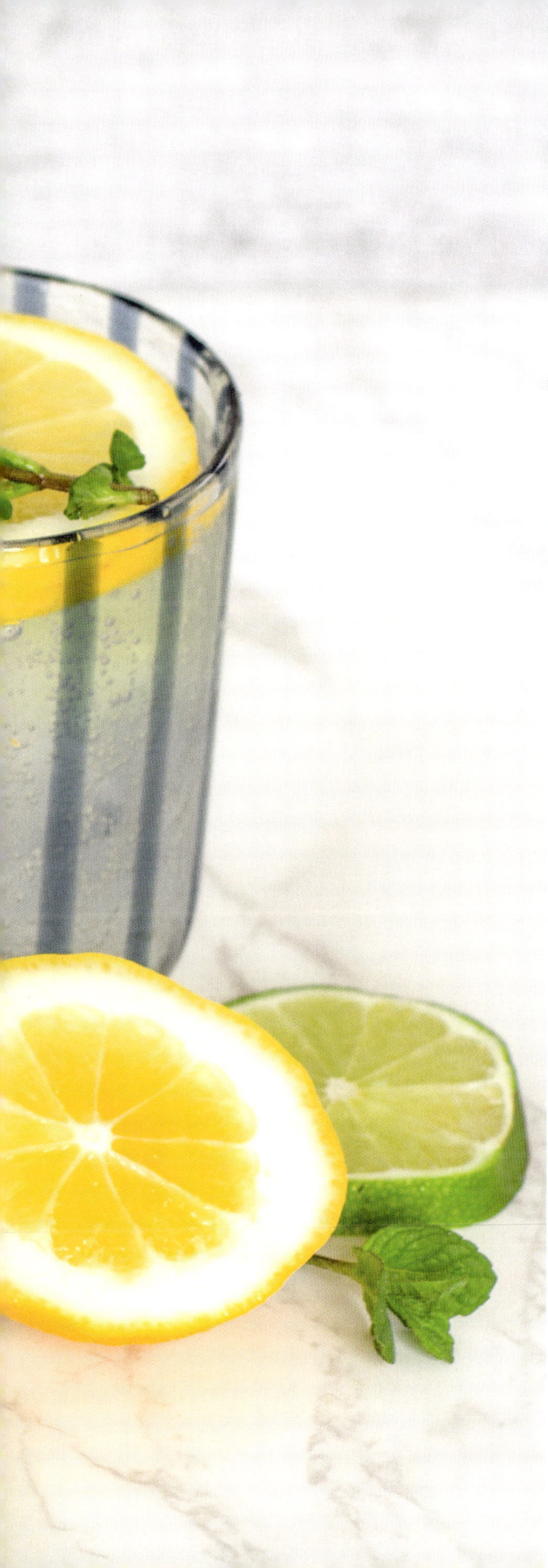

GINGER LEMON TEA

SERVES 2

PREP TIME 2 minutes

COOK TIME 10 minutes

Ginger is one of the few foods that naturally turn on the migrating motor complex (refer to page 6). This system flushes out left-behind food and bacteria, which is really important for preventing bloating and promoting gut health. My husband and I sip on this warm drink every night after dinner to take advantage of the health perks. I also recommend it to my clients and those following my gut-healing protocols. Simmering the tea for the full 10 minutes helps to extract even more of the ginger goodness, so don't rush it!

1 inch fresh ginger, thinly sliced (no need to peel)

1 lemon, cut into quarters

Pour 5 to 6 cups of water into a small pot. Add the ginger and lemon and bring to a boil, then reduce to a simmer. Allow to simmer for 10 minutes before serving.

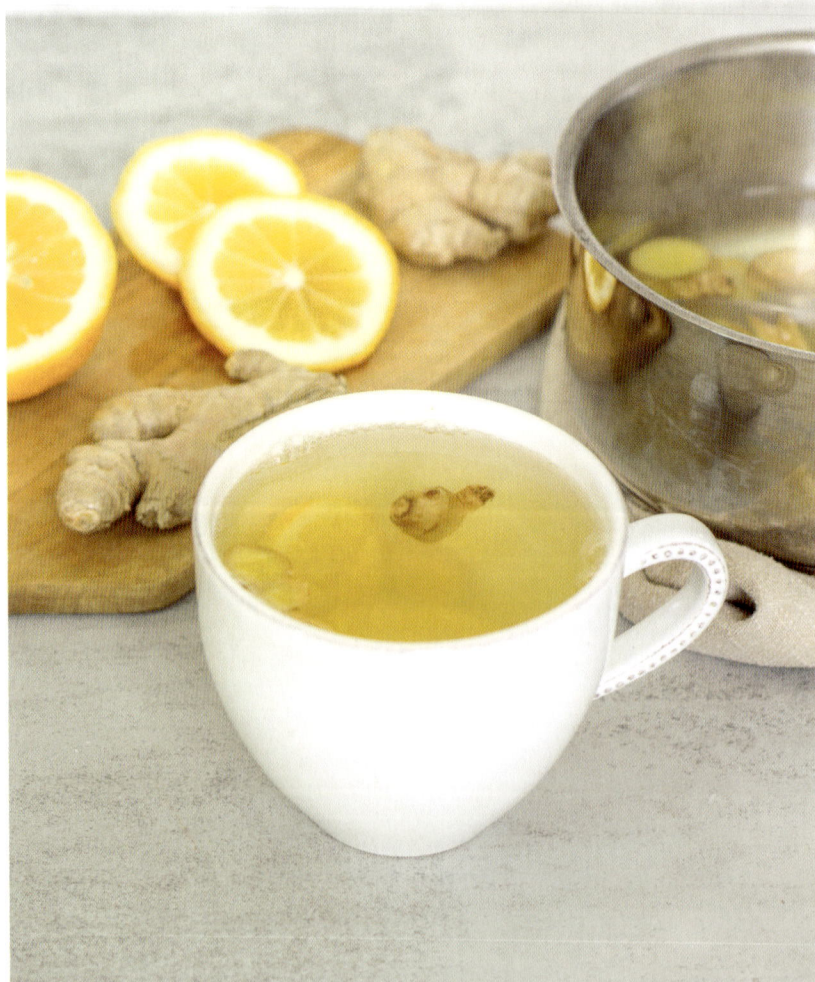

STRAWBERRY KEFIR

SERVES 1

PREP TIME 5 minutes

Kefir has an incredible number of known health benefits. It even contains more beneficial probiotics than yogurt! I personally like the taste of plain kefir, but occasionally I like to switch it up and add some flavor. Unfortunately, most flavored kefir comes packed with added sugar too. To solve this problem, I make a simple strawberry kefir at home that uses zero added sugar.

1 cup plain kefir

2 fresh strawberries

¼ teaspoon vanilla extract

Put all of the ingredients in a blender and blend until smooth. Enjoy immediately.

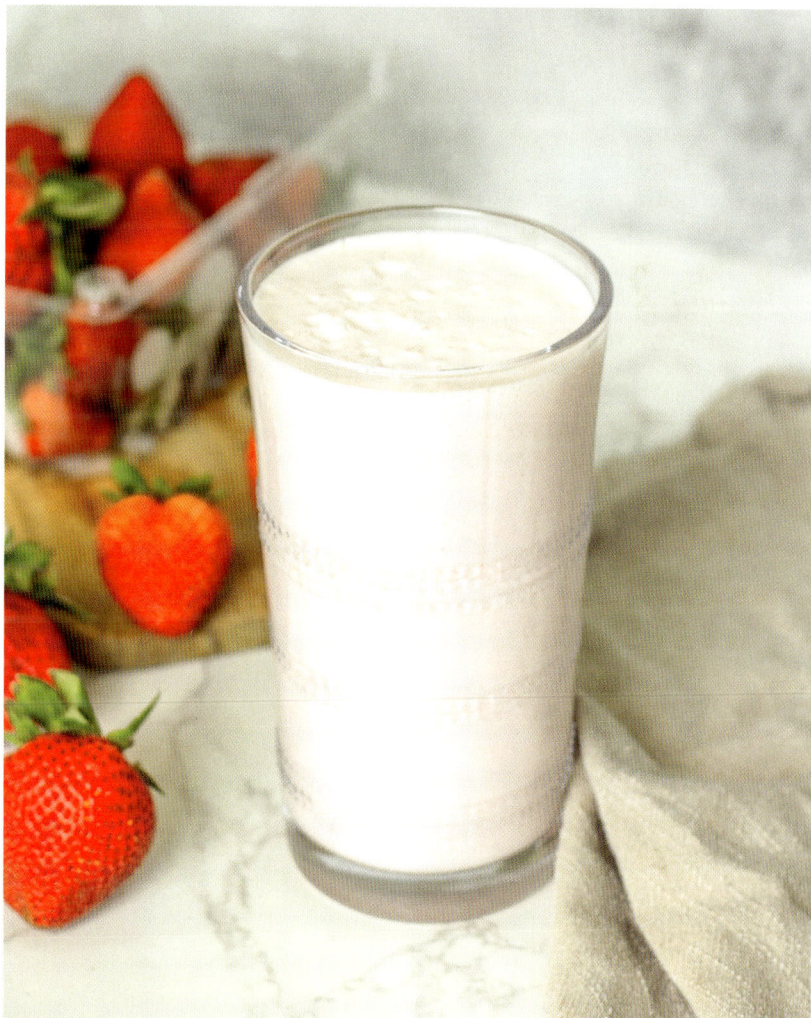

ACV SIPPER

SERVES 1

PREP TIME 1 minute

This recipe is used and recommended in every single one of my meal plans. Apple cider vinegar (ACV) has been found to stabilize blood sugar levels. To take advantage of this benefit, I like to sip on diluted ACV before my first meal of the day. This drink also massively helped with the acid reflux that I experienced during my first pregnancy. I would drink it before every meal to promote digestion and reduce reflux.

1 cup water

1 tablespoon apple cider vinegar

Pinch of sea salt

Pour all of the ingredients into a cup and stir to combine. Drink immediately.

Note If you can't tolerate apple cider vinegar, lemon juice has similar benefits. You can swap out the vinegar for lemon juice.

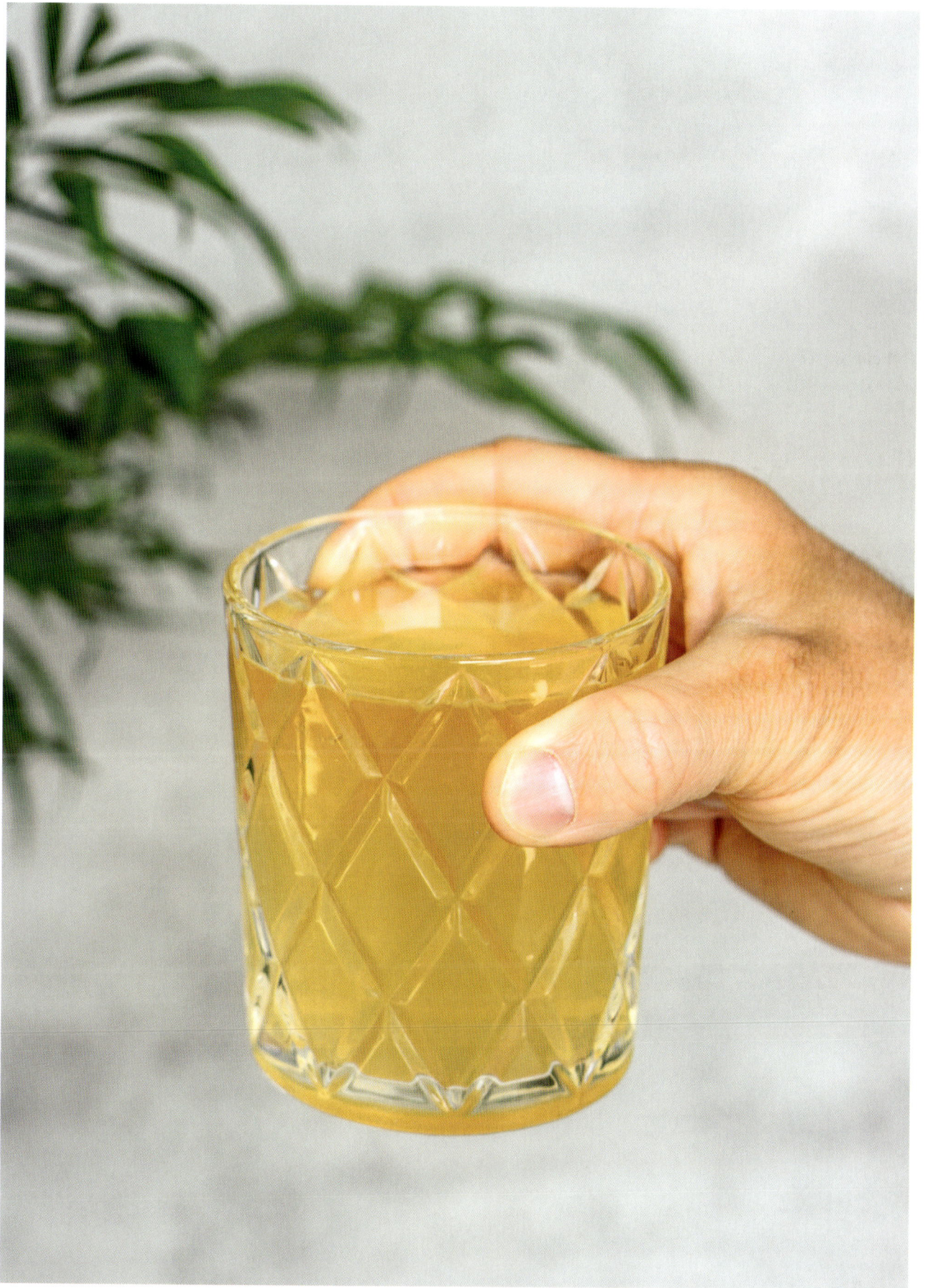

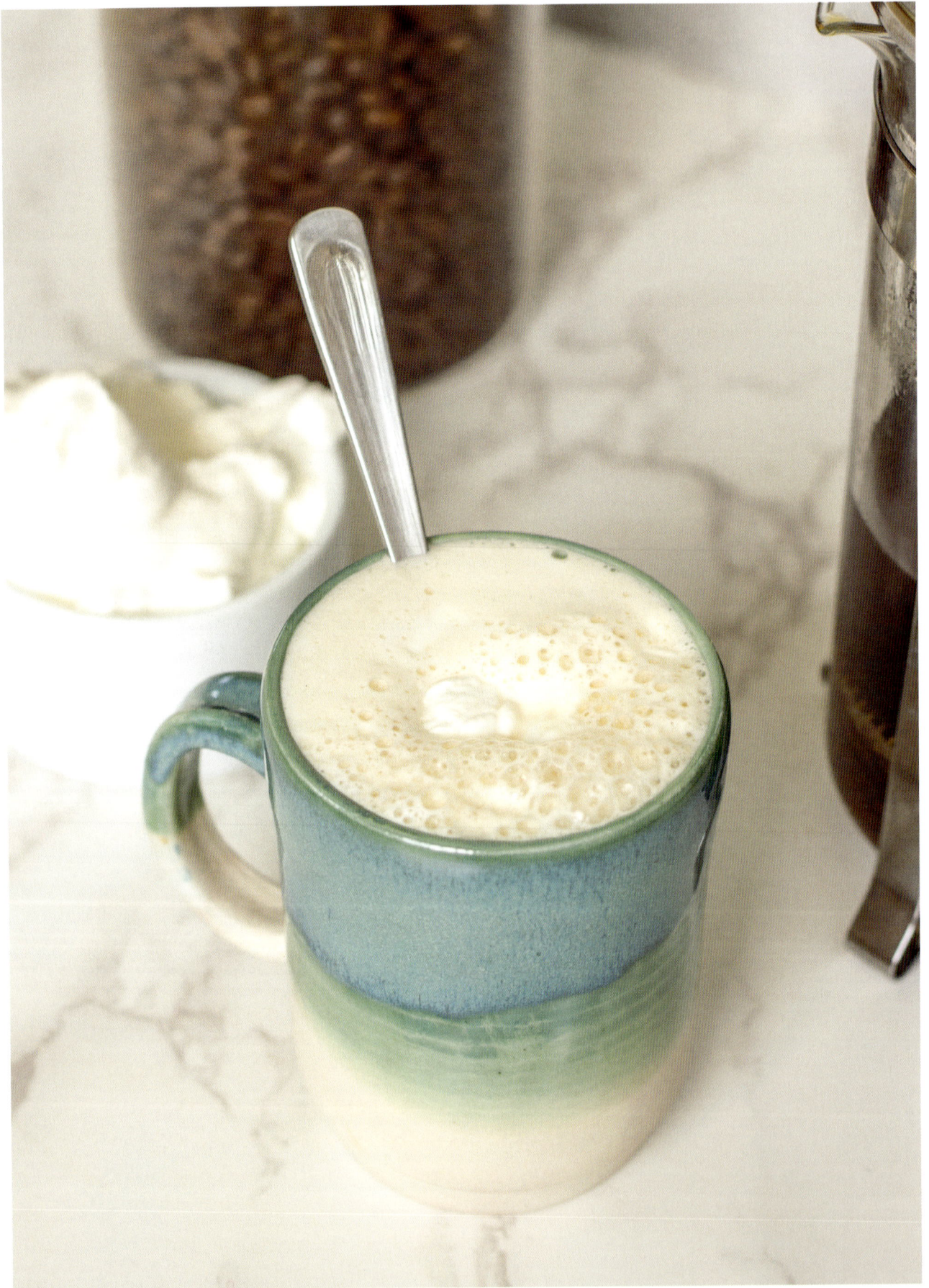

INSTANT VANILLA LATTE

MAKES 1 latte, plus enough whipped cream for 4 or 5 more coffees

PREP TIME 5 minutes (not including time to brew coffee)

I used to make a lot of homemade whipped cream for desserts. It's actually super easy to make and doesn't require any sugar to taste like a decadent sweet treat (especially when you dip strawberries into it). One day, I had some leftover whipped cream from the night before, so I decided to add it to my coffee, and WOW. The homemade whipped cream made my regular black coffee taste like a vanilla latte. I was so in awe of how well it turned out that I decided to share it as a YouTube short video...and it blew hundreds of thousands of people's minds on there too.

½ cup heavy whipping cream

½ teaspoon vanilla extract

1 to 1½ cups hot brewed coffee

1. Pour the cream and vanilla extract into a stand mixer, or use a medium-sized bowl and a hand mixer. Start the mixer on low, then slowly bring it up to medium speed. Whip the cream until firm peaks form. Be careful not to overmix, or you'll make butter instead! Transfer the vanilla whipped cream to a sealable container that you can store in the fridge. Whipped cream will keep in the fridge for up to 4 days.

2. When ready to drink your coffee, put 1 to 3 tablespoons of whipped cream in the bottom of your coffee cup, then pour the coffee over the cream. This allows the coffee to blend with the whipped cream without you having to stir it. Enjoy immediately.

CITRUS MINT SPARKLING WATER

SERVES 1

PREP TIME 5 minutes

Sparkling water is a nightly ritual for my family. My daughter, Sage, is particularly obsessed with sparkling water and will down multiple toddler-sized glasses before her dinner is over. I could drink plain sparkling water all day, every day, but during the summer I find myself craving citrus flavors too. This recipe might look deceptively simple, but it can elevate your water-drinking experience from "meh" to "oh wow."

1 sprig fresh mint

Juice of 1 lime (about 2 tablespoons)

Juice of ½ lemon (1 to 1½ tablespoons)

Ice

2 cups sparkling water

Lemon and/or lime slices, for garnish (optional)

1. Use your hands to gently roll and crush the mint before dropping it into a tall glass. This step helps release the minty flavors into your water faster.

2. Add the lime and lemon juices. Drop in a few cubes of ice before pouring in the sparkling water. Garnish with lemon and/or lime slices, if desired.

Tip If you drink a lot of sparkling water, I highly recommend investing in a SodaStream or similar sparkling water maker. We were spending close to $100 a month on sparkling water before we had the revelation that making our own would be a much more cost-effective route. Plus, you get better control of the quality of the water you use as the base of your sparkling drink. We have an intense reverse-osmosis system in our house that we like using for sparkling water, and having a SodaStream makes this possible!

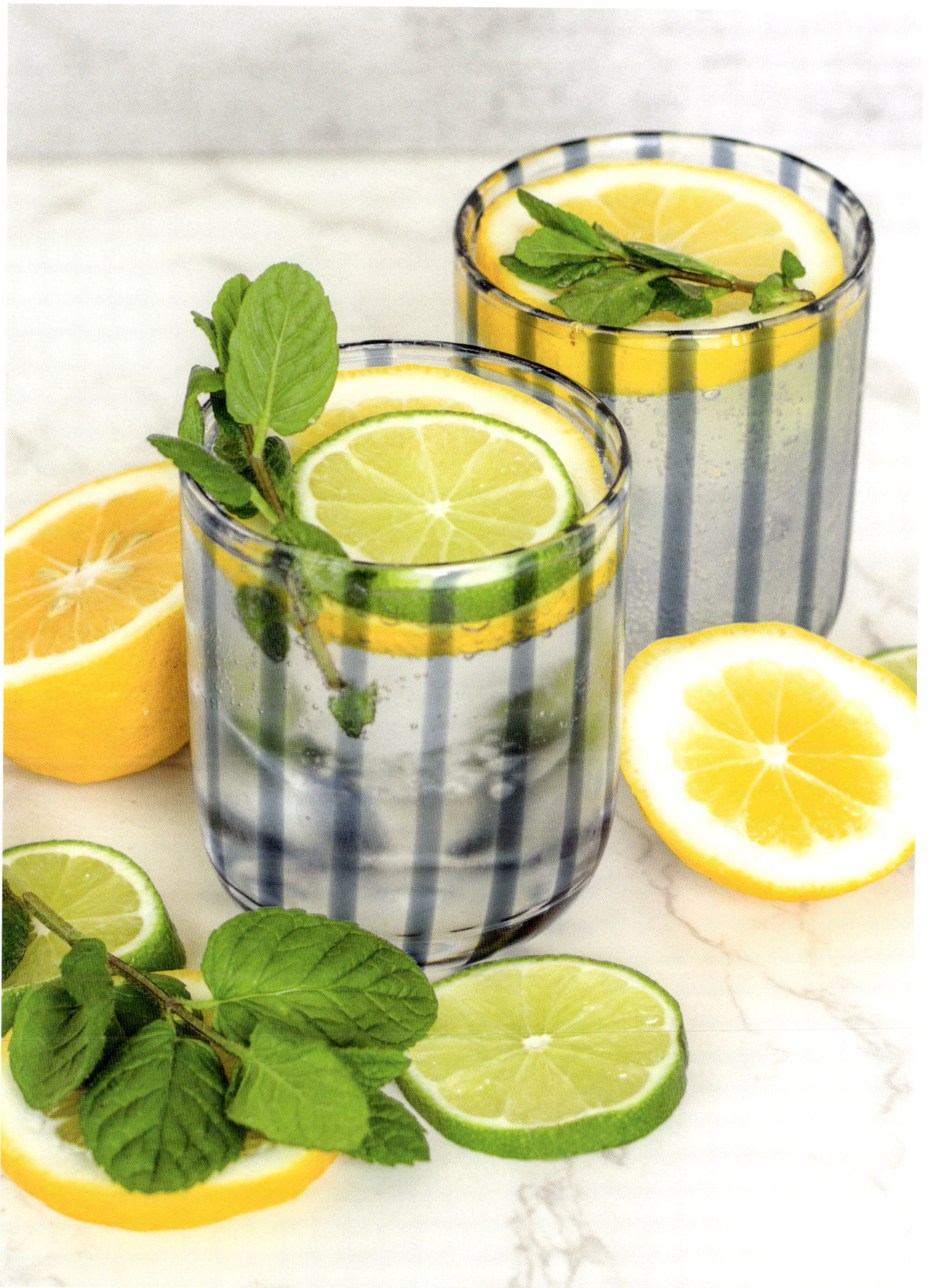

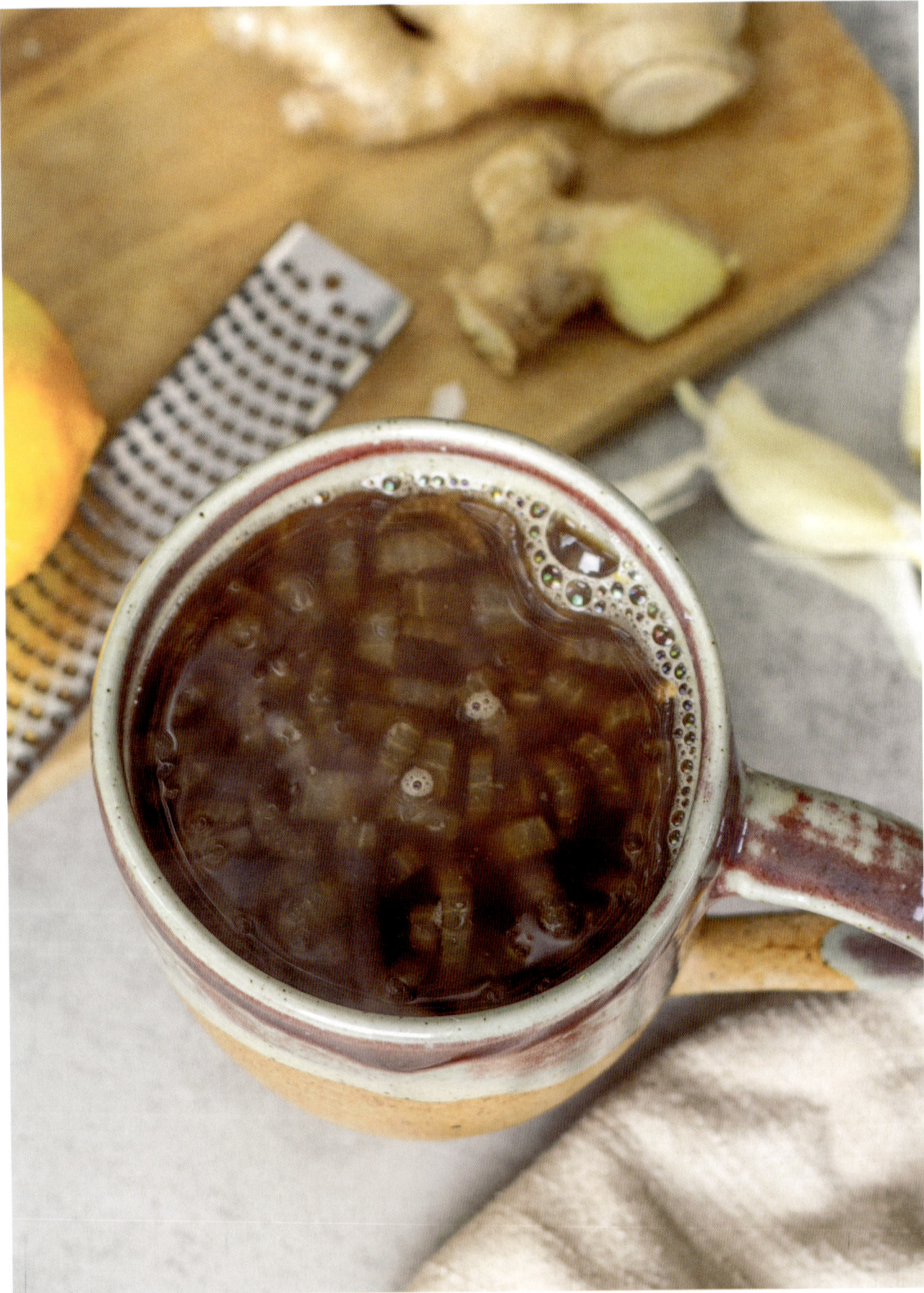

TRULY DRINKABLE BONE BROTH

MAKES 7 cups

PREP TIME 5 minutes

COOK TIME 30 minutes

It always bothers me a bit when people talk about how you can just "sip" on bone broth. I love bone broth for its variety of health benefits. It also adds great flavor to meals like chili and soups. But just *sipping* on plain bone broth isn't really the tasty treat that people have made it out to be. When I lived in Manhattan Beach, I used to get a delicious veggie broth from the local farmers market that was loaded with flavors like ginger and garlic. Now *that* was a sippable broth! I developed this recipe to mimic the amazing flavors of that veggie broth while still using bone broth for its incredible health perks.

8 cups chicken bone broth

3 tablespoons tamari

2 teaspoons rice vinegar

1 teaspoon honey

1 cup finely diced yellow onions

4 cloves garlic, minced

1 tablespoon minced ginger

Grated zest of ½ lemon

½ teaspoon red pepper flakes

¼ teaspoon salt

1. Put all of the ingredients in a medium-sized pot. Bring to a boil, then reduce to a simmer for 30 minutes. After simmering, taste the broth and add more salt if desired.

2. From here, you can either cool and strain the broth into mason jars or leave the minced onions, ginger, and garlic in the final product.

3. When ready to drink, heat 1 cup of the broth to your desired temperature and pour into a coffee mug to sip on. Store leftover broth in the fridge for up to 5 days or in the freezer for up to 6 months.

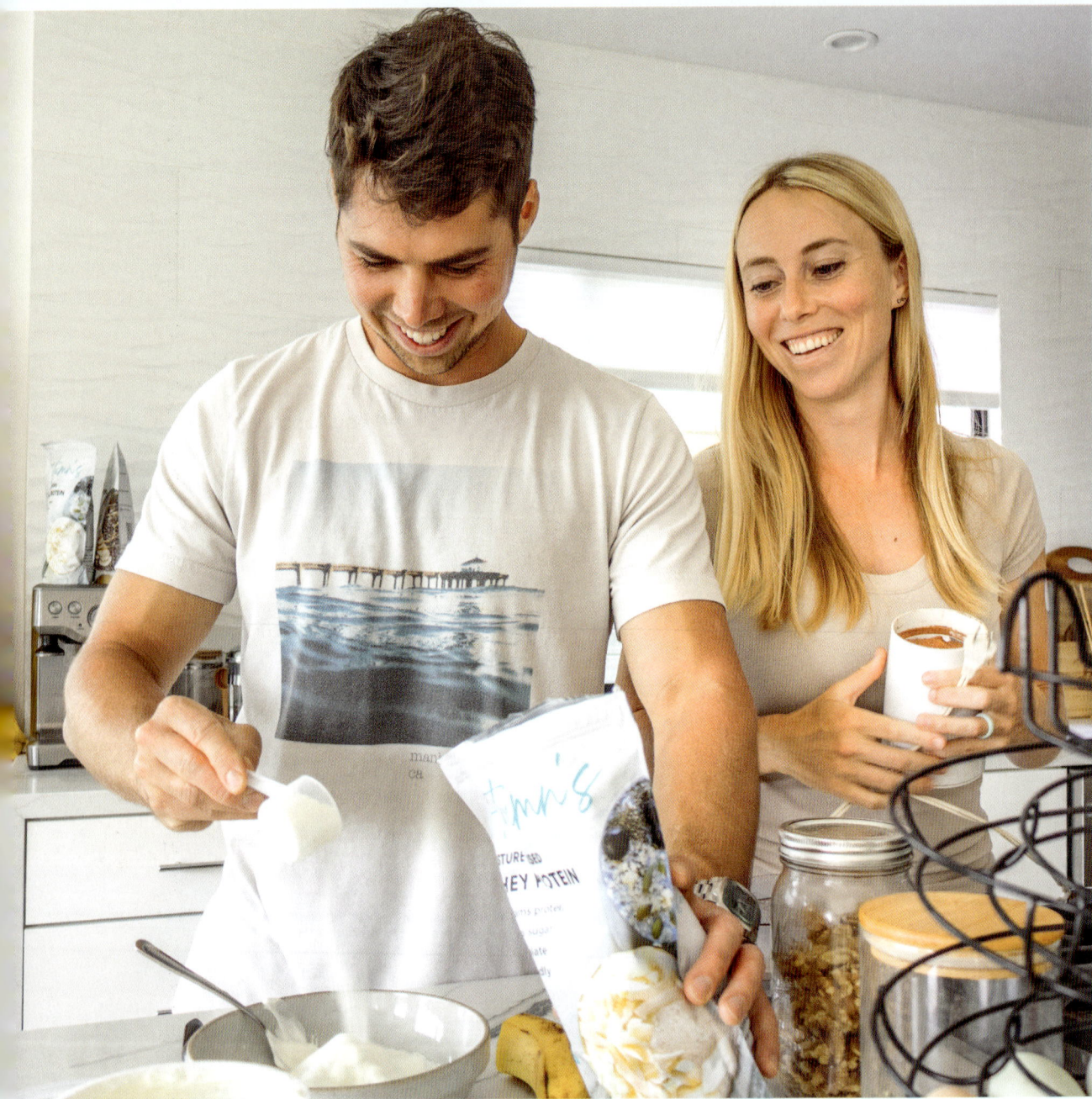

ONE-WEEK MEAL PLAN

The following is a sample one-week meal plan using recipes from this book. This is, of course, just one possible way to put a meal plan together, so feel free to add, subtract, or substitute according to your needs. Make sure to reference "Building Your Plate" on pages 49 to 56 to make any necessary adjustments to best fit your body and goals.

You can also add a dessert from pages 238 to 253 up to a few times per week, depending on your goals. If weight loss is your goal, you might want to stick to no more than one dessert per week. If you are looking to maintain, you can have up to four desserts per week. Find the balance that works for you and your body.

As for drinks, you can add drinks from the last recipe chapter to any of the meals in this plan. For best results, I recommend having any drinks (other than water) *with* the meal to help support gut cleaning between meals.

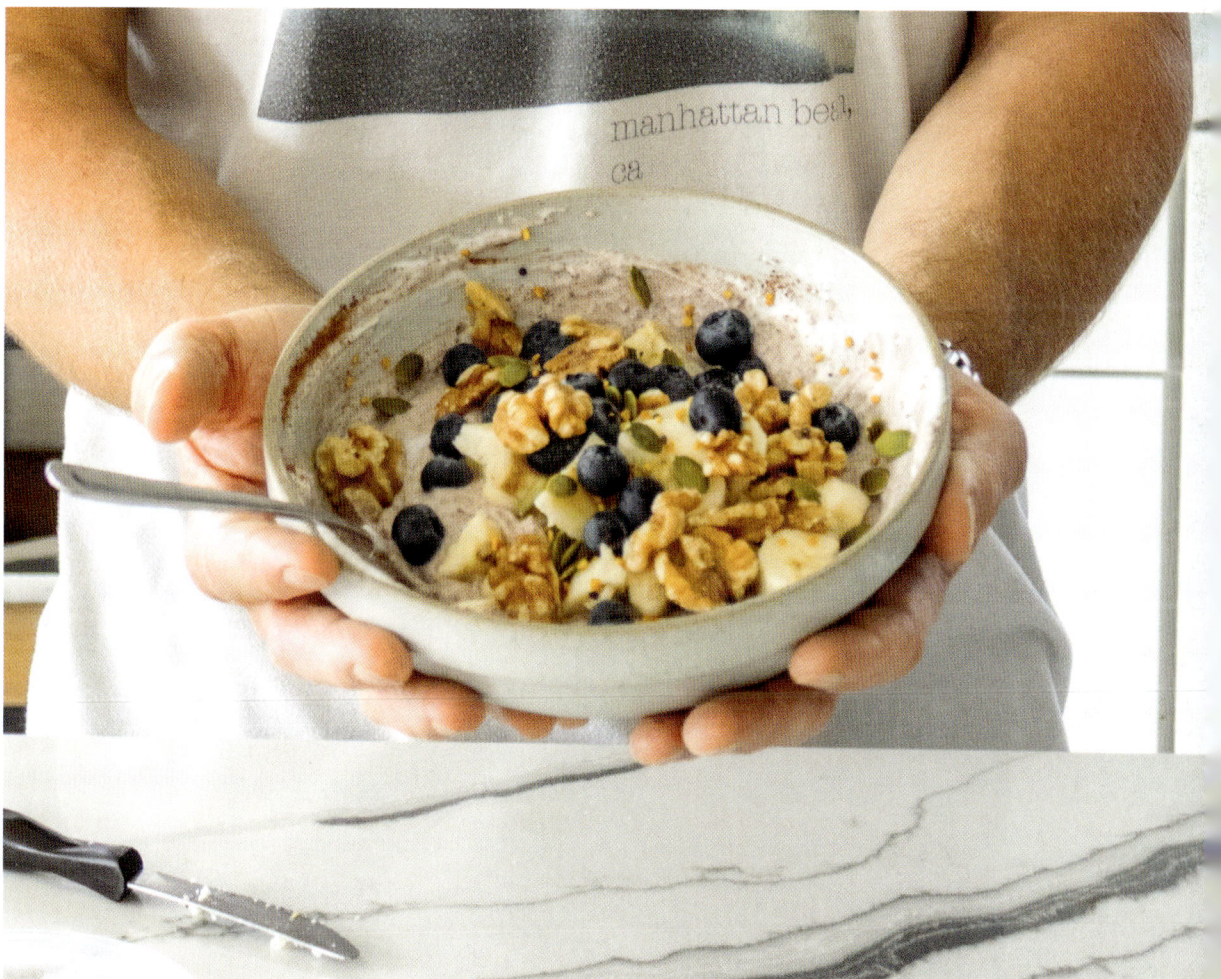

MEAL PLAN

DAY	BREAKFAST		LUNCH		DINNER	
MONDAY	Blueberry Lemon Chia Pudding	105	Quickie Loaded Salad	115	Mini Chicken Enchilada Pies*	164
TUESDAY	Blackberry Chocolate Chip Protein Waffles	93	Tempeh BLT	212	**LEFTOVER** Mini Chicken Enchilada Pies	
WEDNESDAY	**LEFTOVER** Blueberry Lemon Chia Pudding		Salmon Patties with Basil Aioli	196	Beef Chili with All the Toppings*	130
THURSDAY	Trevor's Yogurt Parfait	98	**LEFTOVER** Salmon Patties with Basil Aioli		**LEFTOVER** Beef Chili with All the Toppings	
FRIDAY	**LEFTOVER** Blueberry Lemon Chia Pudding		**LEFTOVER** Salmon Patties with Basil Aioli		High-Protein Mushroom Kale Frittata with Tomatoes* and Roasted Red Pepper Dip*	204 / 229
SATURDAY	Blackberry Chocolate Chip Protein Waffles	93	**LEFTOVER** High-Protein Mushroom Kale Frittata with Tomatoes and Roasted Red Pepper Dip		Jumbo Meatballs with Roasted Veggies* and Garden House Salad with "Buttermilk" Ranch*	146 / 123
SUNDAY	Trevor's Yogurt Parfait	98	**LEFTOVER** Salmon Patties with Basil Aioli		**LEFTOVER** Jumbo Meatballs with Roasted Veggies and Garden House Salad with "Buttermilk" Ranch	

*Each of these recipes serves four, so if you're just making it for yourself, cut it in half to account for just one serving of leftovers.

SHOPPING LIST

SEASONINGS AND EXTRACTS

- bay leaf
- cayenne pepper
- dried basil leaves
- dried dill weed
- dried oregano leaves
- dried thyme leaves
- garlic powder
- ground cumin
- onion powder
- paprika
- red pepper flakes
- salt
- vanilla extract

PRODUCE

- avocados, 3
- bananas, 2 medium
- basil, 1 bunch
- bell peppers (any color), 2
- Brussels sprouts, 2 cups
- carrots, 5 medium
- cauliflower, 1 small head
- cucumber, 1 medium
- curly kale, 1 large bunch
- garlic, 2 bulbs
- jalapeño peppers, 2
- jicama, 1 medium
- lemons, 3
- limes, 2
- little gem lettuce, 8 cups
- mixed greens, 10 cups
- mushrooms (any type), 8 ounces
- parsley, 1 bunch
- radishes, 4
- red bell pepper, 1
- red onion, 1 medium
- romaine or other crunchy lettuce, 2 leaves
- strawberries, 1 pound
- tomatoes, 5
- yellow onions, 2 medium
- zucchini, 2 medium

MEAT, MEAT ALTERNATIVES, EGGS, DAIRY, AND DAIRY ALTERNATIVES

- almond or coconut milk, unsweetened, 1½ cups
- butter, salted, 1 tablespoon
- cheddar cheese, shredded, ½ cup
- chicken breasts, boneless, skinless, 1 pound
- cottage cheese, 1 cup
- eggs, large, 16
- feta cheese, 8 ounces
- Greek yogurt, plain whole milk, 5 cups
- ground beef, 2¾ pounds
- Mexican-style shredded cheese, ¾ cup
- Parmesan cheese, grated, ½ cup plus extra for garnish
- Parmesan cheese, shredded, 1 tablespoon
- salmon, 1½ pounds, or 3 (6-ounce) cans
- tempeh bacon, 8 slices
- whole milk, ⅔ cup plus 3 tablespoons

FROZEN AND REFRIGERATED FOODS

- blackberries, frozen, 2 cups
- blueberries, frozen, 1½ cups
- Ezekiel bread, 2 slices
- sauerkraut, ¼ cup

PANTRY ITEMS

- almond butter, 2 tablespoons
- almond flour, 1 cup
- avocado oil
- avocado oil mayonnaise or organic olive oil–based mayo, ½ cup plus 1 tablespoon
- avocado oil spray
- balsamic vinegar, 1 teaspoon plus extra for drizzling
- bee pollen, ½ teaspoon
- cacao nibs, ¼ cup plus 1 teaspoon
- chia seeds, ⅓ cup plus 1 tablespoon
- chickpeas, cooked, ¼ cup
- chipotle chili peppers in adobo sauce, 1 small can
- chocolate chips, zero sugar, 2 tablespoons
- corn tortillas, 6-inch, 8
- crushed tomatoes, 3 (14-ounce) cans
- hemp seeds, hulled, 3 tablespoons
- kidney beans, cooked, 2 cups
- olive oil
- pine nuts, 1 tablespoon
- pumpkin seeds, 5 tablespoons
- red enchilada sauce, 2¼ cups
- tuna, 1 (4-ounce) can
- vanilla protein powder, 12 scoops
- walnuts, raw, 2 tablespoons

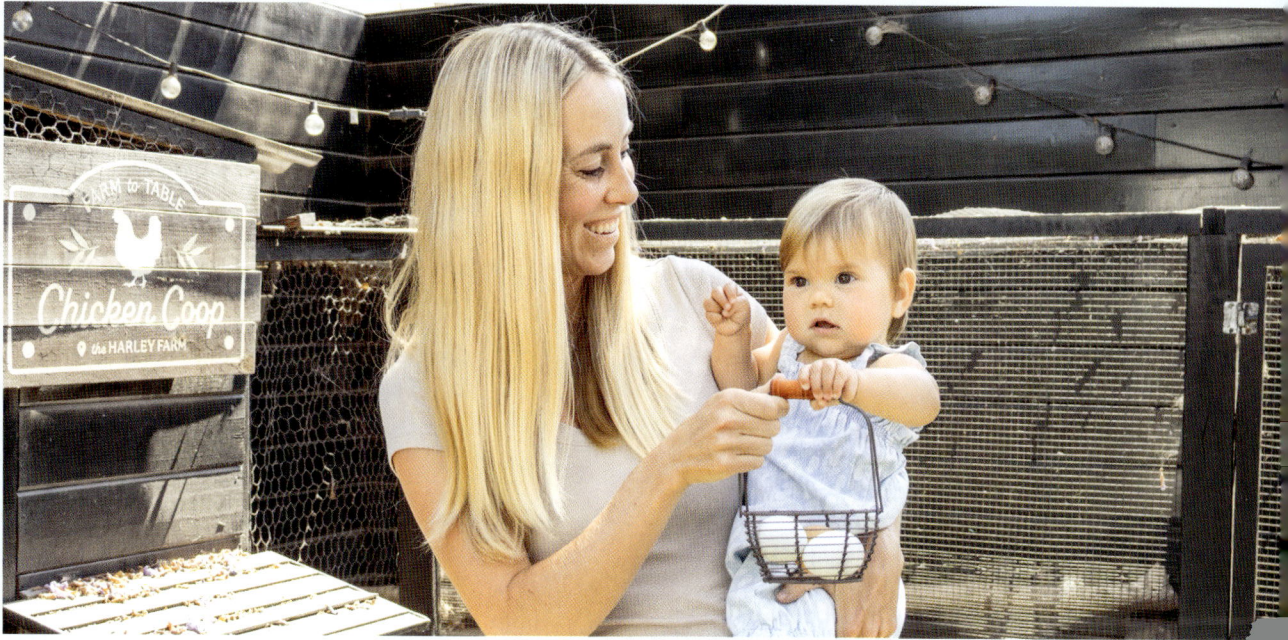

REMEMBER THIS...

Change isn't always easy, even when you're changing habits to make your life easier and more enjoyable. But I want you to remember that the changes you're making aren't just about new meal strategies—they're also about the mindset you're creating. You're no longer eating to fulfill or stay below a certain calorie count. Every bite you take is now intentionally fueling your body, energy levels, gut health, and body composition goals. And you get to do that *without feeling hungry*, which is pretty dang awesome.

Now that you know *How to Eat*, you have the science-backed tools to keep making choices that help you feel your best without being tied to a calorie tracker. It won't always be easy, especially in the beginning, and you won't always get it perfectly right, but that's okay. Every time you make a meal that's in line with your goals, you learn something new about your body and what it needs. Over time, these small learning opportunities will build up into habits, and those habits will build up into your new lifestyle until suddenly everything is *easy*. Pretty soon you'll find that you start to prefer different food groups, no longer need that afternoon snack, and stop craving sugary sweet treats on the daily. Put simply, you'll start to feel *good* again.

I can't wait for you to start feeling your best.

Cheers to the many delicious, satisfying, and nourishing meals in your future!

♥, Autumn

ACKNOWLEDGMENTS

To Trevor: The love of my life, my best friend, and my constant support system. Writing a book while also running a full-time business and being pregnant with our second baby has definitely not been easy. But I would never have been able to stay sane throughout the process without your calming presence (not to mention all your help on Saturdays testing and shooting a zillion recipes with me). Thank you for staying on this wild ride with me and always making me smile even when the days got crazy.

To Sage: My little lady! My firstborn! You reinspire me every day to make the nutrition world a better place. Seeing you grow up eating and loving healthy foods has been my dream come true. You're already so much fun helping me in the kitchen, and I can't wait for you to continue helping me create delicious recipes for the world (and our little family).

To Jack: You've been a constant presence throughout the writing of this book, which admittedly has made things a little tough at times (first trimester nausea set me back a few months during the recipe development process!). But I can't wait to one day share with you the recipes that I created while you were in my belly.

To my parents, Kelly and Rob: This book quite literally would not have happened without your help. To my mom, thank you for watching Sage during the week while I wrote and worked. Sage has no idea how lucky she is to spend so much time with her Gigi. And to my dad, thank you for starting and fueling my interest in natural health.

To Nicole: I'm so glad my friends booked you as their wedding photographer so that I could find you to shoot the cover of my first published book! Your positive, light, and happy aesthetic perfectly match my mission of making food and nutrition joyful.

To Sandy: My talented photographer friend! Thank you, Sandy, for helping me come out of my shell for the beautiful lifestyle photos in this book. You're truly an artist.

To the Victory Belt Publishing team: Lastly, but not least, thank you to the entire team at Victory Belt Publishing. I never would have considered writing a published book, because I was scared that I wouldn't have control over the message I wanted to share. But the entire team has been so supportive of me sharing my simple yet unconventional strategies with the world. Thank you for letting me keep my voice.

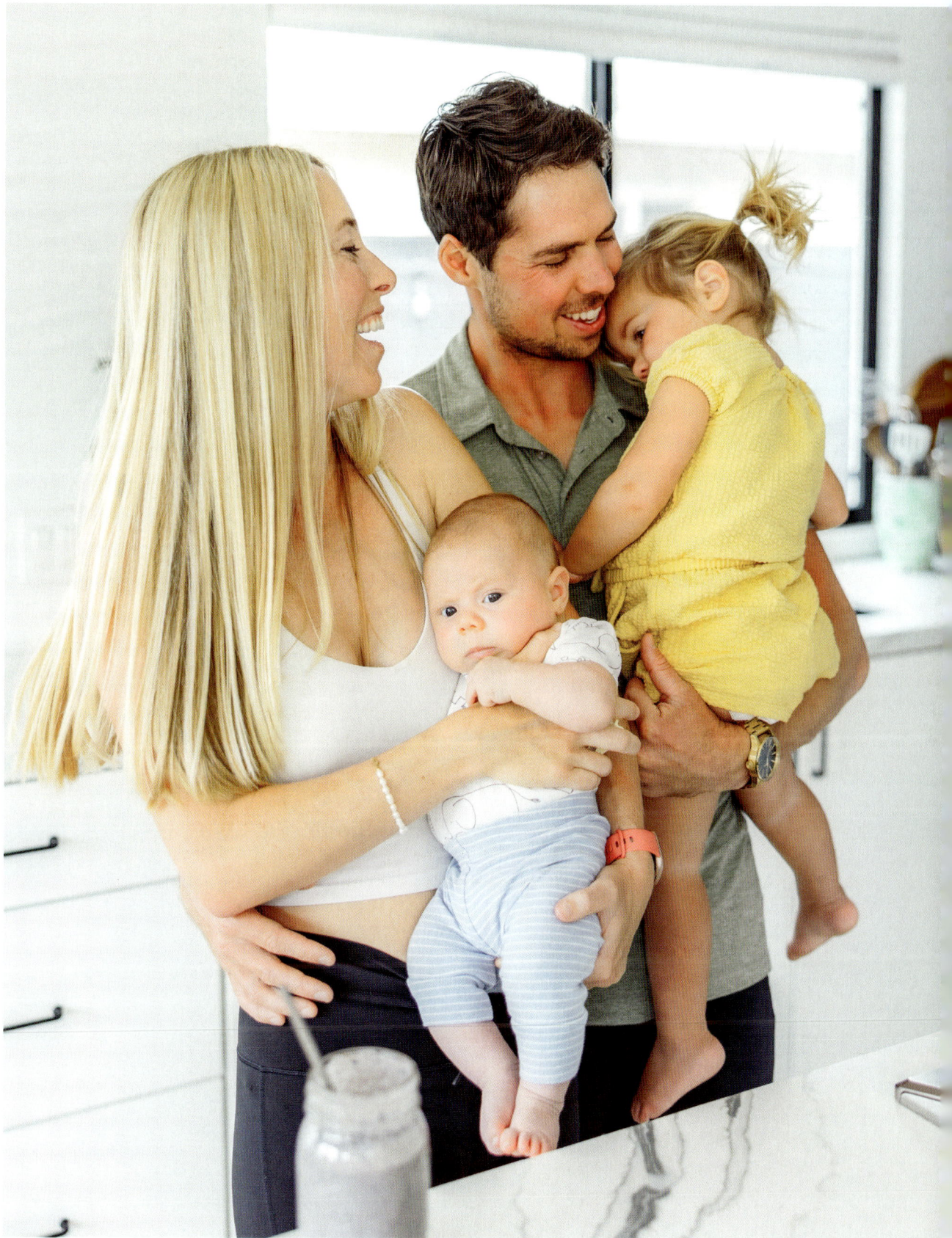

RECOMMENDED BRANDS AND STORES

Finding quality ingredients can definitely be tricky, so here is a list of my favorite brands that I use and that have my stamp of approval.

Autumn's Pasture-Raised Protein Powder (the only protein powder I use!):
autumnellenutrition.shop

Beekeeper's Naturals (bee pollen and raw honey):
www.beekeepersnaturals.com (use code AUTUMN20 for a discount)

ButcherBox (high-quality meats delivered to your door):
www.butcherbox.com

Cultures for Health (heirloom Greek yogurt starter cultures):
culturesforhealth.com

Lily's (zero-added-sugar dark chocolate):
www.lilys.com

Masienda (heirloom masa harina and tortilla-making supplies):
masienda.com

Primal Kitchen (zero-sugar and low-sugar sauces, dips, and mayo):
www.primalkitchen.com (use code AUTUMN for a discount)

Purity Coffee (mold-free organic coffee):
puritycoffee.com (use code AUTUMN for a discount)

Thrive Market (healthy pantry staples delivered to your door):
thrivemarket.com/autumnbates

SAFE COOKING TEMPERATURES AND CONVERSIONS

SAFE COOKING TEMPERATURES

Beef, pork, and lamb steaks, roasts, and chops	145°F
Ground beef, pork, and lamb	160°F
All poultry	165°F
Fish	145°F
Shellfish	Until pearly or white and opaque, or until shells open

CONVERSIONS

OVEN TEMPERATURES

225°F	110°C
250°F	120°C
275°F	140°C
300°F	150°C
325°F	160°C
350°F	180°C
375°F	190°C
400°F	200°C
425°F	220°C
450°F	230°C
475°F	240°C

OUNCES TO GRAMS (FOR PROTEIN)

1 ounce	28 grams
2 ounces	56 grams
3 ounces	84 grams
4 ounces	112 grams
5 ounces	140 grams
6 ounces	168 grams
12 ounces	336 grams
16 ounces	448 grams
20 ounces	560 grams

INDEX